Sheila Kitzinger

The New Good Birth Guide

Penguin Books

Penguin Books Ltd, Harmondsworth, Middlesex, England
Penguin Books, 625 Madison Avenue, New York, New York 10022, U.S.A.
Penguin Books Australia Ltd, Ringwood, Victoria, Australia
Penguin Books Canada Ltd, 2801 John Street, Markham, Ontario, Canada L3R 1B4
Penguin Books (N.Z.) Ltd, 182–190 Wairau Road, Auckland 10, New Zealand

First published 1983

Designed by Yvonne Dedman
Figure drawings by Russell Barnett
Maps by Eugene Fleury

Set in Linotron Palatino by
Rowland Phototypesetting Ltd, Bury St Edmunds, Suffolk
Made and printed in Great Britain by
Hazell, Watson & Viney Ltd, Aylesbury, Bucks

Contents

Birth at home

This book does not attempt to discuss the option of home birth. Less than 2 per cent of women in the UK now have their babies at home, but many more might like to if they realized that it was a possible choice. *It is*. But you may have to be very firm that this is what you want. And you should be sure that there are no special 'risk factors' for you and your baby. You can find out what these are and how to set about getting a home birth in my book *Birth at Home* (Oxford University Press).

Introduction

This book gives a picture of the alternatives available today in hospital birth, based on women's own experiences and on what hospitals are prepared to describe about their policies and practices. It draws on reports of hospital experiences and births from thousands of women who had babies between 1979 and late 1982. It is more than just a 'shopping list', since it also includes some of the research evidence which is likely to affect the reader's choices. Armed with this information, she can look again at routine and not-so-routine hospital practices and different kinds of obstetric intervention and have a basis on which to discuss these things with doctors and midwives and come to her own decision.

Much of the technology used in obstetrics today has been introduced, and become a routine part of clinical practice, without adequate research and without strong evidence of its advantages. It is difficult for a woman who is told 'this is done for the benefit of mother and baby' to query the use of, for example, electronic fetal monitoring or an oxytocin infusion. Moreover, many hospital rites are taken for granted by members of staff and performed as a matter of course, so that to question them seems almost insulting. Shave, enemas and suppositories, putting women to bed during labour, the assumption that a woman will lie down when she *is* on the bed, breaking the bag of waters artificially, not letting a woman eat during labour, urging her to push and to hold her breath in the second stage, and performing an episiotomy are all examples of routines which are so much an accepted part of our Western way of birth that the woman who prefers to do something different may have a label of 'neurotic' pinned to her or be castigated as 'a troublemaker' or 'one of those women's libbers'. Because childbirth is something that only happens to women, their concerns about it, what *they* want, their hopes, fears and anxieties, are often explained away as either irrelevant to the only criteria of success, 'a live, healthy mother and a live, healthy baby', or are seen as parts of a pathological process in the female psyche.

Women in labour usually do not want to be thought 'rude' or aggressive, and as a result when they feel trapped in situations which are entirely out of their control, on territory over which power is exercised by professionals, they become passive and placating. Sometimes they are frightened into obedience because they fear that non-compliance will result in worse things being done to them or their babies. I know that some obstetricians and midwives, giving of their energy, time and skills without stint, to do the best they can for their patients, will urge a gentle approach to change, a willingness to 'cooperate'. Women having babies, too, may warn us 'not to rock the boat', even those who stand beside us in wanting to create the conditions for informed choice between alternatives.

But the evidence is that change does not come, or does not come for enough women, when an expectant mother has a quiet talk with the obstetrician, but only when there is open and public protest. There is a place for quiet talks, but we need more than that if our Western culture of birth is to see any radical transformation. The task calls for knowledge and understanding, the courage to question assumptions and the energy to work together to create a way of birth in our society in which women are recognized as adults and active birth-givers.

A whole section of the book is devoted to new kinds of teaching about birth. These are profoundly affecting women's ideas about what they want. They include the work of Leboyer and Odent, new approaches to labour in which the woman keeps on the move and keeps changing position, a way of working with contractions in the second stage so that pushing is harmonious and there is no long breath-holding, and the new birth rooms which are increasingly being offered in hospitals.

The next section explores the whole subject of how to think ahead to birth and make plans and contingency plans. Women are often told that it depends who is on duty at the time whether they will be allowed to deliver in an upright position, hold the baby before the cord is clamped and cut, whether the father can be up on the delivery table behind the woman and hold her in his arms and whether he will be permitted to cut the cord himself, for example. This is not good enough. It should be possible for a woman to plan ahead for birth with her doctor and midwife so that they understand what she wants, and she knows that she can trust them to do everything they can to make that possible. When intervention is necessary a woman is much more likely to be able to accept it with equanimity if she feels that the people helping her acknowledge and share her goals. A written birth plan, one copy of which is in the woman's hospital records, and which is the result of negotiation and full discussion with those who are going to attend her, is an important step on the way to achieving this.

Section V consists of a directory of hospitals so that readers can discover some of the exciting changes which are taking place and on the basis of these descriptions can find out more. Reading these accounts can give you an idea of what questions to put and things for which you may want to ask. They can also offer clues as to whether a particular hospital is the kind of place in which you would like to have your baby.

Acknowledgements

I want to thank most of all the many women who wrote at first-hand about their birth experiences and those divisional and senior nursing officers, administrators and consultant obstetricians and paediatricians who have sent information about their hospitals. Professor Geoffrey Chamberlain and Professor Gordon Stirrat have been most kind in giving me permission to use illustrations from their own books, *Lecture Notes on Obstetrics* (Blackwell Scientific Publications) and *Obstetrics* (Grant McIntyre Medical and Scientific) and Mr John Studd has provided the partogram. The initial collecting of information from hospitals was done by my research assistant, Rhiannon Walters. She organized the material with great care so that it provided an excellent base on which to link official policies and statistics with mothers' own reported experiences.

My secretary, Margaret Pearson, has been a tower of strength and dogged hard work, and Ann Cook has made herself cheerfully available to take over extra work when the going got too hard.

My family puts up with a lot. I want to thank Tess, Nell and Polly, the daughters most likely to have been at home during this time, for tolerating my absorption in work, and especially Uwe for all the encouragement and emotional support he gives me. My stamina is based entirely on his love.

Sheila Kitzinger
The Manor, Standlake, nr Witney, Oxfordshire

A New Awareness

Rapid and far-reaching changes are taking place in many hospitals today. I believe it is important that women having babies are aware of what is happening and keep in touch with the new developments. In some hospitals groups of women who have had babies there are forming advisory committees consulting with obstetricians, midwives and administrators to effect change. This would have been almost inconceivable even ten years ago.

Such an entirely new climate means that there are new responsibilities. We cannot remain passive, simply accepting whatever care is offered without comment – we now have the responsibility to consider alternatives and to speak out about what we want. It means also that we have to bear in mind the needs of the women who have no voice, those who have not had the same educational advantages, who do not know how to express their feelings in ways which are easily understood by hospital staff, and those who come from other cultures and who cannot speak English. We have to remember that not all women want the same thing and need to listen to what others are saying too.

In the hospitals of the future I hope that doctors, midwives and mothers will be collaborators in change, pushing forward the frontiers so that more and more institutions designed to serve women having babies really offer the environment which women themselves seek.

Section I

The Medical Way of Birth

1. Pregnancy as a Disease State

What are antenatal clinics for?

In most societies there are rules about pregnancy, strict regulations about what the woman may and may not do and what she must eat and avoid. In this way each culture stresses the marginal nature of the pregnant state and surrounds it by *rites de passage*. We have always done this in the West, and our 'old wives' tales' are vestiges of a complicated network of beliefs which controlled the behaviour of the pregnant woman. Today new elements of social control have replaced those imposed by older women, grannies and aunts, and these have to a large extent even taken over the power and aura previously invested in the priesthood.

The new system is controlled by doctors. They lay down the rules and a woman looks to medical experts to tell her how she should behave. If she attends antenatal clinics early in pregnancy, keeps on going regularly and obeys the doctors, it is implied that she has done everything she possibly can for a safe childbirth and for the benefit of her baby. If she breaks the rules she is a 'defaulter', a term used to describe women who do not turn up for clinic appointments, the penalty for which, it is suggested, may be a difficult labour, and a deformed, handicapped or dead baby.

In fact, we have only just started to investigate the cost-effectiveness of antenatal care. We do not really know how soon or how often a woman ought to go to an antenatal clinic, or even whether a healthy woman need go at all. We do not know if there are some tests, such as the presence of protein, sugar and bacteria in urine, which could not be done in her own home by the woman herself and whether there are others which would be best done by a midwife rather than a doctor. Nor do we know whether the things done in the clinic are, for the most part, worth while or not. It is true that women who do not attend antenatal clinics early in pregnancy are most likely to lose their babies, but then they are also most likely to be unhappy about the pregnancy, to be unmarried, still in their teens, at the bottom of the social scale, to have a nutritionally inadequate diet and to be living in poor or overcrowded conditions, and may find it difficult to find out about the social services available.

The chart on p. 16 gives the tests most often done in antenatal clinics. The only one of these tests which has to be done in a hospital clinic or somewhere where sophisticated equipment is set up is the scan.

Doppler ultrasound for recording the fetal heart could be easily used outside a hospital; it is a box about the size of the average cassette player. It requires a 13 amp electric plug. It produces very powerful ultrasound, and since we do not yet know whether there may be some long-term effects of ultrasound on the baby, it should be used with discretion and when the benefits apparently outweigh any hypothetical risks.

Tests routinely or commonly done

Test	Time	Purpose	Involving sample of
Pregnancy test	any time from 2 weeks after missed period	to know if pregnant	urine
Blood group	booking clinic	to test haemoglobin level in case of need for blood transfusion or to reveal a rhesus incompatibility	blood
Sexually trans-mitted disease	booking clinic	so that it can be treated	blood
Weight	every visit	to assess growth of fetus, reveal possible pre-eclampsia	—
Nipple inspection	booking clinic	see if nipples retracted	—
Albumen	every visit	reveal pre-eclampsia	urine
Bacteria	every visit	so that bladder infection can be treated	urine
Glucose	every visit	reveal pre-diabetic state	—
Ultrasound scan	16/17 weeks	confirm length of gestation, locate placenta	—
Palpation of abdomen	every visit	confirm height of top of uterus, position and size of fetus	—
Listening to fetal heart by Doppler ultrasound, stetho-scope or trumpet	12 weeks and after	confirm pregnancy, fetus alive, heart rate and any abnor-malities	—
Blood pressure	every visit	reveal hypertension, pre-eclampsia	—
Vaginal examina-tion	booking clinic 36 weeks plus	confirm pregnancy; reveal state of cervix, position of fetus	—

Here are some of the tests which are not done routinely in most clinics, but which may be done as a matter of course in some hospitals:

Tests sometimes done

Test	Time	Purpose	Involving sample of
Cervical smear	booking clinic*	to rule out pre-cancerous condition of cervix	cells from cervix
Ultrasound scans	early middle or throughout pregnancy	as before and to watch fetal breathing movements, often for research purposes	—
Doppler ultrasound	various times throughout pregnancy	as before, often for research purposes	—
Antenatal cardiography	after 30 weeks	to assess fetal heart rate, often for research purposes	—
Stress test (ultrasound providing stress and fetal heart rate)	after 30 weeks	to assess likely reaction of fetus to labour contractions, often for research	—
Oestriol	any time after 30 weeks, if 'overdue'	to assess placental function, often for research purposes	over 24 hours urine or blood
Kick chart	last weeks of pregnancy if 'overdue'	assess fetal well-being, often for research purposes	—

* In many clinics in the UK this is done as part of the postnatal check up.

The only test which the mother may be asked to do for herself from this list is the last one, keeping a chart of the baby's movements at particular times of the day. Women are usually put into hospital for testing of urinary oestriol, though urine could be provided at home.

Here are some other tests which may be proposed in special cases:

Special tests

Test	Time	Purpose	Involving sample of
Amniocentesis	16/17 weeks	to rule out some fetal abnormalities, e.g. spina bifida, microcephaly, Down's syndrome. To tell fetal sex when there are inherited sex-linked handicaps	amniotic fluid, drawn off through needle pushed through mother's abdominal wall and into uterus

Test	Time	Purpose	Involving sample of
Amniocentesis (cont.)	24 weeks*	to assess state of fetus when there is rhesus incompatibility	amniotic fluid, as above
	30–38 weeks	to assess state of fetal lungs before induction or Caesarean section	amniotic fluid, as above
Amniocentesis should be immediately preceded by ultrasound scan		to locate positions of placenta and fetus	—
Antibodies	24/32/36 weeks	to diagnose rhesus incompatibility	blood
Pelvic X-ray	end of pregnancy	to assess pelvic size and shape, size and position of fetus, fetal abnormalities, more than one fetus	—
Fetoscopy	16 weeks*	to see fetus, take blood sample	fine tube with light passed through mother's abdominal wall and uterus to obtain fetal blood
Human placental lactogen	30 weeks*	to assess placental function	blood
Amnioscopy	36 weeks*	to note signs of fetal distress	tube with light introduced through vagina into cervix to see if meconium in amniotic fluid

*These tests may also be done at other times in special cases.

Women's experiences of antenatal care

I joined the queues for this, that and the other, and then came the examination. 'Take everything off and put the robe on,' said the nurse. 'And then get on to the table.' All the tables were in a row, with a partition between each one.

The nurse came and whipped back my robe. There I lay like a fish on a fishmonger's slab, starkers, waiting for the doctor, with people milling past all the time.

Pregnant women often find attendance at antenatal clinics an ordeal. Even in hospitals which they praise without reservation for the care and understanding given during labour, antenatal clinics are described as badly organized, 'chaotic', 'a shambles', with long, boring waiting times in dreary surroundings with crying children. Women sometimes wait for three hours or longer, being shifted from location to location to wait their turn in front of yet another door. Toddlers and older children are under foot, tired and fretful:

I waited three hours before being seen. The normal wait was between 1½–2 hours and then one was given an extremely swift examination, with no time or encouragement to ask questions. A couple of the doctors had difficulties in speaking and understanding English, which made any attempt at discussion embarrassing. I felt sorry for mums with toddlers. No provision was made for them except for a broken rocking horse. The fretfulness and boredom of these poor little kids made the waiting harder for everyone.

Women write of feeling 'depressed', 'humiliated', 'degraded', 'frightened' and even 'terrified'. They say they feel 'trapped' in a 'sausage machine', depersonalized – 'just a number on a card' or 'like a tin of beans on a conveyor belt'. They come out anxious, feeling exhausted and sick, and on getting home burst into tears. They dread the next visit. In fact, antenatal clinics provide a grim view of our maternity services.

Even when sparkling new units have been built or clinics redecorated and refurbished, the old system of organization and old attitudes have often remained. The answers are not to be found in architecture and interior decoration but in the quality of relationship between providers and users of the service, and probably also that between the providers themselves.

One of the most obvious problems from the expectant mother's point of view is *the fragmentation of care*. She is often bewildered by the number of different people she sees, does not know their names or whether she will ever meet them again, hears comments made by one about the progress of her pregnancy which do not tally with another's and may be given advice which is then contradicted by the next. Conflicting advice and clinical comments are specially worrying concerning weight gain, the estimated size of the baby and length of gestation. A woman whose membranes were found to be leaking after vaginal examination wrote:

Five young doctors came to see me. They all stood round talking amongst themselves as though I wasn't there. One of them said the baby was far too early to be born and just try not to go into labour but wait until the proper time. Another said if it was born now it would be very weak and would probably have to go into an incubator as its lungs would be damaged, and a third doctor said he thought this was the right time for it to be born.

Women who have specific anxieties, or who hope for a chance to have as natural a birth as possible, find it difficult to know who to ask. If they do ask they often say they were 'made to feel like a naughty schoolgirl', or 'a silly child', are told, 'it depends who is on duty at the time', or 'this is a very nice place', get a 'vague answer in a don't-you-worry-we'll-take-care-of-everything tone of voice' or a startled and indignant response which makes them fearful that they are being 'labelled as a troublemaker'. As a result women learn that it pays to be passive. Even when breast-feeding advice is offered in the antenatal clinic and a lactation sister is available to give encouragement, women sit in rows waiting their turn, afraid that if they seek information or do anything different from all the other patients in the waiting-room they will lose their place in the queue or get singled out for treatment which prolongs the wait. Women move from chair to chair, from door to door submissively, smile back at the doctor when they are smiled at even though they are anxious or depressed, and usually try to fill the role of the good and grateful patient who does not interrupt the routine. The main task of nurses is simply to maintain the work flow.

The larger the clinic, the busier it is and, above all, the greater the extent to which sessions are themselves fragmented – taking place with different members of staff, who are *task*-centred rather than *patient*-centred, and in different parts of the clinic – the more the woman is likely to feel that she is being 'processed' through pregnancy:

I felt like one of a large herd of cows being passed through various inspection points – check in, weigh in, blood pressure, urine test, thumb prick, blood sample – and every one with a different nurse, and then a long, uncomfortable wait for the humiliation of the examination room. Feeling hot and nervous I lay legs apart while a retinue of long-haired students gathered round and a doctor whom I had never seen before without warning slipped his hand into my vagina, just as though he was going to clean out a chicken.

The sheer pressure of numbers in antenatal clinics means that obstetricians have insufficient time to give to patients. A frequent complaint is that there is no chance to talk to the doctor, who seems interested only in the lower end of their bodies:

I was really scared and a bag of nerves because no one told me anything.

The doctor just grunted at me. He didn't even look my way and when he did speak it was via a nurse as if I were a retarded child.

Even when an obstetrician appears sympathetic a woman may be reluctant to 'bother' him because she knows there is a queue of mothers waiting outside. She does not want to produce a hiccup in the routine. Moreover, it is difficult to initiate discussion with a male stranger standing over you as you lie naked from the waist down.

When a woman is fearful and worried the clinical examination itself may give rise to further anxiety: 'Why didn't he say anything?' 'What did he mean when he said that to the nurse?' 'He frowned: is there anything wrong with my baby?' 'He said, "We must keep an eye on you." Why?' 'He said there's a big baby there. Does that mean I've got to have a Caesarean section?' . . . 'I felt,' wrote one woman 'like a lump of meat on a butcher's slab.'

Priority must be given to reorganizing the ways in which the time is used in antenatal clinics, not only for the well-being of expectant mothers but for that of the staff too, who themselves may be under stress from the assembly-line system. There needs to be radical re-examination of the work that is done in the clinic to discover whether its doctors, nurses and midwives are doing the work that they can do best, and whether they are doing it under optimal conditions.

When an antenatal clinic is not within walking distance of the pregnant woman's home arrangements have to be made to get there and this can be complicated if she already has children. Clinics are often a long distance away from the women they are intended to serve. With the simultaneous running down of rural bus services, the axeing of train services, and the rise in the price of petrol many mothers of young children have to run a marathon to get to the antenatal clinic.

Two schemes which developed independently of each other appear to be working well in Salop and West Berkshire.[1] The Dial-a-Midwife scheme in West Berkshire is based on the principles that an integrated midwifery service should provide a telephone which is manned twenty-four hours a day, 365 days a year and that midwives go to the woman's home to give advice and help whenever needed, day or night. Every patient booked for delivery anywhere in the division has a home visit from a midwife, when the system is explained to her and the midwife makes a 'home assessment'. The phone number of the midwife attached to her GP's practice and that of the GP unit is written on her 'cooperation card'. Midwives stress that this is not an 'off-duty' service and that a woman should ring however trivial her problem.

Salop has a twenty-four-hour phone-in service to the GP units serving the Shrewsbury and Telford area.[2] A duty rota of community midwives serves a week at a time on nights. Every pregnant woman is visited three times at least in her home. A midwife working with this scheme comments: 'The patient was more relaxed, asked many questions and aired her anxieties, querying points she felt to be too trivial to mention at clinic sessions.' The midwife also learns about the woman's social conditions and is alerted to any social stresses and special problems in the family.

The future of antenatal care
A working party on antenatal care which I set up for the National Childbirth Trust in 1980 made recommendations for change which, if implemented, would have far-reaching effects. The group consisted of midwives, general practitioner obstetricians, hospital obstetricians, a hospital administrator, sociologists and mothers. This is what they recommended:[3]

RECOMMENDATIONS

Pregnancy is not a medical condition. Eighty per cent of women have completely normal pregnancies and labours. Twenty per cent of women are at some risk. Only half of these are discovered to be at risk during pregnancy. The other 10 per cent appears during labour, but with the best of care might be predicted antenatally. So the whole system of antenatal care is designed to identify, at most, 20 per cent of women.

Adapting clinics as they are at present and hoping that by introducing more comfortable chairs and redecoration they will look more welcoming is some improvement but may only delay the fundamental change in the whole system which is urgently necessary. The system needs not modification but a complete and radical rethinking, bearing in mind that the present system fails most where the need is greatest – with those women who come from backgrounds where there is an increased risk of bearing a stillborn or handicapped baby.

1. We call for the progressive abolition of large, centralized antenatal clinics. Work could be done more effectively in smaller, dispersed clinics and also in mobile units, with consultants going out into the community to examine those patients referred to them by midwives and GPs because they are thought to have problems. We accept that, in the present financial climate, immediate implementation of these ideas may not be possible. However, this should not stop us moving as fast as we can in that direction by utilizing opportunities for change with which we are presented. Do existing clinics need upgrading or can we use the capital instead to develop a mobile service? Do we need such large clinics in new hospitals? Has the Area Medical Committee discussed alternatives to large antenatal clinics?

These are questions we can and should be asking locally and nationally – now.

2. We call for a new recognition of midwifery. A midwife is *fully qualified to give total antenatal care*. In the long term we should like to see midwifery extended to concern with women's health care generally, as in some women's clinics in the USA, so that there is a continuing relationship before, during and after pregnancy.

3. A woman should usually be able to see the same midwife throughout her pregnancy, whom she knows as *her* midwife. Wherever possible future bookings should be made for times when it is known that this midwife is on duty.

4. We believe that the continuation of GP obstetricians may be significant for the GP's own skills as a *family* physician. Where GPs are involved in shared care with hospital obstetricians the relationship between them is critical for the well-being of mother and baby. Obstetricians should go out from the hospital into GPs' practices rather than the GP going to the hospital clinic, where relationships tend to be organized in a hierarchical system and where discussion on hospital territory is likely to be about the latest monitoring equipment or other procedures and the GP feels s/he lacks the knowledge possessed by senior students. When a GP is on his own ground he is in a better position to see birth as a significant event in the life of a family and to be concerned with family counselling than one who simply hands over responsibility to the hospital. If there is to be a revitalizing of the role of the GP in obstetrics, and he or she is to give intranatal as well as antenatal and postnatal care, the work must be given adequate financial reward.

5. At present it is not worth it financially for a GP to attend deliveries. A GP earns more by making a home visit to a woman who is miscarrying and sending her into hospital than from giving twenty-four-hour care in childbirth. We call for adequate remuneration for GP obstetricians and a realistic reward for providing continuity of care.

6. It is important that women shall have choice and that there should be a variety of models in which care is given, all in small, intimate groupings of people in a home-like setting. Sometimes the person primarily responsible for care will be the GP, sometimes the midwife and sometimes the hospital obstetricians. But whoever it is, there should be viable alternatives. We recognize that it is much easier to operate a cut-and-dried system and put the woman on a conveyor belt at one end to come out at the other with a baby, but this model produces inadequate and apparently uncaring super-vision of pregnancy. Women should be asked their preferences at the beginning of pregnancy and an opportunity given for discussion about the kind of care each would like. We believe that choices about care are important.

Where the Need is Greatest

7. Up till now antenatal clinics have developed piecemeal from the early years of the century and though there has been much discussion about the needs of women at greatest risk, on the whole the practical application of this awareness has been restricted to those presenting with well-defined medical or obstetric problems, such as diabetes or hypertension. Women whose social backgrounds or lack of education put them in the highest risk categories have often actually received *less* care than educated, middle-class women able to express their preferences and with whom a doctor may find it easier to talk. We call for a new deal for those mothers whose babies are most at risk, many of them from social classes 4 and 5 and unsupported mothers, and for concentration of resources where the need is greatest. We doubt whether the obstetrician is always the right person to take on responsibility for women from deprived backgrounds since it is often the midwife who can establish the most effective communication with a woman. Heré again, flexibility is needed and arrangements should be made which are most acceptable to the individual expectant mother.

8. The booking clinic is of major importance and we urge that ample time is given not only for physical examination but also for the start of a relationship between the pregnant woman and her obstetrician or midwife and for full discussion of any problems and anxieties. It is an important part of the role of the midwife to give emotional support at this stage of pregnancy and nurses who are not midwives are not trained for this work.

9. Yet time alone is not enough to allow communication between all pregnant women and their caregivers. Women from other cultures, and especially those who speak little or no English, are among those at greatest risk and at present may be receiving inadequate care because they cannot express themselves or understand what is said to them.[4]

   Preference should be given to the appointment of multilingual staff members in all areas of immigrant concentration and there should be lists of staff speaking different languages, or of people in the local community able to act as interpreters, in every antenatal clinic.

   We recognize too that understanding is not simply a matter of speaking the same language; it is important that doctors and midwives are aware of the cultural backgrounds from which their patients come and understand something of the value system concerning birth and the family and women's concepts about their bodies which most profoundly affect attitudes and behaviour. There should be much more awareness of the need for this in the training of doctors, nurses and midwives, both before qualification and afterwards, on an in-service basis. The nursing and non-nursing managers of the units containing antenatal clinics have an important role here. They should be encouraged to take a close interest in the area of communications and to ensure that all possible support and assistance is given to staff to establish good communication with women.

What Kind of Midwife?

10. We believe that it is important to attract into the midwifery service women who have personal experience of birth and babies. Direct entrance to midwifery should be seen, not as an inferior form of training, but possibly as the saving of the profession, since it encourages women with experience, commitment and maturity to train as midwives. If women who have themselves borne children are to practise midwifery they must be able to dovetail work with family commitments. We urge consideration of projects in which working times could be made more flexible in the same way as is now being done for women doctors. Autocratic and authoritarian systems prevent midwives from evolving more flexible methods which ensure greater continuity of care for women. Such flexibility is already operating among community midwives in many areas,[5] and is a noteworthy aspect of the Isle of Dogs project, but has rarely been introduced into hospital practice.

We believe that nurses and midwives need opportunities for awareness of and sharing their feelings about the work they do and that counsellors should be available to give emotional support. They are witnessing acts of such enormous significance in the life of the individual and the family that they need to be able to express their feelings about birth and death. It may be that this can best be done within small groups of midwives and students, and we believe that it should be an integral part of professional and in-service training. There is a strong case to be made for something of the kind also being available for obstetricians; teaching rounds and case conferences cannot provide enough opportunity for sharing and for exploring together qualitative aspects of the work that they are doing. The small group is probably the best forum for this.

The older primigravida

When women write about their hospital experiences those who are older – in their late thirties – and having their first babies often say that they appreciated the continuity of care which was provided by being in the 'high risk' clinic. But they were often very anxious about all the tests that were being done and the concern which suggested to them that they would be most unlikely to be able to have their babies naturally. In those hospitals where there was good communication the extra care did not seem to have this effect, but in others, where the woman felt she was being passed along the assembly line and where she could not ask questions or get detailed information, the special care seems to have had a bad psychological effect.

Sometimes it appears to have been assumed that an older primigravida would hand herself over for all modern techniques of investigating and augmenting labour to be used, when in fact she was keen to 'do it all herself' if possible. When modern techniques were used, she tended to feel trapped, or at least disappointed.

A woman having a baby in her late thirties or her forties may also have been trying to conceive for a long time. This often renders her very vulnerable; she feels that she is reproductively inadequate. Her partner may share this feeling, and they may both become very dependent on medical advice and become caught up in a 'medicalization process' involving a 'special' clinic, amniocentesis and other investigations and a series of tests which turns the physiological events of pregnancy into a medical case study. 'Medicalization,' say Fresco and Sylvestre,[6] 'is like a running train from which it would be dangerous to jump. Men and women react differently to this medicalization. The men tend to take up the scientific discourse so as to compensate for the feeling that they have somehow been evicted from *a new couple of genitors: woman–doctor* (my italics). The women . . . try to resist medicalization and the knowledge revealed by prenatal diagnosis, sometimes by refusing to know the child's sex before birth . . . which enables them to turn their pregnancy into an (almost) normal one.'

Since they are going to have to bring up the child themselves and cannot rely on experts to do that for them, it can be especially important for the woman who has suffered a long period of infertility to develop confidence in herself and to feel that she can actively give birth. Even if she needs obstetric help, there may be a good case for her learning all she can about her own body and the physiological process of labour so that she can discuss things with her doctor and can be as awake and aware as possible.

The challenge of childbirth is just one of the hurdles confronting parents. It is important that the pregnancy and birth form part of a continuum in which they are enabled to feel their way into a satisfying, developing relationship with the baby. It seems that many women need a chance to talk over this kind of thing with an obstetrician or a midwife who understands something of the stresses which they are facing, and that this kind of counselling is rarely available.

The sonar scan

In most consultant units obstetricians now do routine scans some time after the booking clinic, probably at around sixteen weeks. In many hospitals everyone has at least one scan and in some the patients of certain obstetric 'firms' have two or three. Scans are used to confirm pregnancy and can in fact do this even before the first menstrual period is missed, since even at that early stage they show a fluid-filled sac surrounded by the solid, muscular uterine wall. Six weeks after the missed period the baby's heart movements can be detected by ultrasound and three weeks after that the placenta can be seen too. If you have bleeding in early pregnancy and a scan shows that the fetal heart is beating this is a very good sign that the pregnancy is likely to continue. A scan early on often shows the placenta down over the cervix and consequently 'placenta praevia?' is written on the record card. But a placenta which is diagnosed as low-lying at ten or eleven weeks is often found to be in a good position in the upper part of the uterus in later pregnancy.

A scan can also show if there is more than one baby and can do this as early as about six weeks. A scan done if there is acute pain after a missed period sometimes reveals that the pregnancy is in the fallopian tube rather than the uterus. In both early and late pregnancy it can detect a small-for-dates fetus, but results are not always accurate. A scan is used before amniocentesis to identify the position of the placenta so that the obstetrician can avoid piercing it with the needle. It is also used to check for certain abnormalities in the fetus. When scans are used to assess gestational age and work out when the baby is due, they tend to be fairly accurate before about twenty-four weeks but are very unreliable after thirty-four weeks. The most usual method of assessing fetal maturity is to measure the width of the baby's head and estimate the growth between one scan and the next.

Ultrasound can be a very useful diagnostic tool, though its reliability depends on the skill of whoever is interpreting the data. One happy chance side-effect of the introduction of ultrasound has been the joy which women experience when they first see the image on the screen and realize, sometimes for the first time, that there actually is a baby in there.[7] Unfortunately not all technicians are aware of the importance of this first meeting with the baby for many expectant mothers and fathers.

In spite of the undoubted advantages of getting a window into the womb, we do not yet know whether there might be long-term effects on the baby and only time will tell whether the claim made for ultrasound that it is absolutely safe is proven. Chamberlain states unequivocally, 'This is a safe investigation which can be repeated often in pregnancy.'[8] It used also to be thought that X-rays of the fetus were safe and it was only after many years of enthusiastic use that it was discovered that they had long-term effects and were carcinogenic.

Some women feel that scans are used by doctors today rather like St Christopher medals or magic talismans. A woman who wants a home birth, for example, may be told that there is no chance of this unless she agrees to an early pregnancy scan. Apart from diagnosing twins (which could be discovered in a few months' time anyway) just what this is supposed to reveal that would make a home birth safe is difficult to guess.

If scans do have a deleterious effect on the fetus it seems likely that this would be greatest in the first twelve weeks of pregnancy, during the time when we know that environmental factors and teratogenic substances generally can most affect fetal development.

Amniocentesis

This is a method of finding out about the state of the fetus by drawing off some of the liquor in which it floats in the uterus. This is done through a long needle introduced through the mother's abdominal wall and into her uterus. It may be offered to women who want to rule out the possibility of certain genetic disorders. These occur more frequently after the mother is aged forty than before. It may also be suggested when a previous baby has been affected by such a disorder or close relatives have suffered it. It does not prove that a baby is normal, but it will detect certain disorders reliably. The test cannot be done before about sixteen weeks, and this means that the woman has usually passed through several months of anxiety, not knowing whether her pregnancy will continue, and often feels unable to announce her pregnancy to friends and relations. It can be a time of great stress.

There is no point in having amniocentesis unless the parents have discussed the possibility of abortion should the fetus be affected and have decided that this is what they would want. There is a very slight risk that amniocentesis itself may trigger off a miscarriage, but for those women who come into categories which are most likely to be affected this is less than the risk of bearing an abnormal baby.

Before amniocentesis is performed the doctor first finds out the position of the baby and monitors the heartbeat. It is important to avoid puncturing the placenta, so a sonar scan is usually done. An injection of local anaesthetic is given before the needle is inserted. The needle is carefully introduced and some of the amniotic fluid slowly drawn off. The fetus is very unlikely to be pricked by the needle, as it moves away immediately the needle touches it. The baby's sex can be told from the cells in the fluid. Results do not come for two to three weeks, and sometimes even longer. This means that if the fetus is affected and you decide to terminate the pregnancy you have a late abortion, which is like a mini-labour without the joy.

Amniocentesis can also be used to test fetal maturity when induction is planned for a baby who is at risk in the uterus but who is still very small. To test this, the liquid which has been drawn off is shaken and the bubbles counted to see if there are sufficient enzymes to keep the baby's lungs inflated when new-born.

The Shirodkar suture

The Shirodkar suture or circlage is a stitch which is inserted into the cervix to prolong pregnancy. It is often done when a woman has had a previous mid-pregnancy miscarriage, though some obstetricians use it for mothers in their late thirties or early forties who have had previous miscarriages even when there seem no special indications that a Shirodkar suture is necessary. The stitch is put in under anaesthetic and removed under anaesthetic at thirty-eight weeks. The woman often goes into labour then and some obstetricians advocate induction of labour following the removal of the stitch. There are many differences of opinion among obstetricians about the importance of cervical circlage. Some employ it in less than five per 1,000 births and others do more than 30 per 1,000. Internationally the range is wider still and it is a very common operation in parts of France.

One problem is that actually putting in the stitch may make things worse for some women, since it may stimulate the production of prostaglandins which start uterine contractions. Another difficulty is the risk of introducing infection and that always associated with giving general anaesthesia to a pregnant woman. You should know that there have been so far no randomly controlled prospective trials[9] of cervical circlage, though one is at present under way. Though many claims are made for the Shirodkar suture there is no clear evidence that it is effective.

2. Childbirth as Clinical Crisis

Western culture has surrounded birth by hospital routines, many of which are ceremonial procedures functioning to turn a woman into a patient, and then processing her through the system to emerge at the other end as a mother with a new baby. These rites serve to reinforce the power of the hospital as an institution, and that of the professionals who bear responsibility for the outcome of birth, as against the mothers, who are merely the objects of their care.

Many of these ceremonies are similar to puberty rites in primitive societies. One is the purging of the initiate. In our Western way of birth this is done by an enema or suppositories.

Enemas and suppositories

In most labours enemas and suppositories are pointless. Though emptying of the lower bowel as part of the admission procedures in labour is a procedure hallowed by time, you can refuse to have one. The enema is an ancient practice. It became an established part of hospital routine in the nineteenth century, when it was thought that faecal contamination might be a cause of puerperal fever. In the United States, for example, William Goodell devised a special system for eradicating fever which included admission of women to hospital well before delivery, doses of quinine, enemas, amniotomy, forceps delivery, the forced expulsion of the placenta by pressure on the abdomen, and then more quinine until, he said, the woman's ears rang.[1] At the beginning of the twentieth century in New York patients at the Sloane Maternity Hospital had an enema followed by a vaginal douche with bichloride of mercury. Then the woman's head was washed with kerosene, ether and ammonia and her breasts and abdomen with ether. In that hospital women had an enema every twelve hours while in labour and the vagina was douched during and after labour with saline solution to which whisky or bichloride of mercury was added.[2]

The enema thus became an almost sacrosanct part of 'clean' childbirth on both sides of the Atlantic, without being questioned again until very recently. Midwives, especially, believed in its efficacy. But obstetricians, too, have been shocked when women have asked not to have an enema. A woman told me recently that when she said that she would prefer not to have one, her obstetrician exclaimed: 'Not have an enema? There will be shit on the walls, shit in me boots, shit everywhere!' (She stood her ground, did not have an enema and there was no mess at all.)

In 1981 an important study was published in the *British Medical Journal* by Romney and Gordon.[3] The research project was difficult to start because staff opposed it, disliking the idea that a group of women would not receive enemas: 'Most objected strongly to managing patients in labour unless an enema had been given and the bowel emptied.' They thought that without an enema labour would be prolonged and the incidence of instrumental delivery increased. They foresaw faecal contamination of the baby and thought that offensive odour would embarrass both staff and patient.

Women who had enemas were compared with those who had no bowel treatment and it was found that there was no significant difference between the degree of contamination by faeces during first and second stages of labour. In fact, if a woman had an enema and then passed matter from the lower bowel it was much more difficult to control since it was likely to be fluid. Labour lasted about the same length of time in the two groups. Women in the group who had an enema disliked it, however, and only accepted it because it was claimed that they would have a clean delivery, though there is no evidence to support this claim. The authors conclude that enemas should only be used with women who have not been able to open their bowels in the past twenty-four hours and who have a loaded rectum.

One particularly interesting feature of the study was the attitude of the midwives, who started off being very hostile to the trial but during the project changed their opinions radically, so that the study had to be terminated prematurely when midwives objected to subjecting women to enemas without good reasons.

The authors point out that it is not easy to challenge a procedure which has been an integral part of obstetric practice for over three hundred years, but nevertheless advise that 'rectal assaults on women in labour should be discouraged'.

Shaving

Shaving of the pubic hair started in maternity hospitals created for the indigent poor. The original idea was to get rid of pubic lice, which were common in women living under the appalling social conditions which these first maternity hospitals were designed to ameliorate. When Queen Charlotte's was founded, in 1752, for example, middle-class women would not have dreamed of going into an institution to have a baby.

Shaving, together with the enema, was used in Queen Charlotte's as a part of 'clean midwifery' and of the general de-lousing of the poor which was done in workhouses throughout the country. Few women have pubic lice nowadays but shaving has become an established part of the admission procedure in childbirth. Women are sometimes told it is done so as to have a bald area for episiotomy and suturing of the perineum. Over the years the area shaved has become smaller, and a 'mini-shave' of the perineum is now the one most commonly used. Though many women accept it as a necessary part of childbirth, there is an increasing sense that it is a needless and often humiliating and degrading element in modern childbirth ritual. The re-growth of hair after the baby's birth causes extreme discomfort, particularly since it is over an area which may be bruised and tender.

Research at a large London hospital shows that women are right to question it.[4] In this study one group of patients had a complete shave, another a partial shave and a control group was left unshaved. It was discovered that there was no significant difference in the incidence of infection in the three groups. There was, however, much more bruising among the women who had been shaved and even where to the naked eye shaving did not seem to have been traumatic, when high-power photographs were taken of the skin it was clear that there were multiple small abrasions, especially around the hair follicles.

Fifty per cent of the women who had complete shaves complained of a burning sensation after the procedure and all the women who were shaved complained of embarrassing itching when the hair began to grow again. It is clear that, even in skilled hands, a truly atraumatic shave is impossible. Ninety per cent of the women who were shaved disliked it. The conclusion is that there is 'no evidence to support the current and widespread practice of perineal shaving; it increases patient discomfort without reducing infection or improving healing. We believe that perineal shaving is an unjustified assault and should be abandoned.'

Preparation	Infected	Not infected	Total
A. Unshaved	4	221	225
B. Complete shave	4	224	228
C. Perineal shave	7	233	240
Total	15	678	693

Mona Romney, the author of this study, comments that perhaps the popularity of shaving owes more to the development of the safety razor than to any established medical indication and says that 'It is likely that perineal assault with an old-fashioned cut-throat razor would have provoked an earlier and more vigorous patient response.'

Nil by mouth

In strong labour women do not fancy food and would not be able to digest it. It seems as if the whole body is working to get the baby born. They do appreciate occasional drinks, however, and in the hot atmosphere of many delivery suites particularly need cold drinks in order to keep well hydrated. If they are breathing through their mouths they also find that mouth and lips get dry unless they have frequent sips of liquid. Iced water and ice chips to suck between contractions are probably the best for this, with some light grease such as lanolin or Lipsyl to put on the lips.

Some hospitals have a rule that no patient should have any food by mouth during labour in case general anaesthesia for Caesarean section should prove necessary. A patient who has general anaesthesia without the stomach being empty first of all may vomit stomach contents.

Many women now believe that to treat every woman in labour as if she were about to have a surgical operation and subject her to virtual starvation over what may be a long period of hard physical work and mental concentration is unnecessary and could be harmful. If you do not eat anything over a long period of time fat reserves start to be broken down to provide energy and acetone appears in the urine. This is a sign that you have not had sufficient carbohydrate.

In some hospitals it is more or less routine for an intravenous drip to be set up so that the woman can be given carbohydrate in the form of a glucose solution straight into her bloodstream, but the routine giving of intravenous fluids is now being questioned since it sometimes means that a woman suffers from water intoxication and her electrolyte balance is disturbed.

It is common sense to realize that if you do not have food throughout a long labour you are likely to become very tired and emotionally low. Lack of food can also cause secondary uterine inertia, with the contractions becoming weaker and irregular. With this in mind, it is probably a good idea to eat something light and easily digested in early labour. This should be high in carbohydrate, such as an omelette with a baked potato in its jacket and perhaps bread and butter with honey to follow. Some women also take in barley sugar or other glucose sweets to suck between contractions in labour and others like a small pot of honey into which they can dip. Glucose or sugar added to fresh orange or lemon juice is also refreshing and gives energy. The advantage of glucose is that it requires no digestion, passes straight across the membranes of the mouth and stomach and its effects are obvious almost immediately. If you are having a trial of labour with the possibility of a Caesarean section, however, do not take any glucose or glucose drinks, since if this is vomited and inhaled it is highly irritant to the lungs.

Artificial rupture of the membranes

It is common practice nowadays for the doctor or midwife to break the waters at some time during labour. This is called *amniotomy*, or artificial rupture of the membranes (ARM). It is often done when the woman is first admitted to hospital, when she may be only 2–3 cm dilated. There are three reasons for routine amniotomy: first it allows the attendant to see whether there is any meconium in the waters. This is the substance in the baby's bowels before birth and when fresh meconium is present in the water it can be a sign of fetal distress. The second reason, and an important one nowadays, is that an electrode can be attached to the fetal scalp so that continuous electronic monitoring can take place. Thirdly, it is believed that rupturing the membrane stimulates uterine contractions, so making labour shorter.

It used to be thought that the amniotic fluid around the fetus was just a stagnant pool, but research now shows that the bag of waters has important functions not only during pregnancy, but also in labour. In pregnancy the fluid provides a constant, steady temperature for the baby, protects it from pressure and being jolted and allows it to move freely; because it is automatically changed every three hours, it also aids the removal of the baby's waste fluids, and, since it has some nutritional properties, when the water is swallowed it may be an additional means of fetal nutrition. The fetus practises breathing and swallowing movements inside the bag of waters so that it is ready for taking on these important activities immediately after birth.[5]

Because the membranes rupture spontaneously during labour, often at the end of the first stage, they have come to be thought of as something getting in the way of the progress of labour. It is easy to see how this association of ideas came about. If the membranes usually rupture when the most obviously active phase of labour takes place, maybe rupturing them artificially will bring that about more speedily. And it is certainly true that there is a point just before full dilatation of the cervix when, if the waters have not gone spontaneously, rupturing them artificially can often result in quick progress to full dilatation and the onset of the second stage. It is true, too, that if a woman is lying down, artificial rupturing of the membranes at some time during the active phase of labour shortens it. In one study women who had early amniotomy had a labour which was fifty minutes shorter than a control group of women who did not have amniotomy.

The fetal head acts as a better wedge against the cervix than the bag of water and this pressure also encourages the release of oxytocin into the mother's bloodstream (Fergusson's reflex).[6] Nevertheless, labour could be shortened equally efficiently if the woman was free to walk around and the membranes left intact. It appears to be the horizontal position which slows down labour.

When membranes are ruptured early there is more moulding of the baby's head, indicating that far more pressure is put on the baby when the waters have gone.

In his classic study of the patterns of normal labour[7] Friedman shows that early amniotomy does not help and points out that it exposes the baby and the uterus to invading pathogens; infection is directly related to the length of time which has elapsed between amniotomy and delivery. Electronic fetal monitoring also reveals some of the effects of amniotomy. Artificially removing the protective cushion from the baby's head tends to result in more type 1 dips in the fetal heart rate. The heart beats more slowly at the beginning of each contraction. This occurs whenever the membranes have ruptured before 5 cm dilatation of the cervix, whether artificially or naturally, and the effect is greater when oxytocin is also used to induce or stimulate labour. This is attributed to pressure of the fetal head against a resistant cervix.[8]

No one is suggesting that these type 1 dips are dangerous for the baby. But they do indicate that the baby is subjected to more stress than if the membranes were left intact. Most babies can cope with this stress well. There is some evidence that when the membranes have been ruptured there is a greater chance of interruption of blood flow in the baby's umbilical cord[9] and disalignment of the parietal bones as a result of pressure on the baby's skull. One sign of this is the formation of a caput, a big bump on the baby's head often to one side or the other, depending on the position in which the head was coming down through the cervix. The baby's head is not hard bone all over; there is a suture right along the middle, and two soft spots, or fontanelles, one between the parietal bone and the occipital part of the skull and the other between the parietal bone and the frontal part of the skull. When there is a great deal of pressure on the occipital and frontal parts of the skull the soft spots close up and may actually slip under the edges of the parietal bone.

Other studies of the effects of amniotomy look at the chemical balance of the baby's blood immediately after birth. It has been discovered that babies born when the membranes have remained intact until full dilatation or beyond have a better acid–base balance than babies whose mothers have had an amniotomy.[10] One explanation of this is that loss of amniotic fluid may result in compression of the fetal surface of the placenta during powerful contractions, resulting in reduced blood flow in that part of the placenta. The same thing may occur when there is compression of the cord between the baby and the wall of the uterus.

It looks, then, as if one of the commonest reasons given for rupturing the membranes artificially – to put an electrode on the presenting part so that the fetal heart can be continuously monitored – may sometimes produce the conditions which the electronic fetal monitor is designed to record, and that it would be safer to leave the membranes intact until they rupture spontaneously. If your obstetrician routinely employs electronic fetal monitoring you may wish to say that you do not want an internal electrode used until, and only if, the membranes rupture of their own accord.

Fetal monitoring[11]

We have long practised fetal monitoring; all over the world, in different times, midwives have listened to the baby's heart through the mother's abdominal wall, either by simply applying an ear or by using some device to magnify the sound. Midwives in the past, as today, used a hearing trumpet pressed against the mother's abdomen. But human monitors are now being replaced by electronic apparatus. In increasing numbers of hospitals continuous fetal monitoring is used, involving an electrode being strapped to the mother's abdomen. About 20 per cent of readings do not register properly with this method. Once dilatation of the cervix is great enough, the electrode is inserted through the vagina and cervix to be clipped on or screwed into the baby's head.

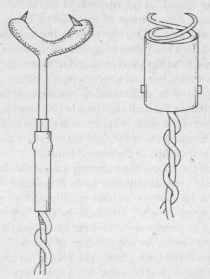

Figure 1 Fetal skin electrodes (from Geoffrey Chamberlain, *Lecture Notes on Obstetrics*, 4th ed., Oxford, Blackwell Scientific Publications, 1980).

Some obstetricians believe that every woman in labour should have electronic fetal monitoring.[12]

The baby gets its oxygen from its mother's blood passing through the placenta. The normal fetal heartbeat varies a great deal, but it is usually 120 to 140 beats per minute. (If the midwife is monitoring with her ear trumpet she may listen for a quarter of a minute and then multiplies by four. If you are in advanced pregnancy your husband or a friend can probably do the same thing using an upturned glass tumbler or the cardboard middle of a lavatory paper roll, at least if you can discover where the heart is.)

When the heart is very fast it is called *tachycardia*. If the fetal heart gets slow this is called *bradycardia*, and if it drops below 100 it is reckoned that the fetus is in distress. It may be that the placenta is not functioning well, so that insufficient oxygen-bearing blood is getting through to the baby, or that there is pressure on the cord which is preventing free flow. If this seems to be the problem it can often be cured by the mother changing position and lying on her side, getting up and moving around or being on all fours, when the weight of the uterus is automatically lifted off the big blood vessels in her body.

When oxytocin is used to induce or accelerate labour continuous monitoring should always be done, as oxytocin is a powerful drug which when used without caution can lead to massive uterine contractions which are too powerful for the baby and distressing for the mother. Continuous fetal monitoring is nearly always used when a woman is on an oxytocin drip.

If continuous fetal monitoring is not being used it is normal practice to record the fetal heart at least every 10 minutes in strong labour and between every contraction of the second stage, and this does not mean that anything is wrong.

When continuous monitoring is done the heartbeats are recorded on a print-out, a long strip of paper a bit like ticker tape, which rolls off the machine. There may be a flashing light and there is usually a switch which enables the fetal heart to be heard in the room. If this is reassuring for the mother it can be left on. If it is offputting it can be switched down.

These machines record the strength and length of uterine contractions at the same time as the fetal heart so that it can be seen how the baby is doing in relation to the work undertaken by the uterus. Many women like to be able to see the strength and length of contractions and find it reassuring to hear the baby's heartbeats. The baby's heart often gets fast at the height of contractions, as the uterus presses on the baby and 'massages' it strongly, but sometimes it becomes much slower. The obstetrician is especially watching for 'dips' in the heart. If the dip does not correct itself when a contraction is over, the obstetrician suspects fetal distress and is ready to hasten the labour, usually with a forceps delivery or a Caesarean section.

From the woman's point of view there may be four drawbacks with continuous fetal monitoring:

1. Before the cervix is sufficiently dilated to put a clip on the top of the baby's head with which to record heartbeats, the only way of recording them continuously is by putting a monitoring corset tightly round the mother's abdomen. For the electrodes to pick up the fetal heart clearly this has to be firmly applied. Unfortunately pressure around the abdomen during contractions can cause unnecessary pain.

2. It is difficult even to change position in bed when the most widely used kind of continuous monitoring is employed. Lying in one position for a long time can be uncomfortable and cause back pain even when one is not in labour. When a woman is in labour it can cause acute discomfort. Monitoring by radio waves, similar to that which is used for astronauts, is only just beginning. This kind of monitoring, known as *telemetry*, allows the mother to walk about in labour. In a controlled trial women who walked about in labour while being monitored needed less analgesia than others who were monitored in bed, and also were more likely to enjoy their labours and later to breast-feed successfully.

3. When an abdominal monitor is used, it is difficult or impossible to do light abdominal massage – which often helps during contractions – since the electrode is dislodged or the massage interferes with the recording.

4. The other problem is that machines sometimes go wrong. It can be alarming when the baby's heartbeat apparently stops, or when the room suddenly fills with people who are checking what is happening. Some women also find it disturbing when electrical engineers come to mend the monitor.

There may also be some negative effects of continual fetal monitoring on the fetus which, although they should be weighed against the obvious advantages of having a 'window into the womb' during labour, are not necessarily negligible.

The first and biggest problem, one which affects both mother and baby, is that because the normal variations in fetal heart rate are not yet fully understood, delivery may be accelerated with forceps or an emergency Caesarean section may be performed when in fact the baby is all right.

The use of continuous fetal monitors has usually meant that both the forceps and the Caesarean section rates have gone up in those hospitals which rely on this method for detecting fetal distress. Some obstetricians believe that it is so easy to make mistakes and intervene unnecessarily that when the monitor points to the possibility of fetal distress a drop of blood should always be taken from the baby's scalp and analysed to see if there are chemical changes which indicate distress. Even when there are late decelerations of the fetal heart rate (towards the end of each contraction and in the interval between contractions) which are considered the most severe type, only in about one third of cases is the blood chemistry abnormal.

The immobility of the mother may affect the baby, particularly if she is lying flat or almost flat in bed. Many kinds of obstetric intervention are associated with this *dorsal* position in labour, since obstetricians are used to having women lying supine and easily accessible. The trouble is that it tends to put pressure on big blood vessels and to reduce blood flow to the baby. So continuous fetal monitoring may occasionally actually produce the variations from normal which it is designed to record. If you are being monitored, it is a good idea to lie on your side or to sit up well, and to change position occasionally. If the electrode gets dislodged it will have to be refitted after this.

Because the clip has to be firmly fixed to the baby's scalp it is pricked through the skin and this leaves a small mark. Occasionally this becomes infected later, and sometimes hair never grows over this tiny patch. This is a small price to pay if there are indications that a baby needs to be monitored. It is an unnecessary price when monitoring is not used selectively.

Some very big firms produce fetal monitors and it is a highly competitive market. Some obstetricians are getting wary of high-pressure salesmen for monitors. In 1976 one firm alone sold 800 monitors and made £2 million. Steer[13] points out that the fetal monitor is no longer simply a research instrument and is now big business.

There is another subtle and invidious effect of electronic fetal monitoring. It is that the focus of interest is removed from the woman who is having the baby to the machinery. Staff may come into the room and look first at the print-out, only afterwards at the mother. Even the father may trust what the machine shows rather than what the woman says she is feeling. It is almost as if the baby itself is in that machine, as if its very essence is represented by the moving needle and the jagged shapes which testify to life inside the uterus. When the mother looks at the print-out it is as if she is watching her baby, no longer inside her body but out there, in the unceasing activity of the machines. We do not know what effect this scenario may have on the way in which the mother, and the father too, thinks about the baby. We do know that the very space taken up by electronic machinery means that everything else seems to be crowded out and of less importance than the monitor, and that sometimes the father may find it difficult to get in physical contact with the labouring woman because there is simply no space for him to be close to the bed. The machinery is central and he is squashed in beside it. The emotional effects on self-image, on the relationship between the couple during labour and on their perception of the baby have yet to be explored.

Fifty per cent of babies who produce apparently abnormal fetal heart readings in labour have nothing wrong with them. This means that half of all babies delivered by forceps or Caesarean section in some hospitals simply because of a worrying print-out need not have had an operative delivery.

Professor Richard Beard has publicly stated that one reason he dislikes human monitoring is because a midwife listening to a baby's heart can convey her anxiety to the mother. He therefore seeks to move midwives into the background and relies on machines to do the work instead. Anyone who has had electronic fetal monitoring, however, is aware that machines can cause anxiety in doctors, midwives and the parents. When they go wrong they may generate anxiety in the whole delivery 'team'. When they work, but the print-out shows unexplained variations in the fetal heart rate, they also cause anxiety.

Figure 2 is a print-out of a 'normal' fetal heart, between 120 and 160 beats per minute. The mother's contractions are shown at the bottom. No

Fetal heart

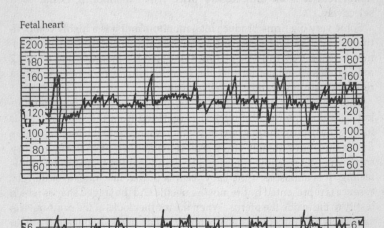

Figure 2 Print-out of normal fetal heart.

Fetal heart

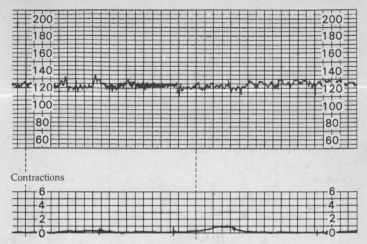

Figure 3 This baby's heart rate is on the slow side and the trace is rather flat; contractions are still slight.

baby's heart is absolutely regular. It is normal for it to vary by about 10 beats a minute.

Contractions squeeze the baby and the healthy fetus responds by a variation in heartbeat. If the heart does not change with contractions there is a flatter print-out. The baby may be drowsy because of shortage of oxygen – *hypoxia*.

Deep dips indicating a slowing-down of the heart – bradycardia – during contractions may be a sign of hypoxia, but are usually of no significance. Only 7 per cent of babies with deep dips at the height of contractions suffer from shortage of oxygen. In the print-out in Figure 4 the baby's heart gets much slower at the start of each contraction, but it picks up beautifully again as the contraction wears off.

In the next print-out (Figure 5), however, there are *late* decelerations. The heart rate is fast – tachycardia – except that it dips dramatically at the peak of each contraction and stays down a while after the contraction has finished. The combination of tachycardia with late dips is a warning sign.

A very rapid heart rate is more likely to indicate shortage of oxygen than a slow one, but even then only 20 per cent of babies have oxygen deprivation. Figure 6 shows a print-out of a fetal heart which shows tachycardia.

Fetal heart

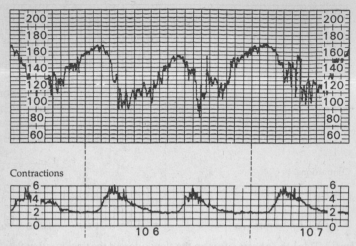

Figure 4

Fetal heart

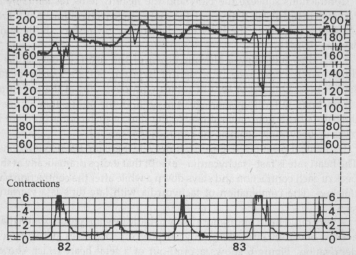

Figure 5

The fetal heart sometimes dips alarmingly in response to oxytocin used to induce or accelerate labour. The heart is dropping to 60 in the print-out in Figure 7. The baby is at risk. The oxytocin drip should be stopped. The mother would probably be best kneeling or crouching forward or on all fours to help the flow of blood to the baby.

The obstetrician who is anxious about the fetal heart rate can either intervene immediately and deliver the baby by forceps, vacuum extraction or Caesarean section, or he can do fetal blood sampling. This is done by making a small cut with a sharp-bladed knife in the baby's scalp. Some obstetricians believe that blood sampling before intervention eliminates unnecessary forceps deliveries and Caesarean sections. The disadvantage of this is that since there is a good deal of pressure on the baby's head before delivery it is unlikely that the pH of scalp blood accurately reflects the baby's general biochemistry. In effect, the blood being analysed is blood from a bruise. So even then unnecessary operative deliveries may be done.

If your labour is induced or accelerated with an oxytocin drip there is a case to be made for continuous fetal monitoring, since the contractions produced by the drug may be so great that they interfere with the flow of oxygenized blood to the baby or cause direct pressure on the baby's circulation. If vaginal *prostaglandins* are used, however, there is no proved benefit from electronic monitoring. Research comparing labours after prostaglandin treatment in which continuous electronic fetal monitoring was used with others which were monitored by human attendants has shown that there is no advantage from electronic monitoring. There is, in fact, an obvious disadvantage because the rate of Caesarean sections is significantly higher when electronic monitoring is employed. With intermittent human monitoring the Caesarean rate is 3 per cent, which is low, but with electronic monitoring it shoots up to 47 per cent. Babies show no benefit from the electronic monitoring when their one-minute and five-minute Apgar scores are compared.[14]

Randomized controlled trials have been considered unethical by some obstetricians because they felt that the benefits of fetal monitoring were so obvious that their patients should not be exposed to the risk implicit in *not* using monitoring. However, all the studies that have been done point to an increase in the rate of Caesarean sections by anything from a third to a half. This was not because there were more indications of fetal distress. Either something to do with monitoring introduces an unknown hazard or the very fact that women are being monitored makes obstetricians more likely to intervene.

One of the things that emerged from women's accounts of their hospital experiences was that very often monitors do not work correctly

Fetal heart

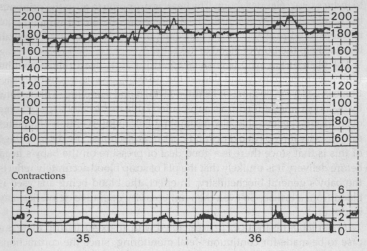

Contractions

Figure 6

Fetal heart

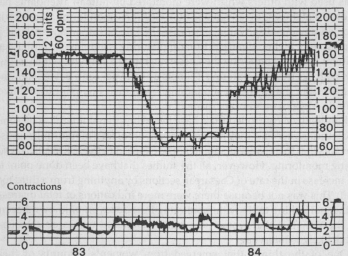

Contractions

Figure 7

or break down completely. They also describe situations in which doctors and midwives are uncertain how to use the machine or ignore its findings because they do not know how to interpret them. Often the sounding of an alarm or a print-out showing that the fetal heart rate was dropping was ignored and the mother might be told, 'Oh don't worry, it's always doing that.' Quite often someone kicked the machine. Sometimes too, the mother's heart, rather than the baby's, was being monitored and this was likely to result in unnecessary intervention. In one case, for example, in a famous London teaching hospital, the monitor indicated fetal distress whenever the mother pushed. So she was urged to push still harder and longer to get the baby born more quickly. She strained and struggled and held her breath for still longer periods. Preparation was made for a forceps delivery. It was then pointed out that the monitor was recording *her* heart changes during strenuous bearing-down efforts, not the baby's. Any equipment that might be advantageous in the hands of people who know how to use it is clearly not going to be of benefit, and may actually be harmful, when in the hands of someone who does not understand how to use it or how to interpret the squiggles on the print-out.

Continuous fetal monitoring obviously has a place in obstetrics and seems likely to be beneficial for women to have known risk factors. But to conclude that because something is right for 10–15 per cent of women it must therefore be right for all women and for all labours is a dangerous generalization and is likely to lead to the misuse of monitors and to the devaluing of clinical skills.

If electronic monitoring is strongly recommended in your case but you are not happy about being 'wired up' a compromise is to agree to have the external monitor some time at the beginning of your labour for a period of not more than an hour. If all is well during that time the monitor is removed and is only used again if dilatation is slow or there are other reasons for thinking that the baby may be under stress.

Active management of labour

This term includes all kinds of obstetric intervention to ensure that the pattern of labour relates to a norm, devised by obstetricians, of how labour should be. The intervention is planned to prevent rather than to cure. It is based on the concept that birth is always potentially hazardous and should be conducted in an intensive care situation. Practice varies but an active approach may include induction of labour, which contributes to a 'regular and orderly turnover of work in a planned manner and rationalizes work flow in delivery suites which usually are "bottlenecks"';[15] continuous fetal monitoring for every woman, with monitors placed centrally at the nursing station so that observers can see the state of the fetus without needing to stand beside the patient's bed; and the management of labour so that it is short (not more than six hours from 2 cm dilatation in women having second and subsequent babies, and eleven hours in those having first babies, is one model). 'The active management of labour necessitates that obstetricians take over, not just a single aspect of delivery, but responsibility for the whole process of parturition. Our control of the situation must be complete.'[16]

Some studies of active management do not show the good results, in terms of the reduction of perinatal mortality and morbidity, which are claimed for it. Chalmers and others[17] analysed 9907 deliveries which took place in Cardiff between 1968 and 1972, where two obstetric teams had different ways of conducting labour, one doing active management and the other having a more conservative approach. There was no difference in the state of the babies, but more urinary and genital infections in the actively managed mothers, and the authors concluded that active management had not improved 'perinatal outcome'.

Professor A. C. Turnbull, commenting on the way in which maternity units vie with each other to utilize new techniques, remarks that 'because the national rate [of perinatal mortality] fell steadily over the period when the use of new techniques was increasing, a cause-and-effect relationship was assumed which may well have engendered a false feeling of security about the value of obstetric intervention'.[18]

A large proportion of obstetricians, however, see active management as a major advance in obstetrics and believe that all mothers and babies benefit from it.

Some believe that it is important to limit the duration of labour, both for the mother's and the baby's health, but that induction is usually unnecessary and may actually extend the period of stress to which a fetus is exposed.[19]

Again, they may believe in careful monitoring of the baby, but base this on observation of the waters in which the baby floats in the uterus rather than on continuous fetal monitoring with electrodes. Normally the liquor is clear, but sometimes it is stained with *meconium*, the baby's first bowel movements, and this *may* indicate that the fetus is under stress. O'Driscoll, in the paper quoted above, indicates that clear liquor early in labour virtually ensures the birth of a healthy baby, provided labour does not last too long and the delivery is straightforward. One way of observing the liquor is to do an artificial rupture of the membranes (ARM) as soon as labour is diagnosed, if spontaneous rupture of the membranes has not occurred already. Another way is to use an *amnioscope*, an instrument which allows the obstetrician to direct a tiny light on the membranes while still unruptured. Since other obstetricians again believe that the membranes should be kept intact as long as possible because they protect the baby's head and the umbilical cord,[20] amnioscopy may be the preferred method of observing the state of the liquor. Another way of finding out about the state of the baby is by taking a fetal blood sample, some drops of blood being drawn from the baby's head, and often results show that there is no need for further intervention. In this way unnecessary Caesarean sections can be avoided. O'Driscoll uses this technique if the liquor is meconium-stained, to discover whether the baby really is at risk.

Since policies regarding the management of labour vary between different consultant obstetricians in the same hospital it is a good idea to discuss this with your general practitioner before you are booked in with a particular 'firm', or to ask the obstetrician about it when you attend the antenatal clinic if you are already booked in.

Induction of labour

Induction means that labour is started artificially. This has been done, in one way or another, for hundreds of years. But it is only in the last twenty years that a really efficient method for doing so has been invented. Because it has become so easy to do, some doctors rely on this technique to initiate labour at the time they think best for the baby, the mother and the organization of the hospital. This is particularly marked in some Scottish hospitals where women are admitted from very wide areas and where it may be difficult for them to get to hospital in labour when the weather is bad.

Different hospitals and different doctors in the same hospital have varying ideas about whether induction is desirable in any particular patient. A few adopt the view that most women should be induced, because labour should take place in the daytime, when doctors, midwives, anaesthetists and paediatricians are available. Some doctors feel that everyone is at their freshest and most efficient during ordinary nine-to-five working hours, and that it is best to arrange for all babies to be born then. Some attribute the drop in perinatal mortality rates to the greater incidence of induction. This argument does not really hold water however, because there has been a corresponding decrease in perinatal mortality in countries like Norway, which have not increased their induction rate as we have in Britain.

Many hospitals do some inductions purely for the convenience of the mother. She may want to plan the birth because she has a toddler whom granny is going to look after, or because her husband's business is taking him abroad. A great many women are weary of pregnancy by about thirty-eight weeks and welcome the opportunity of being induced.

But the contrast between social or 'convenience' reasons for induction on the one hand and 'medical' reasons on the other, does not really present a true picture of what is happening. For there are *pressing* medical reasons, such as severe toxaemia, or a baby whose placenta is no longer functioning well, and *minor* medical reasons, which some doctors think indicate that induction ought to be done and which others believe do not call for interference.

Expectant mothers can feel bewildered. Some prefer to leave all the decisions to the doctors. Others, however, would like to be given the facts, to discuss the advantages and disadvantages of induction with the doctor, and share in the decision-making. Still other women believe that, in the last resort, whether or not to have the induction must be their own decision, not the doctor's.

Weighed against this is what doctors consider to be 'professional responsibility'. Some feel that they cannot be expected to continue to take responsibility for a patient who rejects their advice and who appears to question their professional competence. It is important that women bear this in mind when discussing induction with their doctors.

Why inductions?

Effective induction is a great technical advance in obstetrics, and one which, if used with discretion, can save the lives of many babies. It does not mean that all babies need to be induced or that most would benefit from it. Because some children need their tonsils out does not indicate, as used to be thought, that *most* children benefit from having their tonsils removed. In fact, if unnecessary tonsillectomies are performed, more harm than good is done. The same applies to labour. This is why induction for social or administrative reasons is usually unwise. The conditions for which induction may be advisable are:

Toxaemia or *pre-eclampsia* (they mean the same thing) in the mother. This means that her blood pressure is up all the time, not just when she goes to the clinic. She also has albumen (protein) in her urine, and is retaining fluids so that her fingers, ankles, and possibly her face, may become swollen. She often has a sudden excessive weight gain too. This condition is a clear indication for induction before the placenta ceases to function. If she develops severe pre-eclampsia the placenta which nourishes the baby inside her, provides its oxygen and excretes its waste products, will not be able to function well, so there is a risk to the baby.

Very high blood pressure (hypertension) alone is also an indication for induction. Puffiness and retention of water in the tissues, however, or a rather large weight gain, are not in themselves signs that induction ought to be done.

Diabetes in the mother means that her baby may be very large and that it may be subjected to added risk in the uterus after thirty-six weeks or so. So labour is usually induced two or three weeks early, so that the baby does not get so big that vaginal delivery is impossible.

Prolonged pregnancy is often considered an indication for induction, although obstetricians do not always agree on what constitutes prolonged pregnancy. Dates should always be supported by other evidence that the pregnancy is really longer than it should be. One way in which doctors discover this is by measuring at intervals in pregnancy a hormone called *oestriol* in the mother's bloodstream or urine. Another way is by taking a series of 'pictures' of the baby by means of a sonar scan.

Many women go past their dates. The date given by the doctor is only a statistical average. Hospitals may have a rule that when an expectant mother gets to EDD (expected date of delivery) plus one week or two weeks, she comes in to be induced. But it is important that you are sure of your dates and really remember when you had the first day of your last period before pregnancy. This is easier said than done for many women, and what is presented to the doctor is often a convenient fiction.

It can be more complicated still if you were on the Pill, as many women conceive without having regular periods after coming off the Pill. It is always a good idea to use some other contraceptive method immediately after stopping the Pill until a regular rhythm of three periods has been established.

There may be other good reasons for inducing labour, and these should be fully explained to the woman in terms she can understand. For example, if her pelvis is small there may also be a case for inducing before the baby gets so large that she is likely to need a Caesarean section.

One woman wrote that she much preferred induction to the spontaneous start of labour. 'It is,' she said, 'the only civilized way.' Similarly, a midwife said to a woman in one of the high-tech-hospitals listed in this book – 'Oh, but you wouldn't want to have your baby in the middle of the night, would you?'

Women who are taken into hospital early for bed rest and observation also long to see an end to the pregnancy. In some larger Scottish hospitals where women are told to go in from country areas and the Isles often several weeks before their babies are born, they beg to be induced.

You should know that if you are having your baby privately there appears to be a much greater chance of being induced than if you are having it on the NHS. In Ann Cartwright's study of induction[21] she revealed that private patients, though only 2 per cent of all obstetric patients, had a 44-per-cent chance of induction as compared with a

24-per-cent chance for NHS patients. This is odd, because women who can afford to pay for private care are clearly not in the lower social classes and in theory, therefore, should require less, not more, induction, because they have fewer risk factors.

What happens?

The term 'induction' actually covers a number of different methods. There is the old OBE (castor oil, hot bath and enema) which only works if the woman is really ready to go into labour. Then there is artificial rupture of the membranes (ARM) which involves puncturing the bag of water surrounding the baby. This is a painless procedure if the uterus is already slightly open (dilated), but it can hurt if the uterus is tightly closed.

Much of the debate which surrounds the subject of induction now, however, concerns the use of oxytocin. This is usually introduced straight into the bloodstream through a drip into a vein in the woman's arm, which remains in place throughout labour, and often for an hour or two after to make the uterus contract tightly and reduce bleeding. Artificial rupture of the membranes (early in the morning) followed immediately or a few hours later by controlled infusion of oxytocin into a vein in this way is usually a successful method of inducing labour. If the woman is right-handed it is best for the left hand to be used, so that her other hand is still free, or vice versa.

The oxytocin is dripped in slowly at first and then the rate is gradually increased. The aim is to simulate normal labour, starting off with contractions which are three or five minutes apart and which last one minute or a bit longer. In fact, contractions often start coming every two or three minutes and each may last two minutes. If they are longer than this the woman should tell the obstetrician immediately.

Other substances can be introduced through the same apparatus, and it is common practice to give glucose as well. This acts as a pick-me-up straight into the woman's bloodstream, and is considered useful in long or exhausting labours.

Induced labours tend to be short and sharp, and the woman needs to adjust quickly to powerful and frequent contractions. Some women have labours like this anyway, and cope well.

Increasingly prostaglandins, substances found in many body tissues and first discovered in semen, are used to soften the cervix before other methods of induction are employed. With a woman having her first baby this softening is achieved by introducing pessaries of prostaglandin into the vagina overnight. With a woman having her second or subsequent baby a few hours is usually sufficient. Sometimes induction is done with prostaglandins alone. This means that the woman does not need to have an intravenous drip and can be much more mobile. If the cervix is already soft before induction takes place there is a 95 per cent chance of vaginal delivery. If the cervix is unripe, however, there is only a 65 per cent chance of the baby being delivered vaginally within forty-eight hours. This is why the use of prostaglandin gel to ripen the cervix is so important.

Some possible hazards of induction

It would be surprising if what the *Lancet* in an editorial called a 'wholesale interference with this delicately balanced physiological process' (i.e. labour) did not produce some deleterious side-effects.[22]

Because contractions are strong from the beginning, the woman whose labour is induced may feel the need of pain-relieving drugs early on, and may require more of them than she would in spontaneous labour. One study, in Glasgow,[23] showed that women had the same amount of drugs for pain relief whether induced or not. Women who have been to National Childbirth Trust classes, however, need much less pain relief when they are not induced. In my own study, *Some Mothers' Experiences of Induced Labour*,[24] it was found that only 8 per cent of these women, all of whom were highly motivated to have as few drugs as possible, coped without drugs in induced labour, whereas 50 per cent managed without drugs (apart perhaps from Entonox over a few contractions) in spontaneous labour.

Obstetricians are not agreed as to whether induced labour is really more painful. In one German study, where 25 per cent of women complained about excessive pain as compared with earlier labours which were not induced, doctors concluded that the pain was largely 'an organic correlate of unconscious feelings of guilt'![25] Whether or not this is true, most obstetricians would probably agree that women who are induced require more analgesia. Since we now know that *all* pain-relieving drugs can affect the baby, unnecessary induction should be avoided.

The most effective form of pain relief is an epidural, and the rate of epidurals has paralleled the increase in inductions. Since it can be difficult to push a baby out when the woman has little or no feeling from the waist down, there has been an increase in the number of forceps deliveries, though these are, for the most part, simple 'lift-out' forceps. A baby delivered by forceps is often sent automatically to the special care nursery and does not stay with its mother. Psychiatrists and some paediatricians are becoming very concerned about the number of babies in intensive care who are separated from their mothers at birth, since this can interfere with the relationship between mother and baby and lead to difficulties in breast-feeding.

Babies are also more liable to be jaundiced after induction, and sleepy and difficult to feed.[26] It may be a combination of the use of oxytocin and the baby not being quite ready to be born.

A study in Oxford showed that when labour was induced other forms of intervention are more likely to be used too. When a group of healthy women having their labours induced were compared with a matched group starting labour spontaneously, it was found that the induced group had more electronic fetal heart monitoring, more epidurals, more forceps deliveries and Caesarean sections, and that more of their babies needed resuscitation.[27] Because oxytocin-stimulated labours are often more painful, pain-relieving drugs, as we have seen, are more likely to be used. The baby is then exposed to the combined effects of two different kinds of drug. And once the mother has been given effective pain relief, more oxytocin can be introduced into her bloodstream at a faster rate, since she is now out of pain and is not aware of the strength of contractions. Avis Ericson, Professor of Pharmacy for Obstetrics and Gynecology at the University of Kentucky puts it succinctly:

Any drug which artificially changes the mother's blood chemistry or alters the intrauterine environment can jeopardize the fetus. Any drug which interferes with the normal oxygenation of the fetus by shortening the recovery intervals between uterine contractions or by increasing the length and intensity of the contractions beyond the physiologically normal range can damage the fetal brain.[28]

Some induced babies are discovered to be unexpectedly premature. In the United States a new term, 'iatrogenic prematurity' (that is, doctor-produced prematurity) has been coined and it is said that it constitutes a major perinatal health problem.[29] The greatest risk for any baby is to be required to start life before it is mature enough to cope with the challenge of existence outside the uterus. Fetal maturity should always be tested before labour is induced. There is now sophisticated technology to date pregnancies. (Even so, in one study of nearly 1,000 births in Wales it was discovered that the use of these techniques did not really reduce the proportion of women who were classed as 'gestation uncertain').[30] Babies born prematurely may suffer from the *respiratory distress syndrome*, when, because of lack of surfactant (like the bubbles in detergent) their lungs do not inflate properly and collapse between each breath. Respiratory distress is the greatest single cause of perinatal death.

One of the reasons why some babies are born prematurely is misjudgement by the obstetrician of gestational age and resulting induction of labour.[31] As we have seen, a mother and baby are more likely to be separated after induced labour. Though this may seem unimportant, in some ways it could be the most significant finding of all. The hours and days following delivery may be significant for bonding of both mother and baby and father and baby, and separation then can produce problems in the subsequent relationship between the parents and their child. In my own study of women who had induced labours I discovered that as many as 42 per cent were separated from their babies, either because the baby was in the special care baby unit or because the mother was drugged to the eyeballs and was not interested in the baby, or sometimes did not even know that she had had it. This last condition I called 'pharmacological separation'. It seems to me important, because there is little point in a baby being beside a mother's bed if she is unable to relate to it. So it is not just a question of the couple being physically separated but sometimes of drugs adversely affecting the mother and the baby so that their relationship is not a going concern.

Thus it is not just a question of induction, but of a train of events that may be set in motion when labour is started off artificially, which may affect not only the mother, but also her baby. These effects have to be weighed against the obvious advantages when induction can save babies' lives.

If you are concerned to avoid induction unless strictly necessary, it is important to let your doctor know politely that you would like an opportunity for discussion with him, perhaps when your husband can come too, and then time to consider it together. Work out together the questions to ask, and write them down.

There may be good reasons why you should accept the offer of induction and you should give the doctor's explanation your serious consideration. But if you are not convinced of its value in your case, go home and talk about it and then let the hospital know your decision.

To be able to make a decision, however, you may need to ask for information and also for time in which to consider the facts given you. In Ann Cartwright's study of induction,[32] 80 per cent of women wanted more information than they received. It certainly was not just those in the 'vocal minority' who sought more understanding of what was being done to them, and why. It was so for women from all social classes. In my own study[33] two thirds of those who reported no discussion about induction before it was done had unhappy labours, but when they felt that there had been full discussion less than a quarter had unhappy labours.

Should new medical indications for induction develop – such as your blood pressure shooting up – you must, of course, be prepared to take fresh advice. Ultimately whether or not to be induced can be your own, informed decision.

Certainly some babies, probably some 10–15 per cent, although Roberto Caldeyro-Barcia believes that the rate is 'less than 3 per cent of labours,'[34] can be born safely only if labour is induced. It really would be a pity if women whose labour ought to be induced did not benefit from this advance in obstetric technique. Equally, it is a pity to be induced when it is unnecessary and when induction may itself introduce some hazards for the baby.

Acceleration of labour

Labour can often be speeded up by doing an artificial rupture of the membranes. Contractions may become stronger and more effective after this is done.

Acceleration of labour which involves an ARM has, however, come under fire from some obstetricians who have done research on the effect of loss of the waters, which act as a protective cushion for the baby's head, on the baby's condition at birth. Type 1 dips in the fetal heart rate, with the heart beating more slowly at the beginning of each contraction, occur when the membranes have ruptured before 5 cm dilation of the cervix, and are made more severe when oxytocin is also used to induce or accelerate labour. This is attributed to pressure of the fetal head against a resistant cervix.

There is also increased risk of infection when the woman labours for a long time after the membranes have ruptured, one reason why an oxytocin drip to accelerate labour may be recommended.

But acceleration of labour usually nowadays 'means that an oxytocin drip is also used after labour has started naturally.

Some obstetricians consider that labour should never last longer than ten to twelve hours, or even less, and speed up and intensify contractions to shorten labour, an approach sometimes called 'enhanced labour'.[35] They say that long labours are tiring for the mother and believe that all women prefer to have short labours. This assumption does not take into account the fact that many long labours begin very gently. If the woman is happy and relaxed, and, above all, if she is in the familiar surroundings of her own home, she can continue her everyday activities, and let gravity help press the baby down against the cervix by walking about. Not only can lying in a hospital bed cause compression of the *vena cava*, so reducing oxygenation of the fetus, but it is also a poor position for getting contractions going and for ensuring efficient uterine contractility.

Very prolonged labours can be helped by an oxytocin drip. There is, however, a kind of slowly unfolding labour which lasts a long time, but which a well-prepared woman who is given adequate emotional support and encouragement may cope with well.

Problems arise when a woman who 'always has slow labours' or who perhaps says that 'all the women in my family have slow labours' goes into hospital early, or is in there already because she is in the antenatal ward for observation, and is not allowed to take longer than the norm.

Women who are aware of this often plan to labour as long as they are comfortable at home and hope that when they go into hospital they will already be 5 cm dilated. Your own comfort is a pretty good guide. If you feel you want to be in hospital it is one of the best signs that you should be there. If you are happy at home, continuing to do things around the house perhaps, and stopping to breathe through each contraction, it is one of the best indications that this is where you should be.

You should be asked if the obstetrician proposes to set up an intravenous oxytocin drip and it should not be done if you do not agree. If you are told that something is going to be done and you do not demur it is taken for granted that you have agreed to the procedure.

Being upright and walking around for a while may get a labour going and it can be a good idea to try this first, a practice which midwives have favoured since antiquity in many different countries. Michel Odent (see p. 132) advises a woman who is having a long, slow labour to try the effect of relaxing in warm water. Much of the debate about the ways in which labour is managed today is about who is in control, the obstetrician or the woman having the baby. Changing your position, kneeling in water or walking around are ways in which you control your own labour.

If you agree that you would like labour induced or augmented with oxytocin, you can make sure before the catheter is inserted in the back of your hand that you are in a comfortable position and as upright as possible. This helps the descent of the baby's head and avoids pressure on the big blood vessels in the lower part of your body. You may like to sit out of bed in a chair or be in bed well supported by pillows. Some hospitals have wedges and other means of back support too. Be certain that there is a sufficiently long lead to the drip stand for you to be able to change position when you wish and that the sticky tape is firmly fixed so that you are not frightened about moving your arm lest you detach the drip. If you are right-handed you will probably prefer the drip in your left, and vice versa, so that it interferes as little as possible with normal mobility.

If it is difficult to relax your legs, see if a pillow under each thigh helps you to release the muscles on the inside of your legs. To prevent the pillows becoming wet or bloodstained, slip them into large polythene bags – pack two in your case for the hospital.

Oxytocin is introduced slowly at first and gradually increased. If you are getting very long, painful contractions the drip can be slowed down.

If the possibility of acceleration is being discussed you have the right to be kept fully informed and to share in the decision-making.

In some hospitals in this book 40 per cent of women have labour induced. In some, a further 30–40 per cent are reckoned to need acceleration. This means that 70–80 per cent of women having babies in these hospitals are attached to an oxytocin drip. It stretches the imagination to believe that this proportion of women has something so wrong with them that they cannot be permitted, for their own or their babies' sakes, to labour naturally. Obstetricians who favour these high rates of oxytocin stimulation imply that women are incapable of giving birth without intervention and that they must depend heavily on doctors if birth is to be safe.

The partogram

The partogram is a graph depicting labour in linear form and representing the normal progress of dilatation of the cervix. There are different forms of partogram, but they are all based on the idea of an optimum length for each phase of labour and that deviations from this norm should be corrected by active management and the use of intravenous oxytocin.

The earliest phase of labour is called 'the latent phase'. This is the phase preceding 2–3 cm dilatation. During the active phase dilatation is supposed to take place at 1–3 cm per hour in women having their first babies (primigravidae) and at 1–6 cm per hour in women having second and subsequent babies (multigravidae). If a woman does not meet this standard her labour is considered abnormal and intervention takes place.

Zero time is usually considered the time when she is admitted to the labour suite and from then on a point is marked on the graph every two to four hours and the points connected to make a curve. An 'alert line' is drawn from the time when the cervix is 3 cm dilated (or the woman was admitted) to a point six hours to the right on the top line. Thus, if she was 3 cm at 4 a.m. the alert line starts at 4 a.m. and shoots up to 10 a.m. Two hours to the right of, and hence below this, another line is drawn, the

Figure 8 (opposite) One kind of partogram showing the details of prolonged labour (from J. Studd, in *Management of Labour*, Proceedings of Third Study Group of Royal College of Gynaecologists and Obstetricians, 1975).
This partogram is a record over a twenty-four-hour period. The top section shows the fetal heart rate; the narrow band beneath, the point at which amniotomy was performed; the next section the descent of the presenting part of the baby through the cervix and deep into the pelvis, the angle at which the head is presenting – it changes from LOP (left occipito posterior) to LOT (left occipito tranverse) – and the points at which fetal blood samples were taken. The next narrow band records when an oxytocin drip was started. (It can be seen that this corresponds with deep dips in the fetal heart rate) and, in the next band, with non-stop contractions. The next section shows that the mother had a mixture of pethidine and sparine early on, another two doses later and then, before the oxytocin infusion was started, an epidural. Finally there are two sections which record maternal condition.

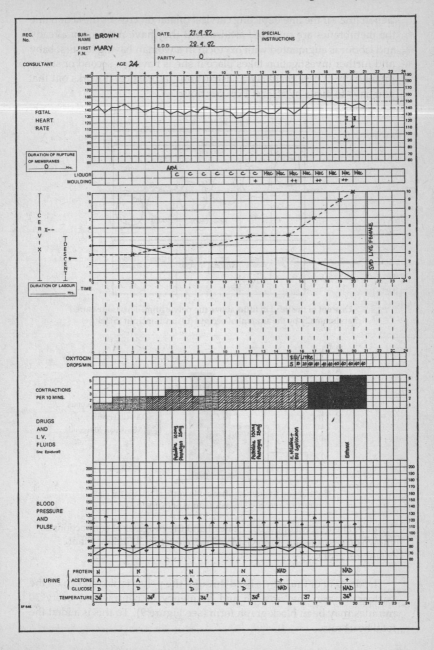

'action line'. If the line depicting cervical dilatation crosses the action line the membranes are ruptured artificially if they have not broken already and labour is augmented with oxytocin in a woman having her first baby and further investigation takes place if she is having a second or subsequent baby in case there is an obstruction. In practice, it works out that you have to dilate by at least 1 cm per hour.

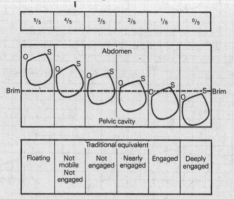

Descent of the head in fifths above the pelvic brim. This is measured abdominally by the amount of occiput (O) and sinciput (S) felt.

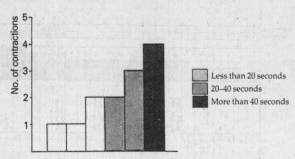

Contraction frequency: Shade one vertical square for each contraction recorded in last 10 mins of every ½ hr.

Figure 9 The descent of the baby's head and the progress of contractions as shown on a partogram (from G. M. Stirrat, *Obstetrics*, London, Grant McIntyre, 1981).

The descent of the baby's head through the pelvis is also shown on the partogram, and the strength and frequency of contractions every 30 minutes may be in block graph form (see Figure 9). To this is added the fetal heart rate.

When the waters have gone the condition of the amniotic fluid is also noted on the partogram: C for clear; M for meconium-stained; B for blood-stained: if the membranes have not yet ruptured an I stands for intact membranes.

The moulding of the fetal head as it is pressed down like a grapefruit through the cervix is also recorded, O standing for no moulding and the degree of moulding being assessed by +, ++, +++, or ++++ (most moulding).

If the woman is given an infusion of oxytocin this is recorded on the chart in milliunits (mu) per minute or drops per minute (dpm). Her blood pressure, pulse, temperature, urine analysis and any drugs she receives for pain relief are also recorded on the partogram.

Pain-relieving drugs used in labour

It is probably worth asking the obstetrician at an antenatal clinic the proportion of women who have different kinds of pain relief, at least for pethidine and epidurals. This will give an indication of hospital practice in that particular hospital. He may even know if the obstetricians in different 'firms' have varying practices in this respect. The main types include:

Regional anaesthesia (that is, sensation is removed from part of the body) such as epidurals, caudals and paracervical blocks and pudendal blocks. Caudals and epidurals are injected into the spinal area and a catheter is left in place so that the anaesthetic can be 'topped up'. A pudendal block is an injection into the birth canal or sometimes just around the vulva.

Narcotics given by injection, such as pethidine, morphine, heroin, Omnopon, Fortral and Talwin. These cause drowsiness and tend to make the woman feel drunk.

Sedatives which make the woman drowsy or get her to sleep, such as Welldorm, chloral, Seconal, Amytal, Nembutal, Soneryl, Tricloryl, Mogadon, Melsedin, Doridan and Mandrax.

Tranquillizers which reduce anxiety, such as Sparine, Phenergan, Valium.

Inhalation analgesia, which is a gas which the mother administers herself: Entonox (gas and oxygen), Trilene and Penthrane.

Questions you may like to ask about drugs used in labour are:

- What is the likely effect on the woman taking it?
- What are the possible side-effects on her?
- How quickly does this drug go through the placenta to the fetus?

- What is the concentration of the drug in the fetus as compared with the concentration in the mother's blood?
- What are the possible effects on the baby at birth?

The answers to these questions allow a woman to make her own choice.

Pethidine

Pethidine – Demerol in the United States – is one of the most commonly used drugs in obstetrics. It is often combined with phenothiazines, a class of drugs which tranquillize and sedate. Pethidine is usually given in doses of 100 mg or 150 mg, though when it was first introduced the manufacturers advised 50 mg to 75 mg, and if you want to try the effect of a small dose it is wise to ask for only this amount. Some obstetricians prescribe doses as high as 200 mg in labour. It is usually given as an intramuscular injection, though lower doses can be given intravenously. One disadvantage is that if given during the last three or four hours of labour the baby is likely to be very doped from it, since the liver cannot easily cope with the breakdown products of pethidine. There may be both breathing and sucking difficulties with the baby and muscle tone may be poor. If pethidine has been given to the mother in the last four hours before delivery an antagonist drug is usually injected into the baby.

Pethidine can also produce problems for the mother, nausea and vomiting, disorientation and restlessness being the most common, and sometimes a woman has hallucinations. In fact, she often acts as if she is very drunk. In up to 40 per cent of women the pain relief received from pethidine is not enough to cope with contractions. The woman who has a very heavy dose of pethidine at the end of the first stage may be unable to cooperate with her attendants or work with her body to push the baby out in the second stage. Some women give birth and do not realize or cannot remember for more than a few seconds at a time that they have had a baby. This, of course, interferes with the important process of bonding with the baby immediately after delivery. There is now a general realization that it is bad practice to separate a mother from her newborn, so babies are left with their mothers for at least a short time after delivery. But we have already seen that pharmacological separation can be as severe an obstacle to the creation of the initial relationship with the baby as physical separation. O'Driscoll describes the effects of pethidine on a woman who has had no previous experience of hard drugs as 'little short of horrendous'.[36] Though he uses pethidine in the Rotunda, Dublin, it is only in small doses and as few as 5 per cent of the women there receive as much as 100 mg. He criticizes present practice, saying that 'It is difficult to avoid the conclusion that no serious attempt is made in most hospitals to assess the requirements of patients in respect of analgesia in labour on an individual basis.'

If you decide that you need something more than gas and oxygen to take the edge off contractions, and do not want to have an epidural, you can choose to have a dose of 50 mg of pethidine to assess its effects during the next half hour and then to have another small dose if needed; 50 mg of pethidine is usually enough to help you achieve complete rest *between* contractions and you may even drop off to sleep. You will need somebody with you to help you wake up as the uterus contracts so that you can use your breathing and relaxation.

Epidurals

Epidurals were first used in the United States more than twenty-five years ago, and were introduced to Britain in the late sixties. The idea is to block with local anaesthesia the two spinal nerves which send messages from the uterus. The result is complete or partial loss of sensation in an area of the body roughly equivalent to that which would be covered if you had on a pair of old-fashioned long-leg bloomers. Legs and feet may feel 'dead' too. Epidurals reduce the woman's blood pressure, which may be a good idea if it is high. They prevent a woman becoming exhausted during a long and difficult labour. They may also help if she has heart disease or severe asthma.

If delivery has to be by forceps or a Caesarean section this can be done under an epidural so that the woman does not have to have other drugs and is less likely to vomit. Episiotomies and stitching and, if necessary, manual removal of the placenta, can also be done under an epidural without the need for further pain relief. So epidurals have many advantages when labour is not straightforward. Some obstetricians believe that they should not be used when a woman has had a previous Caesarean section, as the risk of uterine rupture if she has no feeling below her waist is too great. Nor should they be used when it looks as if the baby's head is too large to be born through the pelvis – *cephalo-pelvic disproportion*. Facilities for resuscitation of the baby should always be available when an epidural is used, as with any anaesthesia. There are some other conditions which rule out epidurals: a septic area where the epidural has to be inserted, haemorrhagic disease, anti-coagulant therapy, neurological disease, and various spinal abnormalities.

A woman should always be asked whether or not she wants an epidural before it is given, and should not be put under pressure to have one if she declines.

In some hospitals a woman has to decide in advance whether she wants an epidural. In others she can make up her mind as labour advances. In some the epidural is inserted as soon, or almost as soon, as she is admitted to hospital. In others the epidural is given once contractions are getting uncomfortable. In others still, the epidural is not given until the very end of the first stage of labour, when contractions are strongest and most frequent, a time when it can be difficult to sit still in one position for a long time while the epidural is inserted, and when for many women the labour ahead is plain sailing even if they do not have an epidural.

First a local anaesthetic is given in the lumbar area and then a long needle is inserted in the epidural space between the spinal cord and the ligaments which lie directly under the skin. Pain relief comes in about 10 minutes. It is very important that the anaesthetist avoids penetrating the dura and entering the space immediately over the spinal cord, or a full spinal anaesthesia is given accidentally, which can produce disturbing side-effects, including a crashing headache which may last for three days afterwards. This happens in 1–2 per cent of women in a teaching hospital, probably more in some other places.

Some anaesthetists are skilled at giving epidurals so that the woman's legs are not numbed and she can still wiggle her toes and move slightly. This feels better than being 'paralysed'. An epidural may slow down contractions at first, but the oxytocin drip can usually produce strong contractions very soon.

The fine 'topping up' catheter is usually taped into position and draped over the woman's shoulder or chest. Since the blood pressure tends to drop it is important that her blood pressure is checked 15 minutes after the epidural is given and again 15 minutes after that, and that it should be carefully watched throughout. If it drops rapidly she should turn on to her left side or sit well up, when the pressure on big blood vessels will be lifted. If blood pressure drops, the woman may feel suddenly giddy, sick and faint and may become unconscious.

The numbing effects of the epidural are likely to spread upward towards her chest if she is lying flat on her back, and this could be dangerous, so an epidural is often given with the woman sitting up. The effects spread downward towards the perineal area and her legs if she is sitting. After the injection is given she is often turned on to her left side and told to remain in that position. Her bladder will have to be emptied with a catheter as she will have no urge to pass urine. She may still not feel that she can empty her bladder some hours or even days after the epidural has been given, so a catheter may be left in position. Some women do not recover feeling in their legs for some time after having an epidural, so they are not able to walk for a few hours, or even longer, following the delivery. Some obstetricians believe a woman should never be left alone when she has had an epidural.

In many hospitals where epidurals are available it is possible to discuss them with an anaesthetist beforehand and to ask questions about side-effects. One of the most important subjects to talk about is the rate of forceps deliveries with elective epidurals (epidurals which are performed because women want them, not because labour is difficult anyway). In some hospitals the forceps rate is much higher when epidurals are given.[37] One study, done in Oxford, revealed that nearly 60 per cent of women who received epidurals had forceps deliveries, compared with 11 per cent of those who did not have them. The baby was also more likely to get stuck in a bad position (21 per cent, compared with 6 per cent who did not have epidurals). The rates of forceps and malpositions in the second stage were not related to the *timing* of the epidural.

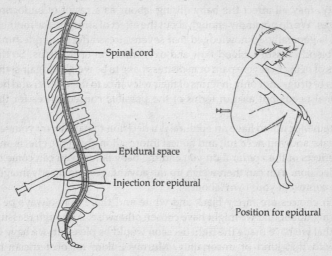

Spinal cord

Epidural space

Injection for epidural

Position for epidural

Figure 10 Epidural.

A well-managed epidural eliminates all pain, though, as we have seen, the forceps rate with epidurals is some five to ten times higher than in births where no epidurals are given. Anaesthetists often try to let the epidural wear off before the onset of the second stage so that the woman feels her contractions and is able to cooperate with them in pushing the baby out. This involves very careful timing and does not always work. With an epidural a mother can be fully conscious while her baby is born and watch the delivery, even though she feels little or nothing. Most babies born after epidural anaesthesia are in good condition and the epidural does not seem to have affected them in any readily measured way.

But it must be remembered that all drugs given to the mother go through into the baby's bloodstream. Some research workers have found that after babies have had large doses of bupivacaine, a drug often used in epidural anaesthesia, they are more likely to be unresponsive to their surroundings: 'Adverse effects of bupivacaine levels on the infant's motor organization, his ability to control his own state of consciousness and his physiological response to stress were also observed.'[38] Long-term effects of the drug are more doubtful, though Brazelton believes that epidurals can introduce the same risk of neurological damage to a baby as if he or she had been born to a mother subjected to semi-starvation during the first seven months of pregnancy.[39]

On the other hand the mother's emotional state, her anguish, fear or anxiety, may all affect the baby during labour as a result of endocrine changes. We do not know enough about the effect of stress on the mother, but it is generally acknowledged that severe stress affects uterine function, blood pressure, blood flow and oxygenization of the fetus. So the effects of being in severe pain or in distress have to be weighed against the effects of drugs, not only in terms of their relevance to the mother and her personal needs but also in terms of the possible consequences for the baby.

Whether or not to have an epidural is a decision that only you yourself can make and you need full and honest information about the effects and side-effects of the epidural on you and the baby before you can come to that decision. You can then weigh up the advantages and disadvantages in the context of your own labour.

Such choices are rarely black and white and there may always be a lingering doubt that we might have chosen otherwise. Although reassurance that we have made the right decision would be pleasant, we have to live with that kind of uncertainty. Murray Enkin, an obstetrician in McMaster University, Hamilton, Ontario, puts it this way:

Pain, suffering, enjoyment, control, sense of accomplishment, all have different meanings and values to each childbearing woman. She must weigh the available evidence according to her own value system, her own unique experience. Life is a series of conscious and unconscious weighing of risks and benefits, which each person must make in his or her own way.

Spinal morphine

Spinal anaesthesia is little used in obstetrics in the United Kingdom because of its inherent risks. Recently, however, it has been suggested that spinal morphine might be more effective and reliable than epidural anaesthesia.

In 1980 some obstetricians started using a spinal injection of morphine.[40] A needle is first introduced into the spine and some cerebro-spinal fluid drawn off. Morphine is then injected and pain reduced or eliminated. About half an hour after the injection the woman finds that her nose, mouth, face and eyes itch and this disappears only gradually after several hours. In some women the itching lasts for several days after the baby is born. Also about thirty minutes after the injection a woman is likely to feel suddenly hot and many women feel sick and some vomit. It may be necessary to catheterize urine, since she may be unable to pass it herself. Postnatally patients are nursed lying flat for twelve to twenty-four hours to reduce the risk of a post-spinal headache which occurs in up to 20 per cent of women. The doctors using this technique report a high rate of forceps delivery and Caesarean section, but do not think that this is associated with the spinal anaesthesia.

Handling pain yourself

Pain is not a simple matter. Some people experience it in circumstances where others feel only discomfort, or say that though the sensation is intense it is not something involving suffering. This happens particularly in childbirth. A lot seems to depend on how secure and comfortable you feel with the people around you and whether you feel in control of the situation, not just 'a body on the bed'. Women who enjoy their labours often say that pain was incidental to the main experience, a side-effect rather than something that filled their consciousness. Some feel the pain was 'positive' or 'creative'. Others say that pain is the wrong word for what they felt.

Some drugs which cloud the consciousness, such as pethidine in large doses, given to reduce awareness of pain or to make the patient forget it, actually seem indirectly to cause *more* pain because the woman gets confused. She is unable to handle things her way because everything is experienced in a haze. The result is that though the actual sensation may be less acute, the *experience* gets worse and she is in a state of anguish. In my own study of women's experiences of induction[41] there was some evidence that if a woman already had a poor relationship with those looking after her in labour she had bigger doses of pain-relieving drugs than if she got on well with them. When the relationship between the midwife and the woman was positive a small dose of pethidine (50–75mg) worked well to relieve pain. Unfortunately pain-killing drugs are sometimes used in place of good emotional support in labour. When a woman feels safe and among friends the loving care she gets can often take the place of pharmacological pain relief.

The body has its own methods of pain relief. The brain can produce morphine-like hormones, called *endorphins*, which relieve pain and induce a sense of contentment. These are stimulated by such non-pharmacological methods of analgesia as acupuncture, acupressure and trans-cutaneous electrical stimulation. (This may also explain why inert medicines, called placebos, can often reduce or eliminate pain if the patient believes in their efficacy.) Research has been done with pigs and camels, and in both cases it was found that when endorphins were injected they could block pain.

It has been discovered that blood endorphin levels in women after delivery are high and that these substances also stimulate prolactin secretion, the hormones which are associated with the physiological interdependence of a mother and her new-born baby and which play an important part in breast-feeding. The same thing happens after energetic physical exercise done for pleasure. Kimball,[42] who has done research with joggers, has found that the endorphin level increases by approximately 60 per cent and prolactin by 40 per cent. He comments: 'These findings further support the notion that stress-induced endorphins contribute to the joy of living by satisfying the inborn appetite for physiological opiates.'

Individuals have different capacities to produce endorphins and if a woman experiences a great deal of pain in an otherwise straightforward labour it may be a matter of a combination between the setting for birth, including her relationship with those attending her, and her natural capacity for producing these endogenous opiates. As Rosemary Cogan points out,[43] if pain is difficult to control in labour, it may be that her endorphin system is to blame, rather than her birth preparation or her character.

Episiotomy

'Going to give you a bit of help now dear, just a little cut' . . . 'You'll be sorry if you don't have one – prolapse by the time you're middle-aged' . . . 'Better a nice, straight cut than a nasty, jagged tear' . . . 'Of *course* it hurts, what do you *expect* after having a baby?'

Episiotomy, the surgical cut to enlarge the vagina at delivery, is the most commonly performed operation in the Western world. It is surprising that it has been so little questioned. An American obstetrician, writing in 1978, actually apologized that 5–10 per cent of his patients did *not* have an episiotomy.[44]

In 1742 Sir Fielding Ould, in his *Treatise on Midwifery*, advised incising the perineum at childbirth. The first obstetrician to recommend 100 per cent episiotomy was the famous Dr Joseph DeLee of Chicago, who advised not only episiotomies for all but also, in a paper written in 1920, routine prophylactic forceps.[45] His practice was to sedate the woman, knock her out with ether when the fetus was in the birth canal, then make an incision several inches long through the skin and muscle of the perineum and apply forceps to the fetal head. He claimed that routine episiotomy prevented 'permanent invalidism', epilepsy, idiocy, imbecility and cerebral palsy in babies and that women could be sewn up 'better than new' and restored to 'virginal conditions'.

DeLee believed that in normal childbirth damage to the perineum occurred just as if a woman fell on a sharp piece of metal and injury to the baby's head as if it were caught in a door jamb!

If a woman falls on a pitchfork, and drives the handle through her perineum, we call that pathologic – abnormal – but if a large baby is driven through the pelvic floor, we say that it is natural, and therefore normal. If a baby were to have its head caught in a door very lightly, but enough to cause cerebral hemorrhage, we would say that it is decidedly pathologic, but when a baby's head is crushed against a tight pelvic floor, and a haemorrhage in the brain kills it, we call this normal; at least we say that the function is natural, not pathogenic.[46]

He claimed that very few women could escape injury under natural conditions and suggested that, in fact, Nature might 'deliberately intend women to be used up in the process of reproduction, in a manner analogous to that of the salmon, which dies after spawning'.[47]

In the past midwives did very few episiotomies. An important part of their skill was to avoid the need for incision of the perineum. Today it is just the opposite. Episiotomies are done readily and a midwife who does not do one and whose patient gets a small tear tends to feel ashamed and may be put under some pressure to justify her inaction. The operation is so frequent nowadays that many midwives have never learnt the skill of avoiding the need for one. If the woman has already had several babies and the delivery is gentle there may well be no episiotomy and no tear, but this is almost a matter of chance and nearly all women having first babies are expected to have episiotomies.

The cut can be anything from just a little nick to an incision about the length of one's little finger, and most episiotomies are probably somewhere in between. It should be done with really sharp scissors in a single movement when the presenting part of the baby, which is usually the head, is well down on the perineum (the area between the vagina and the anus) and is bulging like a grapefruit. The skin should be pale and glazed like a balloon which is being blown up too fast and in danger of popping. This distension and shine is the sign that if an episiotomy is not done a tear will probably occur anyway.

The main, and perhaps the most usual reason, for doing an episiotomy, is to avoid a tear, especially a big tear into the anus. This is called a 'third-degree laceration'. There is no evidence that episiotomies avoid tears of this type and some indication that the biggest tears occur when episiotomies are done. It is difficult to see why this should happen, unless doing an episiotomy means that the person delivering fails to exercise other skills and just pulls the baby out.

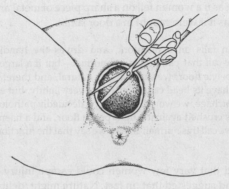

Figure 11 Episiotomy.

Another reason often given is to enable the baby to be born quickly so that there is no delay in the birth canal. Some obstetricians strongly believe the second stage of labour is particularly dangerous for the baby because pressure against the cord and the baby's head reduces the oxygen supply. Any woman who is told that she is having an episiotomy for the sake of her baby and to avoid brain damage will probably be very grateful that she has the opportunity of having one. The authoritative 1970 British birth survey,[48] however, revealed that a long second stage did not damage babies. Though more babies who were delivered by forceps after long second stages tended to suffer from lack of oxygen, those who were delivered naturally were in good condition.

Studies by Caldeyro-Barcia[49] show that very hurried second stages with directed pushing, strenuous bearing-down and prolonged breath-holding, can actually cause fetal distress. It is better for both mother and baby if the woman is left to do what comes naturally, and only holds her breath when she feels that she absolutely must. A forced pace in the second stage is harmful; it tends to result in shortage of oxygen for the baby and almost invariably in an episiotomy for the mother. (See p. 124.)

Another explanation for episiotomy is to avoid stretching of tissues and stress on muscles. The baby comes down through the pelvic floor muscles to be born. These form a figure-eight configuration round the vagina and urethra at the front and the rectum at the back. When these muscles lose tone prolapse may result. This can be caused by very hard and prolonged pushing while holding the breath, either in the second stage of labour or when a woman strains to empty her bowels as the consequence of chronic constipation. Nutritional inadequacies probably also play a part, at least for some women. There is no evidence to show that there is any relation between episiotomy and the subsequent state of the mother's pelvic organs. By the time the baby's head can be seen in the vagina (the usual time for an episiotomy to be performed) any stress on muscle fibres may have occurred already. Moreover, smooth, gentle, rhythmic bearing-down, both in labour and on the lavatory, can be done so as to avoid damage.

In 1958 only 12.5 per cent of first-time mothers had episiotomies. When *British Births, 1970*[50] was published the authors stated that one of the major changes in the management of labour was greater use of episiotomy, but, strangely, nowhere presented the statistics for it. Nowadays episiotomy has become more or less routine for women having their first babies in most hospitals. A study in a large London teaching hospital gave the episiotomy rate for first-time mothers as 90 per cent. In Ann Oakley's sample from another London teaching hospital 98 per cent had episiotomies.[51]

Episiotomy rates vary widely between different countries and at different times, though there has been a clear trend for more and more episiotomies to be performed everywhere. The incidence varies between hospital and hospital and between obstetricians too. In the United States most women have them, whether or not it is the first or a subsequent baby, and overall rates range between 70 per cent and 98 per cent. Dr Pierre Vellay, the exponent of psychoprophylaxis in France, has a 33 per cent rate for women having first babies and a 5 per cent rate for those having later babies.

Most of the British women who wrote to me with accounts of their births had this operation, even though some had asked not to have it unless essential: 'I requested it should not be done unless absolutely necessary. The doctor replied "It is *never* done unnecessarily."' Many had it without being forewarned or asked if this was what they wanted at the time. Midwives seemed often to think that for a woman to have a tear, however small, was a disgrace for them, and did episiotomies readily 'just in case'.

The cut is made under local anaesthetic. When it is done there is often an astonishing sound as if shears are slicing through canvas, or the woman may not notice it at all. It is stitched up (sutured) afterwards, either under the same local or, if it is some time after, when more injections have been given. The anaesthetic takes a few minutes to numb the tissues. If it has not yet taken effect when the first stitch is introduced tell the midwife or doctor.

If a woman has had an episiotomy with a previous labour she does not necessarily need to have one with a subsequent birth, though in some hospitals almost every woman, however many babies she has had, gets an episiotomy. Obstetricians tend to do more episiotomies than midwives. In teaching hospitals women may get episiotomies, and the stitching up afterwards, done by medical students, who have to learn how to do this during their training. You can find out whether this may happen beforehand. In the past midwives were taught to 'guard' the perineum with a hand so that there was less need for episiotomy; some doctors do this too, especially GP obstetricians.

The extent to which episiotomies are done in hospitals depends partly on the obstetrician's views about the right length for the second stage of labour. Those doctors who believe that there should be a strict time limit on pushing instruct midwives to call them to do a forceps delivery after a specified length of time. In the past this was often two hours, but another of the changes that has occurred as a result of a general speeding up of childbirth, with induction, oxytocin stimulation of labour and other forms of 'active management', is that this time limit is often set at one hour and for some obstetricians is 45 minutes or even 30 minutes. A midwife who wants to avoid her patient having a forceps delivery does an episiotomy to get the baby born quickly. One who works in a unit where the rule is 'Call a doctor 1 hour after full dilatation of the cervix if the baby is not about to be born,' says, 'It puts us under pressure. It's obvious sometimes that everything is OK but slow. We cheat a bit. We don't start timing until the woman has the pushing urge. Or if there is obvious, steady progress, though slow, that's fine.'

Midwives in Sweden do not time the second stage until the point where the woman has an involuntary desire to push and cannot help doing so. They treat the part of the second stage which in Britain is often used as a time for coaxing or commanding the woman into pushing, as a kind of bridge between full dilatation and the active second stage and think it is bad midwifery to get women pushing too soon. Even so, they have a high episiotomy rate, largely because pain-relieving drugs are given which completely anaesthetize the birth outlet and pelvic area. The woman cannot feel anything to coordinate her pushing with contractions and must depend on instructions, and since the vagina and perineum are numbed anyway, there seems little point in avoiding episiotomy.

Most episiotomies done in Britain are medio-lateral, that is they start near the midline at the bottom of the vagina and extend out sideways. This is so that if the episiotomy extends it is less likely to result in a tear into the anus and rectum. In North America most episiotomies are mid-line and run from the base of the vagina down towards the anus. Obstetricians there believe that it is better to cut where a tear would naturally occur since healing takes place there more easily. If an episiotomy is done too early, before the perineum is thinned out by the pressure of the baby's head, there tends to be excessive bleeding. Some women who wrote had experienced this.

Many said that they had to wait for long periods before being stitched up. Sometimes they were made to wait the better part of a night until a doctor had come on duty at the normal time in the morning. (There is always a doctor on call, but midwives seem to avoid calling a busy obstetrician who has gone to lie down after having been on duty for many hours at a stretch, which is understandable.) What is not clear, however, is why midwives did not do their own stitching, as they are entitled to do. Since it is women who usually do embroidery and are considered to have skill with a needle, there seems no reason why a midwife who has learned how to suture the perineum should not do so (and thus allow the woman to feel that the birth is really over and that she can get on with being a mother). Lying around waiting to be stitched, and not knowing how painful it is going to be, is a daunting prospect, and is not conducive to rest after childbirth. Moreover, the delay often meant that women had to be given another series of injections in already bruised tissue.

Not all episiotomies are expertly repaired and so may result in unnecessary pain and granulation. Sometimes women are sewn up far too tightly. Medical students have to learn how to do episiotomies, but they need not practise on you without supervision. Some of those who wrote had been sutured by a medical student without anyone there to guide. Sometimes the stitches even have to be cut and unpicked afterwards. You can ask to be sutured by a registrar. One senior registrar in obstetrics says, however, 'If it becomes a rule in our unit that only senior registrars are experienced enough to repair episiotomies in the middle of the night, I'd be removing the Mayo scissors from most of the delivery packs.'[52]

The first few days after an episiotomy or after a tear which has been stitched are almost invariably uncomfortable and the mother may feel as if she is sitting on thorns. Some stitches dissolve by the end of a week. Others are snipped out on the fifth or sixth day. For some weeks or months after the area may be very tender. When intercourse takes place it must be slow and gentle, avoiding the site of the stitching.

Rubber rings on which to sit do not seem to have been available in most hospitals, and many women also complained that the lavatory paper was sharp and crackly. It is worth taking your own roll of soft lavatory paper. The usual treatment for a sore perineum is kitchen salt in the bath or bidet. Sometimes the hospital did not provide salt and women had to take in their own. In some hospitals ice-packs and infra-red treatment were also available. It is a good idea to ask for these if you are in pain. Hygiene was easiest when the hospital had bidets, but mostly only modern hospitals had these.

In 1980 I started a study of women's own experiences of episiotomy and stitching which drew on the accounts of nearly 2,000 women who had been to National Childbirth Trust classes in different parts of the UK.[53] While women who went to antenatal classes do not form a representative sample, they can give us valuable information as a basis for other studies which should be undertaken. The alarming thing about episiotomy is that it is a procedure which has come into general and almost completely uncritical use without ever being properly evaluated and also without women having ever been asked what *they* think. If this can happen with an intervention like episiotomy it raises questions about many other obstetric routines and it is hardly surprising that women are now demanding to be given reasons and to know what research has been carried out.

My study revealed that:

- Episiotomy is more painful than a tear. Thirty-seven per cent of women with episiotomies were in pain, compared with 15 per cent of those with tears, at the end of the first week after delivery.
- Women with episiotomies are more likely to find it difficult to get into a comfortable position to hold the baby than those with tears and are more likely to be distracted with pain during breast-feeding.
- More pain is felt with an episiotomy several months after the birth and there is more likely to be pain with intercourse three months after delivery.
- Twenty-three per cent of those with episiotomies had pain with intercourse, compared with 10 per cent of those with tears and only 2 per cent of those who had an intact perineum. Most women found that nothing helped make intercourse more comfortable except time.
- Two thirds of the women had never discussed episiotomy with a doctor or midwife during pregnancy. Some who tried to do so felt fobbed off.
- Forty-four per cent of episiotomies were done within half an hour of the start of the second stage, sometimes before the perineum had fully fanned out.
- Most women (59 per cent) said they were urged to push harder and longer in the second stage. All their concentration and effort was put

into pushing instead of releasing the vaginal muscles.
- Twenty-two per cent of women said that they were never told to stop pushing as the head was being born. Some felt that the baby shot out like a cannon-ball because they were pushing with all their strength and believed this need not have happened if they had been helped to follow their own instincts.
- Some women (7 per cent) had a double wound, with a tear as well as an episiotomy. These women had the greatest pain of all.
- A number had an infection or other problem with healing, and in some cases the stitches broke down and they had to be resutured. When a woman went back into hospital to be restitched she was sometimes not allowed to take her baby with her on to the ward and this was especially distressing for a breast-feeding mother and baby.
- Most women who had a tear did not know what degree laceration they had, but of the 45 per cent who did know, most had only small tears (first degree).
- Thirty-seven per cent of women said they were never given a reason for the episiotomy either at the time or afterwards. Some said they felt 'violated' or 'mutilated'. Some women had to wait a very long time before they were stitched. Twenty-four per cent had to wait for thirty minutes to one hour and 13 per cent for longer than one hour. Some women had to wait as long as eight hours, until the doctors came on duty in the morning.
- Only 4 per cent of women were stitched by their midwives.
- Some women found stitching painful. When they complained the doctor did not always take any notice of the complaint. Some women said they were told: 'It doesn't hurt. There are no nerve endings there.'

There are situations in which a baby needs to be born quickly. An episiotomy is then one way of speeding the birth. But an intervention which is right in an emergency should never be allowed to become the rule in normal labour and delivery.

Episiotomy often causes unnecessary pain. There is no evidence that it has any long-term benefits for the mother. It has the disadvantage of interfering with the mother's first relationship with her baby and the start of breast-feeding during the all-important days when the two are getting to know each other for the first time. It may also affect the relationship between the parents for a long time after the birth and makes sexual intercourse uncomfortable or painful.

If you are pregnant it is wise to have a plan of action about episiotomy, both how to avoid one, and if you have one after all, how to ensure that it is *your* choice.

- First, pluck up courage and discuss it with a senior member of staff at your next antenatal clinic visit. If you do not want one unless you are given an explanation why you should have it and agree to it, say so and ask for this to be written in your notes. State this quietly, clearly and firmly. It is your body and you have a right to express your wishes.
- Practise pelvic-floor exercises, especially the 'lift exercise' as described in my book *The Experience of Childbirth*,[54] and concentrate on the feeling of letting the perineum bulge down like a heavy bag of soft fruit.
- Practise the 'sheep's breathing' for second-stage contractions described in the same book and rehearse light, rather quick breathing with your mouth open while you feel yourself soft and loose below.
- Massage the tissues in and around your vagina with some warm oil, or get your partner to do this for you. While you do so think of the tissues opening up and spreading like the great petals of a flower as the baby's head passes through.
- Discuss this with your labour companion so that he helps you think 'open up' if anyone tells you to 'push'.

In labour

- 'Listen' to your contractions in the second stage and push only when you most want to and only as hard as that contraction tells you to. (See p. 124.)
- Ask the midwife or doctor if she will help you deliver without episiotomy. The key is *communication*.
- Ask to be in a position for the second stage where you can see your perineum and the birth of the baby's head in a mirror if you wish and where you can yourself see the point at which it is sensible to stop pushing and start breathing.

To have an episiotomy, or even a small tear, need not be an inevitable part of childbirth.

From mothers' accounts of their hospital experiences it seemed that it was possible, providing the woman asked and made it clear that this mattered to her, to try and deliver without need for an episiotomy. Many of these women had episiotomies in the end, however, and it seemed that those delivering did not always know how to help a woman so that she was less likely to need one. There were many instances of women being urged to push harder and harder in such a way that they lost touch with what was happening on the perineum and this made discretion with pushing as the baby's head crowned difficult. They mentioned that they were told to pant as the head was born, but do not seem to have been told to do this with earlier contractions when the pressure on the perineum must have been great. Sometimes they were not reminded to pant at all. So it is important to make your wishes clear beforehand and to keep the lines of communication open with your birth attendant.

Female bodies are well designed for giving birth. The evolutionary argument that because human beings have big brains they can no longer pass through the female pelvis without trauma is a male view of birth and not borne out by many women's personal experience. The obstetric view of birth as entailing inevitable injury is a violent interpretation of delivery, and ignores the woman's capacity for opening up all the soft tissues and the ability of the accordion-like lining of the vagina to spread apart so that the baby literally oozes out. In our culture there has been a great deal of emphasis on delivery techniques and manoeuvres employed by midwives and doctors, and very little on things the woman can do to help herself *give* birth. Learning how to avoid an episiotomy is not just a question of refusing an unnecessary intervention, but of getting to know your body and working with it to give birth without haste.

A study by Reading,[55] at King's College Hospital, London, examined post-episiotomy pain and showed that a great many women still had pain three months after delivery. This pain was not correlated with pain in labour and a woman might have an easy labour but a painful episiotomy scar, and vice versa. The author recommends that women should receive counselling for coping with episiotomy to facilitate their adjustment. Yet should it be women who are doing the readjusting? Maybe obstetricians and midwives should adjust their practices.

In a *British Medical Journal*[56] leader Professor J. K. Russell, after stating that 'We have few objective data to support claims' made for episiotomy, goes on to say that 'It would be a pity if clinical practice were changed on insufficient evidence because of a patient-led protest,' and in effect asks women to give obstetricians time to do research to discover whether or not routine episiotomy was advisable. Two hundred years have already passed since episiotomies first became a standard part of obstetric practice, long enough, one might think, to investigate whether it is necessary. The onus should be on the medical profession to justify intervention, of whatever kind, not on women to prove that it is harmful. With episiotomy, as with induction, it should be a matter of some concern among obstetricians that criticism had to come from outside the profession and from lay people before obstetricians themselves got down to doing research.

It is up to women to refuse to give consent to any intervention unless it can be shown to be necessary and evidence is produced to back up this claim. It is up to those who make this surgical wound to prove that its benefits outweigh its hazards, or to learn how to avoid a practice which is demonstrably harmful to many women and causes a great deal of needless suffering.

Management of the third stage

After a baby is delivered contractions of the uterus continue, though the mother may not feel them. This tightening of the uterus causes the placenta to peel off the lining. When it is fully detached it either slips out when she kneels or stands upright, or slides out when she deliberately takes a deep breath down to expel it. It can take fifteen or thirty minutes for this to occur naturally, sometimes even longer.

Because between 5 and 10 per cent of women bleed heavily in the third stage of labour, the placenta becoming partially but not completely detached, with bleeding from the sinuses, the pools of blood in which the 'roots' of the placenta were fixed, the third stage is actively managed nowadays. A drug to make the uterus contract is injected, usually in the mother's thigh, just as the baby is being born. Having intervened in this way, further intervention is then necessary. The uterus contracts down hard and since this means that the placenta could get trapped in a closed uterus, action is taken to get it out quickly. This involves 'controlled cord traction' or, quite simply, pulling on the cord. It is a dangerous practice except in expert hands. If the placenta has not yet separated there is a risk of breaking the cord and possibly also of the mother needing manual removal of the placenta under general anaesthetic. It is disturbing that in a number of accounts of deliveries the cord has snapped off in this way. (In one case the attendant pulled so hard that the uterus was pulled inside out.)

Another disadvantage of the active management of the third stage is that women are often asked to wait to suckle their babies until after the placenta has been delivered. It is as if the 'housework' has to be done first. Yet if the baby is put to the breast the stimulus produced on the mother's nipple triggers off further uterine contractions. Mothers notice this when they breast-feed in the days after the birth. As soon as they put the baby to the breast they get 'after-pains'. The larger the uterus was to start with, the more these are likely to be felt. A woman whose uterus is stretched by a twin pregnancy, for example, may find these contractions very uncomfortable. Suckling the baby after delivery reduces the risk of third-stage bleeding because it produces contractions of the uterus.

In many Third World cultures a mother is in an upright position at delivery so that the placenta literally drops out by its own weight once the baby is delivered. There is no reason why the same thing should not be done in the West.

The breech baby

Nowadays, since it is common practice for obstetricians to deliver breech babies by Caesarean section, many women become anxious in late pregnancy because their babies are presenting by the breech. They feel that the chance of choosing the setting in which they give birth is being taken away from them.

You should know that at the thirtieth week of pregnancy approximately 30 per cent of fetuses present by the breech. The majority of them turn spontaneously. By the fortieth week only 2.5 per cent are still breech. Some obstetricians try turning the baby. This is called 'external version' and is done at the thirty-fourth week or after, while there is still room in the uterus for the baby to be turned. Some obstetricians do not do it because they do not believe that the procedure is effective and would prefer to deliver by Caesarean section those that do not turn spontaneously.

In some cases a baby cannot be easily turned because the tone of the abdominal muscles and the uterine wall is too high or because the baby has extended legs, with its feet up near its shoulders, which may make it difficult to push the baby up out of the pelvis in order to turn it. Some obstetricians nowadays have never learnt how to do external version.

The first stage of labour is often little affected by a baby's breech position. Seventy-five per cent of breeches have extended legs and when this occurs the bottom acts very much like a head to dilate the cervix, so there is no reason to anticipate a long first stage.

The important thing is that whenever a baby is presenting by the breech a woman should not push until there is ample room for the baby's head to descend through the birth canal and be delivered. Yet because the body can slip out through the uterus and be lying in the birth canal while the head is still inside the uterus, some women get a premature urge to push. Getting into an all-fours position usually reduces this urge. Epidural anaesthesia, of course, will also take away the urge to push, though it also makes a forceps delivery more likely. Being in an all-fours position has the added advantage of tipping the heavy uterus away from the inferior *vena cava*, so facilitating the blood supply to the baby. Because the baby is tilted on to the abdominal wall it may also have the effect of preventing the cord being nipped between the baby's head and the rim of the bony pelvis.

Though many obstetricians deliver the baby's head with forceps after having allowed the body to be born naturally. Michel Odent (see p. 133) believes that the safest way of delivering a breech is to have the mother standing so that the baby's whole body hangs and gravity draws out the head.

Many breech babies are pre-term and so tend to be on the small side; around 2,500 g seems to be the ideal weight for a breech baby born vaginally. When the baby is known to be large the obstetrician may advise Caesarean delivery because there is some uncertainty about the ease with which the birth of the head could be achieved.

If your baby is breech you will probably want to discuss all these matters with the obstetrician around the thirty-seventh or thirty-eighth week of pregnancy. If you find that antenatal clinic visits tend to be very hurried and that it is difficult to raise questions or discuss anything, it is worth asking in advance, by letter, for some extra time for discussion at that clinic visit.

Caesarean birth

Caesarean section rates vary widely in different countries. The lowest are in Norway and Holland, where they occur in about 3 per cent of births, the highest in the USA and Canada, where in some hospitals rates are as high as 40 per cent.[57] It is hard to believe that American women have fourteen times as much need for Caesarean section as Dutch and Norwegian women. Rates are also higher among patients having private care, though we might expect women suffering from socioeconomic deprivation to be in more need of operative delivery.

Throughout the 1970s Caesarean section rates went up internationally. They are highest in the United States, where they increased threefold between 1970 and 1978 and are still going up. Rates of increase in Canada are almost as high. Though in Western European nations there has been a greater reluctance to resort to Caesarean section, there is still a clear trend towards more Caesarean births.

One of the commonest reasons given for doing a Caesarean section is that there is cephalo-pelvic disproportion or dystocia – that is, the baby will not go through that particular pelvis, or labour is long and there is failure to progress. Both these diagnoses are often made without adequate justification. They are 'dustbin' diagnoses, resorted to as a simple explanation of why Caesarean sections should be done, but often with no real proof that disproportion or dystocia exists.

If your labour is taking a long time and dilatation is slow it makes sense to try different ways of getting the uterus to function more effectively *before* resorting to intervention of any kind. Sometimes a woman simply needs rest, a chance to relax and sink into her own fantasies without feeling that she has to put on a performance or reach any goal. Many hospitals are so organized nowadays that women in labour feel that it is a testing time, that they have to show that they are in control and make a demonstration of breathing exercises.

Most of all they feel under pressure of time. Some are told by hospital staff that they will not be allowed to go on beyond twelve hours, for example, and that if labour lasts longer the obstetrician will deliver by forceps or Caesarean section. They are told, too, that an oxytocin intravenous drip will be set up if labour seems long drawn out in order to make the uterus contract more effectively. Many feel the whole thing is a race against time, under threat of various kinds of intervention.

When a woman has the chance to lie in a darkened room and soak in a hot bath, forgetting time, and simply get in touch with her own body and fantasies, a previously ineffective contracting uterus sometimes starts to work efficiently. It does not always happen, but it is worth trying. These very simple ways of helping the uterus to function effectively are often ignored in modern hospitals. Walking around can help too. It is remarkable how just getting off the bed and being in an upright position and perhaps going for a stroll down the corridor can get a labour going again which looked as if it had come to a full stop. Fifty years ago midwives knew this and it was common practice for them to keep their patients walking around during much of the first stage. Some women believe that freedom to move around in labour is a basic right and are prepared to change doctors or hospitals if it cannot be guaranteed.

Fear, anxiety and any kind of emotional distress are also associated with uterine dysfunction. If a woman feels that she is in a hostile environment contractions can be painful but ineffectual and the cervix does not open. Every woman in labour, without exception, however many classes she has attended and however extensive her knowledge, needs emotional support. When this is not given and attendants do not have the sympathy or skills to communicate effectively, unnecessary Caesareans are performed. A peaceful setting, mobility in labour and the feeling that one is among friends are three of the most important elements in creating the atmosphere in which birth is encouraged to be a physiological rather than a medical process and unnecessary obstetric intervention is avoided.

In North America many Caesarean sections are done as repeats and it is sometimes said 'Once a Caesarean, always a Caesarean'. Repeat Caesarean sections account for about 30 per cent of the increase in the section rate between 1970 and 1978. It is rare in the United States for a woman who has had a previous Caesarean section to be allowed to have a baby vaginally afterwards. This started early in the 1900s in order to avoid rupture of the scar during a subsequent labour. At that time the incision made was the 'classical' one, a vertical cut in the wall of the uterus. This cut is only done nowadays when there is an emergency Caesarean section and even then a low-segment or 'bikini cut' is often made. This kind of scar is far less likely to rupture in labour.

Having a repeat Caesarean section carries twice as much risk of maternal mortality as delivering vaginally, even though this risk is still very small. The number of women dying with repeat Caesarean sections has not dropped since 1970. The practice of repeat Caesarean sections introduces risk to mothers while being of extremely doubtful advantage for the babies. A study in New York City showed that low-birth-weight babies were especially at risk when delivered by Caesarean section.

Many obstetricians on both sides of the Atlantic now believe that all breech babies should be delivered by Caesarean. (Breech births are about 4 per cent of all deliveries.) Their concern is that with a vaginal delivery the baby can suffer brain damage as its head is pulled through an opening which has only been made wide enough to deliver the body, which is much narrower.

If the second stage is hurried insufficient fanning-out of the tissues can cause a dangerous hold-up and cause extreme pressure on the head. Since this has been the normal way of dealing with the second stage in many hospitals it is not surprising that it has been discovered to be especially risky for breech babies. If vaginal birth is to be made safer for breech babies the approach must be much gentler. The woman should push to deliver the body only when she really wants to, so that ample time is allowed for the fanning out of the perineal tissue. A supported squatting position is probably best.

There is evidence that it may be safer for a very large breech baby to be delivered by section and that if there is doubt about the size and architecture of the pelvis or if the baby is a frank breech, its legs stretched out straight so that they splint the baby's spine and the chin is lifted up off the chest rather than tucked in, a strong case may be made for Caesarean delivery. But in the study done in New York City babies who weighed 2,500 g or less were at no greater risk if delivered vaginally. Even with heavier breech babies, over the last ten years it has not been possible to demonstrate that lives are being saved by doing Caesarean deliveries and as many of these babies die now as a decade ago.

In the words of an important report, the United States National Institute of Health's *Consensus Statement on Caesarean Childbirth*:[58] 'Caesarean birth is a major surgical procedure with morbidity greater than that of vaginal delivery. Infections constitute the greatest portion of this morbidity; the most common are endometritis and urinary tract and wound infection.' As far as the baby is concerned, 'Caesarean birth, particularly in the absence of labour, appears to be associated with an increase in neonatal respiratory stress at all gestational ages.' What this means is that even if the baby is ready to be born there is still a greater likelihood of breathing troubles after a Caesarean birth.

What, then, have you a right to expect from the people who are giving you care if Caesarean section is recommended? In the absence of an emergency, you should be able to participate in the decision-making and have all the information that you feel you need on which to make an informed decision. You may come to the conclusion, for example, that you would prefer a trial of labour with everything ready for a section should it be needed. It is important to point out that it is not the woman who is 'on trial' but the uterus. For some women, knowing that they really did need a Caesarean section makes it easier to cope with the experience psychologically than feeling that it was all planned for them and out of their hands.

If your uterus does not seem to be working well you may want to use alternative methods of helping the uterus to work better, such as walking around, sitting on a stool under a hot shower, soaking in a bath if one is available (there are often none in modern hospitals) or asking your partner to stimulate your nipples. There is a direct connection between the nipples and the uterus, as breast-feeding mothers know, and their stimulation often results in uterine contractions. This can be quite painful in the days after a baby is born as the uterus returns to its former shape and size, but can be extremely useful in a labour where there is ineffective uterine action.

If it is considered safer to deliver the baby by Caesarean section you should be able to decide with your doctors which kind of anaesthesia you prefer. It can be general anaesthesia, which puts you to sleep, or an epidural. The great advantage of an epidural is that you can be awake and aware and ready to greet your baby as soon as she or he is born. You also will not get the side-effects of general anaesthesia which include vomiting and a sore throat. Those women who wrote who had Caesareans with epidural anaesthesia were often very happy about them. They enjoyed being awake, able to see and touch the baby immediately and not having to suffer the after-effects of general anaesthesia. Being together may be as important for the baby as it is in giving you emotional support.

The National Institute of Health statement, after referring to the very limited research about the psychological impact on parents of a Caesarean birth, states that there is clearly 'an increased psychological and physical burden when compared with a normal vaginal delivery' and that 'The presence of fathers in the operating room and closer contact between mother and neonate appear to improve the behavioural responses of the families after Caesarean delivery. One consistent finding from small-scale studies of these families has been the greater involvement of the fathers with their infants.'

In the United Kingdom few hospitals allow the woman to have her partner with her for the birth. This may be because obstetricians think it will be too much for the father to take, the same objection that used to be raised about fathers being present at forceps deliveries, or even being present at a normal birth. As doctors get more confident with epidural Caesareans they may feel more relaxed about letting husbands in.

The father does not, of course, stand gazing into the wound. He is up at his wife's head, sitting beside her and holding her hand. A screen is drawn across below her chest so that neither watches the operation. Once the baby is lifted out it may be difficult for the mother to hold it because of the drips in her arm, other paraphernalia to which she is attached and the narrowness of the delivery table on which she is lying. If the father is present he can hold the baby immediately and sit with it where his wife can stroke the baby and feel the soft flesh against her cheek. Couples who have done this say that it was a wonderful experience.

It used to be the rule that all Caesarean babies went to the special care baby unit (SCBU) for a check-up and this meant, of course, that they were separated from their mothers. In many hospitals this is no longer the case and it is worth finding out in advance whether it is likely to happen to you. A healthy baby should not be separated routinely from its parents after delivery.

After a Caesarean birth the mother always has some pain as feeling returns, and she is given pain-killers. She may find she cannot empty her bladder at first and has to have a catheter; the bowel function may also be disturbed. About a quarter of mothers have some fever, which makes them feel groggy. Ten per cent need a blood transfusion after the operation and are further immobilized by this. The Caesarean mother also finds it difficult to get out of and back into a high hospital bed. Women who wrote frequently complained about the height of hospital beds, especially those who had injuries to the perineum and those who had a Caesarean section. If you have had a Caesarean section you are usually in a room of your own at least for the first couple of nights. This often means that rules can be stretched a bit and that your partner can stay with you much of the time. For those who had operative deliveries this was of considerable practical help in a busy hospital and meant that they could reach the baby and put it to the breast much more comfortably, quite apart from the psychological advantages of all being together.

Even if a baby is not sent to special care, she is often put in the nursery attached to the ward to let the mother rest. If a woman finds it difficult to move and her partner is not allowed to stay with her the first night (and few hospitals routinely set up a camp bed or couch in the mother's room for the father) the baby may stay there till the mother feels able to care for her. It seems from mothers' letters that some babies get left in the nursery for no other reason than that everyone is busy, postnatal wards are understaffed and that ward routines take precedence over responding to individual mothers' needs. Another problem in some hospitals is that communication between postnatal wards and the SCBU is very poor. A mother may feel trapped on a ward far from the unit where her baby is being cared for and reluctant to interrupt busy nurses with requests to be taken to see her baby. When she does get there she may find the baby has been fed, though she was wanting to breast-feed. If your baby is likely to go to special care it is worth asking if you may meet the sister in charge first of all to let her know your wishes.

If you know you may have a Caesarean section it is important to find out in advance all you can about this kind of birth so that you understand the technical procedures and are able to discuss all the choices open to you. Sometimes in hospitals it is not immediately apparent that there are such choices, but just by raising the questions and being persistent you can often make them available. If you need a Caesarean section you do not have to give up and hand over. You can continue to make decisions about the kind of birth you would like and the way you wish your baby to be treated.

Coping with technology

As I was writing this page I received a letter from someone about the birth of her first baby, describing how she set about making her wishes known, organized her own Birth Plan and ensured that the staff in hospital understood what she wanted. She was booked into a hospital not noted for being progressive or liberal and was very anxious about going to this hospital because of a previous unhappy experience there and of what she had heard from other women. She saw five different doctors during her antenatal care, but asked to see the consultant in order to raise the issues that most mattered to her.

When I was about seven and a half months pregnant and everything was going normally, my husband and I sat down and made a list of what we wanted/did not want during the labour, e.g. no fetal monitoring or sedation unless absolutely necessary, a modified Leboyer birth (no bath), and to have the baby with me all the time in order to demand-feed. I felt the consultant may have been a little taken aback by my list but he was prepared to discuss my wishes. I asked that these requests should be noted on my hospital records, and the consultant was willing to do this. Throughout these discussions I emphasized that I understood the safety of the baby to be paramount: my work has brought me into contact with children damaged by anoxia at birth.

Things were not plain sailing, however:

One serious criticism of my antenatal care concerned the enthusiasm for induction. I had a six-week menstrual cycle so it was reasonable to assume that my expected date of confinement would be forty-two weeks from the date of my last period. I had been in excellent health. However, when I was forty-one weeks there was a great deal of pressure on me to be induced. One factor used was that my weight had dropped by ½kg: I had not had time for breakfast on this particular morning . . . I requested tests to see if my baby was in distress. I suggested a twenty-four-hour urine collection to test placental function and the doctor willingly agreed. They also suggested half-hour fetal monitoring to test the baby's heartbeat, its response to movements and contractions. I went up to the labour ward straight away for this test, which proved perfectly satisfactory. I requested to see the consultant, with my husband present, on my next appointment, if induction was to be discussed. This was also agreed to by the registrar. As things turned out I went into labour two days later, probably brought on by struggling home with the vast glass urine bottle!

The labour
My discussion with the consultant, and the notes on my hospital file following this, proved most useful. I went into hospital when I was having contractions every three minutes. The two midwives who attended me had obviously read my notes and understood my wishes to do without sedation, etc. The junior hospital doctor had gone through my requests with me during a clinic appointment, and the midwives autcmatically dimmed the lights of the delivery room.

In the event, labour was not straightforward:

Two problems arose during my labour:
(i) Ketones in my urine: this was fully discussed with me. The midwife suggested a glucose drip and after further discussion we agreed to this. I must say that I found the drip very helpful: the contractions really began to work.
(ii) Very high blood pressure: when I was somewhere around 8 cm dilated my blood pressure rose to a dangerously high level. The midwife tried taking it at various intervals between contractions but eventually she had to phone the doctor. Again this was fully shared with us, my husband speaking to the doctor on the phone. They suggested a shot of pethidine which brings down blood pressure. They didn't feel that half a dose would be sufficient to achieve this. They also suggested monitoring. Because we were well aware of the possible dangers of high blood pressure we agreed to the pethidine and monitoring. I didn't find the monitoring as obtrusive as I had imagined. Pethidine made me slightly dopey during the first quarter of an hour after my daughter was born but I soon became remarkably alert.

Twice during the first stage my husband discussed my wishes regarding not having an episiotomy unless essential. The midwives helped me to deliver the baby's head very slowly and I had no stitches. The baby was delivered straight on to my stomach, and the cord was allowed to finish pulsating before it was cut. Although we had to compromise on our original position regarding sedation we felt there was a genuine partnership between us and the midwives. They demonstrated a real desire to do what we wanted and they seemed really pleased that we had our modified Leboyer birth and I had no stitches.

We were left alone with our daughter for about an hour and a half. This was absolutely wonderful. During this time I put the baby to my breast and she sucked beautifully. Eventually both of us were washed and we went up to the ward with my husband.

Postnatal care

On our way to the ward my daughter was given a drink of sterilized water to which I did not object. I made it clear that I wished to demand-feed and that she was to be entirely breast-fed because of family allergies. This was put on her cot card.

The important thing about this account is that she did not just hand over when things seemed to be going wrong. She continued to act as an adult.

It is often said that women should not feel guilty, that having any ideas of how you want your birth to be means setting goals and that you are bound to feel a failure if you cannot attain these. But it is unrealistic to pretend that all birth experiences are equally positive for mothers, fathers and babies. Some are obviously better than others. This is not just a matter of whether or not technology is used. Even a forceps delivery can seem incidental to a labour in which a woman has felt that everyone present has been helping her to work *with* her body.

When intervention is necessary, technology need not be used in a dominating way. Fiona had high blood pressure in late pregnancy and was admitted to a large London teaching hospital for bed rest for two weeks. Her blood pressure went down and she was discharged. Then, two weeks later, things started to happen . . .

I had a show, but didn't get too excited or dash to hospital or anything. All through Sunday night I had a slight tummy-ache, like a period pain, which was eased by a hot water bottle. The next morning the tummy-ache continued, but I went shopping and took a bus across London to have lunch with my mother. She was horrified to hear that I'd spent an hour in a bus, in a traffic jam in Kensington Church Street, and after lunch insisted on driving me home again! In the afternoon the tummy-ache got a bit worse, but occasionally it went away altogether for five or ten minutes.

When John got home at 6.00 on Monday, I decided to do some breathing 'for practice'. At 8.00 I had a bubble bath and realized that I was doing deep breathing for a minute and a half, with 1 or 2 minute gaps between each session. I suddenly decided I must be in labour, and we felt we ought to go to the hospital because of the possibility of my blood pressure going up very high again.

The Medical Way of Birth: Childbirth

When we got to hospital, the sister asked me how long my contractions had been going on, and when I said I wasn't sure I'd had any because I had dealt with everything with deep chest breathing, she left me for half an hour to deal with a more urgent case. When she came back at 9 p.m. (John stayed with me for company) she examined me and found that I was 7 cm dilated!! She looked amazed, and asked me how I had coped with the pain, and when John said we had been relaxing and breathing, she said to him 'I can tell you're a doctor.' (He's actually a publisher.)

We were immediately taken up to the labour ward and my waters were broken. A monitor was fixed to the baby's head, and my blood pressure was taken every 15 minutes. I had to sign a form agreeing to an epidural if my blood pressure did go up, which I had already agreed to do after talking to a doctor at the clinic last week. We found the monitor very useful, partly because of the reassurance of hearing the baby's heartbeat, but mostly because John could see the contractions clearly on the print-out, and could say how well I'd done and how strong they were. He could also see contractions coming before I could feel them, which was very helpful.

The cervix dilated quickly to 9 cm, but I began wanting to push before it had fully opened. The sister appeared at this moment and recommended gas and air, and I had one puff of it but immediately realized that breathing was far more effective. I did butterfly breathing and blowing to stop myself pushing, for about 1½ hours, and kept on top of most of the contractions. I didn't feel any pain at all but during that 1½ hours I felt a tremendous frustration about not being able to push, which was nearly overwhelming. Suddenly the midwife said I could push, and immediately the contractions thinned out! I realized I was on your Rest and Be Thankful Pass, and it was very peaceful.

John insisted on staying with me while the midwife gave me internal examinations to measure my cervix. (We nearly had an argument about this, because the nurses didn't want him to stay. They said 'Husbands usually faint', but luckily the doctor looked in at that moment and said he could stay so long as he didn't mind staying on the floor if he did faint.)

I loved the cold wet sponge on my face, and I sucked quite a few tiny ice-cubes. I also had ice-cubes on my tummy. John was absolutely marvellous and I couldn't have managed for a second without him. The nurses looked amused at our sponges and thermoses! We asked for the room to be quite dark – I pushed the baby out easily – but had a small episiotomy.

Sophie came swimming out at 11.50 on Monday night (I could see it all in a mirror which we propped up at the end of the bed) without so much as a whimper, and calmly stared round the room. She lay naked on my tummy for a few minutes after she was born. The cord had to be cut before the body was born, because it was round her neck (breathing and blowing helped me stop pushing then, too).

By the end we were both grinning from ear to ear. The midwife wrote 'normal delivery, no analgesics' on my form. We all felt very pleased with ourselves, and I think the nurses and the sister were genuinely impressed by our teamwork and confidence.

Fiona enjoyed her labour though she had an amniotomy, continuous electronic monitoring, a long transition phase and then an episiotomy. Her positive attitude made it possible for her to cope with all this and to spend most of her labour out of hospital carrying on an active life. One of the important lessons is not to go in too soon.

Another ingredient of this happy labour was that John and she were together all the time. This was important for Fiona and helped her handle the new and stressful sensations. John helped her use the monitor in a constructive way so that she knew where she was with contractions. When asked to go outside he politely but firmly stood his ground. He used ice and sponges for her comfort and, far from surrendering to the technology, he and Fiona made their wishes clear about the delivery. The room was to be dark, the baby delivered up on to her abdomen.

Val had had a previous Caesarean birth. The obstetrician wanted to monitor the fetus continually and do a repeat section if necessary. Yet this did not mean that she was willing to 'sell out' to technology. She discussed with him the kind of birth she wanted and the things that mattered most to her. Val and Paul's little girl was 3½ and they wanted her to be there during the first stage and immediately after the birth. It was agreed that this would be fine if a helper could be found who would be responsible for Debbie, take her out if she got bored, or if a Caesarean operation had to be done, and become a kind of surrogate parent for the duration of the labour.

Paul attended some of the antenatal visits with Val, and often Debbie came too, so she was used to meeting the obstetrician and midwives and seeing the inside of the hospital and the equipment there.

Only when labour was established, with regular, good contractions, did Val get on the bed and fetal monitoring electrodes were attached firmly so that she was able to move around on the bed without dislodging them. Debbie spent a lot of time with her mother and was interested in the monitor and how it worked. Paul turned the sound on so that Debbie could hear the unborn baby's heartbeats.

Val felt she wanted to sit up well with good back support and to be held close by Paul. He sat on the bed and cradled her in his arms.

The baby's head oozed forward, pressing the tissues of the perineum out, fanning and thinning them as it advanced more and more. Then, pop, out slid the top of the head like a grey tennis ball. A pause, then with a whoosh the whole head. It turned sideways and immediately the shoulders and then the whole body slid out into the obstetrician's welcoming hands. A boy! He was lifted gently upwards on to Val's abdomen and she reached down and held him straight away. As soon as the cord was cut she put the baby against her breast. First he just licked and seemed to sniff around. After a few minutes he started to root for the nipple, his questing mouth open and moving from side to side. And then he latched on.

After the delivery of the placenta Debbie was brought in wide-eyed to meet her new brother. She climbed on her mother's bed and sat proudly holding him. Not only a baby had been born, but a new family.

Anne had a long and difficult labour, ending in a forceps delivery. She had all the technology but she also had her husband close, and quiet encouragement from the obstetrician to do it all her own way as long as she wanted to. There was never any question of him making unilateral decisions and then imposing them on her. He was available to give skilled professional advice and the whole team made it clear that they were there to support Anne giving birth, rather than taking over.

Throughout the longest part of the first stage of labour she kept walking about. But as her thirty-six-hour labour went on and on she felt happier on the bed. The obstetrician thought that it would be safer for the baby if he monitored the heart and kept up Anne's strength with an intravenous drip of glucose solution.

Patrick was getting almost as tired as Anne so he got on the bed too, and they either lay in each other's arms or he sat her up and cradled her in a sitting position. She liked her lower abdomen stroked slowly during difficult contractions. Sometimes he did this with eyes closed as they both became wearier. Even though labour was a long struggle, it was an intimate personal experience which they valued because modern technology was not allowed to *dominate* a process which was for them private and full of meaning in their relationship. Everyone was very quiet and respected Anne's wish to be disturbed as little as possible.

The obstetrician talked with Anne and Patrick about having a forceps delivery. He believed the baby ought to be delivered soon and since Anne was getting more and more tired forceps were indicated. The couple agreed. He drew the baby's head out with forceps and then handed the baby immediately to Anne. She was radiant and suddenly fresh energy flooded into her as she took her newborn daughter into her arms.

The technology explosion
Many of the procedures and interventions used in obstetric units today have never been properly tested. Ann Cartwright, in her study of induction[59] asks, 'How did it happen that a procedure, which had not been carefully evaluated, which involved considerable costs and hazards, and was disliked by childbearing women, came to be used so widely and

accepted uncritically?' There is great concern that drugs should be thoroughly tested before going into general use, especially for pregnant women, but interventions which are normal practice in labour have often not been subjected to carefully controlled clinical trials. Also, there is no long-term follow-up of either the women or the children who have undergone these procedures. Research is sometimes done within a specific hospital, almost invariably a centre of excellence (or it would not have the facilities for doing the research in the first place), but numbers are often small and there may be no carefully matched control group. Examples of such procedures and interventions are the Shirodkar suture for cervical incompetence, the use of drugs to stop premature labour, induction of labour, acceleration of labour and continuous electronic fetal monitoring, artificial rupture of the membranes, telling women to push in the second state and the practice of episiotomy. In spite of claims that hospital birth is invariably safer than birth at home there have been no controlled studies of obstetrically matched groups of low-risk women having home and hospital births.

Attention is often drawn to the steady decrease in perinatal mortality figures over the period when modern technology and the purposeful management of labour by the obstetrician have been employed. This proves nothing. All we know is that there is an association. We cannot infer that it is cause and effect. In one famous London teaching hospital where the perinatal mortality rate in one year was 8 per 1,000, compared with a national average of 15 per 1,000, obstetricians tell their patients that this shows that electronic monitoring ought to be used routinely, since electronic, rather than human, monitoring was introduced concurrently with this decline in baby deaths. Many different new techniques and types of intervention and new machines have been introduced in this hospital during this period. Any one or a combination of them might account for the decrease. Moreover to compare figures in a hospital which caters for a large proportion of middle-class mothers with the national average ignores the fact that there is a strong link between social class and perinatal mortality and that the lower down the social scale a woman is the more likely she is to lose her baby. It is twice as safe for a woman to have a baby if she is married to a man in the Registrar General's social classes 1 and 2 (the professional and managerial classes) than if she is married to an unskilled labourer. The perinatal mortality rate generally has been declining steadily. This is partly because of modern methods of contraception and the readiness of abortion. On the whole people have babies because, for one reason or another, they want them and many babies who would be congenitally abnormal are aborted when it is known from AFP testing and amniocentesis that they are handicapped. In the hospital in question there is an excellent genetic counselling service and a pre-pregnancy clinic so that women can prepare for pregnancy and not just wait for it to happen. All these things may be saving babies' lives and meaning that babies who would be less likely to survive never get born. Fewer women under twenty and over thirty-five are having babies and fewer have very large families. It could be predicted that the perinatal mortality rate would fall, whatever new technology was introduced.

The absence of any real understanding of which new techniques (or for that matter old ones) are effective, and how, is particularly worrying when they are seen from a historical perspective. At one time it was believed that people had to be bled by leeches, at another that most children ought to have tonsillectomies and, more recently, that all pregnant women ought to have their pelvises X-rayed. It is not, of course, only a question of whether a procedure allows a correct diagnosis to be made or whether it has an immediate salutory effect, but also one of whether there are dangerous side-effects, either at the time or far in the future.

As a paediatrician, R. E. Pugh, warns: 'The history of neonatal paediatrics has been marred by enthusiasm for new treatments which have been carried out without proper concern for the possible adverse consequences, and without the scientific control needed to evaluate possible benefits.'[60]

It used to be believed in the late 1940s that very small pre-term babies could not cope with food, so they were deliberately starved and as a result many suffered from starvation hypoglycaemia and died. Doctors thought that the retained fluid and puffiness of the pre-term baby was a sign of fluid excess and it took fourteen years before Smallpiece and Davies showed that early feeding helped babies survive and that very small babies urgently need food for brain growth.[61]

When it was discovered that giving babies oxygen in incubators helped those who were having breathing difficulties it was the order of the day to put babies at risk into high concentrations of oxygen. It was only later that doctors discovered they had blinded the babies, who suffered retrolental fibroplasia as a result of too much oxygen. A 12–40 per cent incidence was reported in pre-term babies in 1949, which accounted for 30 per cent of blindness, and in the same year the relationship between this blindness and excess oxygen was established. But it was not till six years later that oxygen use was restricted. Now babies being given more than 40 per cent oxygen usually have their arterial blood concentration monitored by an indwelling arterial electrode.

During the forties and fifties the practice was introduced of cooling pre-term or sick babies with the idea that this would reduce the oxygen requirements. In the late fifties it was revealed that cooling *increased* oxygen requirements in other newborn animals. But babies were still subjected to cooling down until in 1958 a controlled study had to be abandoned because so many babies in cool incubators died.

At about the same time 'contrast bathing' of babies was popular on the principle that newborn babies needed stimulus. So a bath of hot water was prepared and another of cold and the baby was dropped in first one, then the other, back again to the first, and so on. The shock of this treatment must have been too much for some babies, particularly those already shocked by a difficult birth.

Nowadays the problem of cold stress is well recognized, with the result that babies are often overheated.[62] Nurseries and postpartum wards are uncomfortably hot and babies may suffer more than mothers from this. It is not just a matter of a baby coming out in a heat rash. There is evidence from animal and human studies that slight cooling after birth contributes to the establishment of breathing. When a baby is kept too hot or too cold he or she has to use valuable energy to regulate body temperature. Overheating can result in dehydration, accentuated when a baby is cared for under a radiant heater. If incubator heating is not adequately controlled a pre-term baby becomes rapidly overheated, since a very small baby cannot sweat. Problems have also been reported with babies suffering burns from plastic sheeting when under overhead heaters.

The early 1970s were the heyday of the 'scientific' milk formula for babies. Under this régime many babies suffered from dehydration as a result of over-concentrated feeds, too much salt and the early introduction of solid food. Sometimes these babies developed gastro-enteritis, had convulsions, and suffered severe brain damage, acute renal failure and renal vein thrombosis. Many of them died.

Today a surprising number of babies seem to suffer from jaundice. Chalmers[63] showed that there was an association between the administration of oxytocin to the mother for induction and acceleration of labour, and jaundice in the baby. A baby whose mother has oxytocin is at 1.6 times greater risk of developing jaundice.

Phototherapy is the standard treatment for jaundice, since light breaks down bilirubin in the skin capillaries. Unfortunately many modern hospitals have been built with nurseries like boxes, without windows to the outside. In the absence of natural sunlight babies are blindfolded and put under phototherapy lights to treat the jaundice. It is not known whether this deprivation of the stimulus of sight, and often, too, of the mother's touch and handling, could have subtle, and perhaps long-term, effects on babies. Certainly some babies get so hot under the lamps that they suffer a large water loss and become dehydrated.

The skilled care given in special care baby nurseries saves the lives of many who would otherwise die, but in these units too there may be practices which actually cause harm to babies. Measurement of noise levels inside incubators, for example, reveals that sick babies are subjected to a constant barrage of sound (over 70 decibels). It is not yet known whether this, too, could affect the hearing of these babies or have some other, more subtle, influence.

The father – an optional extra?
The majority of women who wrote about their experiences in the hospitals in this book wanted their husbands or some other companion to be with them in labour. Most hospitals described, in striking contrast to the situation even ten years ago, allow a labour companion. Unlike the USA, in Britain it is more or less taken for granted that if a man is there during labour he will wish to be there when the baby is born too.

One hospital described permits husbands for the second stage only, to see the delivery, since its first-stage rooms open on to each other and are inadequately screened. This may also show a lack of understanding of why couples may want to be together in labour. It is not just so that the man can see his child born, but so that they can share in some measure in the hard work and the total emotional experience. Some other hospitals cope with a similar problem of inadequate privacy for women in labour by welcoming husbands and keeping each man working hard with his own wife. The atmosphere in one such labour ward was described by couples as 'fantastic' and 'moving'.

There were *no* accounts of fathers being turned out before delivery, except when it was a forceps delivery. Since with epidurals a forceps delivery is more likely, it would be a pity if fathers, having been accepted in the delivery room, are ejected again because of modern obstetric methods.

In some hospitals it is possible for a father to remain when forceps are being used, but this usually seems to depend on him having achieved a good relationship with the obstetrician. Occasionally midwives said that husbands should not witness forceps deliveries and asked them to leave, but when a man queried this with the obstetrician, and especially if his wife wanted him there, he was allowed to stay. So if couples do want to be together for a complicated delivery it is worth asking the doctor.

Few hospitals prepare husbands adequately for the experience of birth, however. Some arrange special evening antenatal classes for couples together, usually just one in the course, but others offer more. Two London teaching hospitals have excellent systems of antenatal education for prospective fathers which might well provide models for other hospitals. Some men welcomed the opportunity to attend all antenatal classes with their wives and then felt they knew what was going on and could help them more. Very few hospitals make this possible. Classes should be held in the evening. When they did attend classes or lectures men appreciated being able to ask questions and discuss in groups which were not too forbiddingly large, to talk to other couples who had recently had babies and to be shown around the maternity unit so that the surroundings and equipment were familiar and they knew where the lavatory was.

The way hospital staff react to the presence of an expectant father in the antenatal clinic, not only in the waiting area but accompanying the woman to the examination cubicle to talk with the doctor, can give a clue about attitudes to fathers in the hospital. But since labour ward staff are usually different from those in the antenatal clinic, you may encounter quite different attitudes in the labour and delivery suite, and as a general rule midwives and doctors there now take the father's presence as normal.

This does not mean, however, that they know what to do with him, or that the man is not turned out whenever they feel his presence might be inconvenient or embarrassing, often on slight pretexts. In many hospitals when a woman is admitted in early labour, or is having labour induced, the partner is still sent away because 'it'll be hours yet', or is told to go and eat or have a smoke because 'nothing's happening'.

Many hospitals do nothing to welcome positively fathers and help them feel at ease. The man is dumped in a chair which is so low that he cannot put his arms round his wife, or may be offered nothing to sit on at all. He wonders whether he dare sit perched on the labour bed so that she can lean against his shoulder, but it seems that midwives rarely suggest this as something which might give a woman greater physical comfort and sense of security. He may be told to watch the monitor print-out so that he can tell her when a contraction is coming, so even his eyes are taken away from her and focused on to a machine. The assumption is often made by labour ward staff that a man is there to witness the delivery of his child and that he has no positive function before then except, perhaps, to do a bit of hand-holding. These professionals are out of touch with social changes in the last fifteen years or so which are drawing couples to want to experience the *whole* of childbirth together, not just its grand climax. The sharp divisions of labour between men and women, differentiated male and female roles, the ignorance that many have about women's bodies, the guilt and hidden conspiracy about 'female complaints', menstruation and childbearing are fast giving way to a new openness and sharing between a man and woman in partnership together. Pregnancy is often a time when such partnership, sharing of information and awareness of each other's psychological needs, acquires a firm basis. It is also a time when turning a woman into a patient and an interesting medical case can mean that it does not get a chance to start. Richman and Goldthorp[64] have shown how when husbands are allowed in only on sufferance they feel awkward and out of place.

It is not only that they are on alien territory, surrounded by strangers, confronted by machinery and equipment which must not be disturbed, in an institution the rules of which they can only guess at, and trying to think of ways in which they can give support to a woman who is certainly under stress and may also be in acute pain. In the hospital hierarchy consultants are at the top, patients at the bottom, and fathers come even lower than that since they are not 'members' at all, but merely temporary visitors. They are technically the least necessary, socially the most marginal. Many practices serve to further demean the man and to reinforce the power of the institution.

Occasionally a midwife tries to form feminine bonds with the mother by saying, 'We women understand each other – men can't know,' or something of this kind. There is a good deal that could be done in midwifery training to help midwives become aware of the social dynamics of total institutions and about personal emotional needs which may result in rejection of the man in this way, as well as to understand the psychology of fatherhood.

In a disturbing number of hospitals the man is asked to wait outside during a number of minor nursing and obstetric procedures when the labouring woman wants him with her. This includes admission procedures (perineal shave, enema or suppositories, shower, etc.) when the woman is using a bedpan, and for vaginal examinations. Occasionally staff forget to invite him in again. In some it is taken for granted that he will go out as soon as a doctor comes in to make any kind of examination, and this means that discussion about the progress or lack of progress of labour and what should be done takes place in his absence. Sometimes drugs for pain relief or an oxytocin drip to accelerate labour are given without him being informed. If he has been supporting his wife he may then come back to find there is no room beside her because a machine has taken his place, or that she is drowsy with pethidine and he can no longer help her to handle contractions with techniques they have practised together antenatally. This is an area in which there is room for improvement. Other, mostly teaching, hospitals involve the man in all decisions about his wife and baby, consult him fully and make efforts to help him feel a valued part of the team.

Studies done by Roth[65] indicate that protective garments play a ritual role, denoting status in the hierarchy; the lower down the hierarchy, the more protective clothing must be worn. Some hospitals insist on gowns, masks, caps and overshoes for husbands. Others do not make partners wear *any* of this paraphernalia. A great amount of protective clothing seems to produce a barrier between husband and wife. The mask, above all, means that they cannot kiss each other. It has been found that the mask used for longer than 15 minutes is no longer sterile, and hence fails in its protective function. At least one hospital which has done bacterial counts when overshoes are used and not used has found that there is no significant difference, and so have discarded their use. Hair coverings very rarely completely cover the hair. It should be possible in hospitals for husbands to be more familiar figures to their wives, and to appear in their normal rather than a 'medicalized' identity.

Most maternity units now give them cups of tea and coffee, some bring food into the labour room for them, provide a comfortable chair or even a bed to lie down on during a long labour, permit them to take photographs and encourage them to do anything they can to help. This means that it is taken for granted that the man does massage, gives the woman a hot-water bottle if she wants one, sits on the bed, cradles her in his arms, helps her with breathing and relaxation.

More hospitals now also take it for granted that a woman will wish to discuss taking any drugs in labour or whether to agree to obstetric intervention of one kind or another with her partner before coming to a decision. In some a couple are left alone for a short while to decide what course to take.

Both doctors and midwives are skilled at giving emotional support to fathers in some hospitals. Remarks that affirm the husband's right to be there and make him feel valued do a great deal to increase morale and confidence. At delivery, if the woman wishes, or if she is unsteady from drugs, the baby is often first handed to the father to cuddle, and then he gives it to his wife, and women who have had a section and have known that the baby was being welcomed and held by its father until they themselves were ready have been very grateful.

Although Caesarean sections are being done under epidurals in an increasing number of hospitals, few husbands have the opportunity of being present and supporting their wives through this operation, although some couples say they would like this.

Couples also appreciate time with the baby after delivery in which they are left in peace. An increasing number of hospitals have instituted a definite system whereby the staff quietly leave the new family together for anything up to an hour. They are available if help is needed – to get the baby 'fixed' on the breast, for example – but otherwise unobtrusive. In some hospitals the other children and the grandparents can come in to meet the new baby in the delivery room.

Sometimes the father is invited to the ward with his wife and baby to stay as long as he likes. A great many hospitals still separate the family at this point, however. The implication is that, the birth over, he is no longer needed. He has had his 'bonding time' and now the hospital gets on with the real work of caring for mother and baby. He can come at visiting time.

Many couples, especially those who feel that they have been through a peak emotional experience together and have shared something of deep significance in their lives, feel as if they have been cut apart at that point. The experience becomes fragmented and each is alone. During the hours after birth they most want to be together and enforced separation entails psychological deprivation for both partners.

Once the triumphant phoning is over the new father comes face to face with his isolation and expendability. The more deeply involved he has been in preparation for the birth and the birth itself, the more marked his feelings of 'let-down' tend to be. Few men are prepared for this and many are unwilling to acknowledge it to themselves. Those who have a self-image, fostered in many antenatal classes, of invariably being a support to their wives, may find it particularly difficult to cope with the depression they experience then. Western cultural traditions impose on men an assumption of emotional strength and stamina which many do not have. When they feel shattered they are not allowed to say so, least of all when a woman has just gone through childbirth and everyone is asking how she and the baby are. The resulting postnatal depression is as real for many fathers as it is for those women who feel trapped in institutions and worn out from constant interruptions and lack of sleep.

The wonder is, not that some new parents are depressed under such conditions, but that any *escape* depression. It is socially created and treatable by changing hospital attitudes to new mothers and fathers. These changes are coming, but slowly.

Some hospitals have completely free visiting for fathers and couples appreciate this. Many now have special times for the father and other children of the family only, and this, too, is liked. Women welcome visiting for 'fathers only' in the evenings and in many hospitals husband and wife and new baby can be together, the father handling, changing nappies, cuddling and enjoying his child. Some hospitals encourage fathers to share in looking after their babies without restriction and when the demonstration bath is done, select a time at which they can be present too. But in others fathers are still not allowed to cuddle their babies except for the few minutes of prescribed 'bonding time' after delivery and some still insist on them donning gowns before holding the baby. They are inflexible about visiting times, treat fathers as germ-laden intruders disturbing mothers' rest and hampering ward routines. In these women tend to feel isolated and alone, completely taken over by the hospital organization and routine.

Some hospitals have stopped talking about 'husbands' exclusively and refer to 'your partner', making it clear that this can be the father of the child, whether or not the couple are legally married, or anyone else the mother chooses to have as her companion in labour and visiting her afterwards. This term includes a mother or sister or female friend.

Some hospitals have an arrangement whereby the night before the mother and baby leave hospital the couple are invited to go out to dinner together while nurses baby-sit for them. One of the main difficulties for a couple in getting out together when they have a baby is that either they must have a reliable baby-sitter or they must take the baby with them. Although a carrycot at a restaurant table is fine, not all places are suitable for babies. Parents appreciate the thoughtfulness which allows them to do this, and perhaps the idea will spread to other hospitals. It is something couples could ask for.

So the best that is being done to support the relationship between the couple and the formation of the new family is a long way away from the worst. There are still many hospitals where the man is made to feel an ignorant, gauche intruder; there is a good deal that hospitals can learn from each other about how to make a father feel genuinely welcome.

Section II

New Ways of Birth

Questioning the mechanistic view of a woman's body

Modern obstetrics treats a woman's body as a machine which is constantly going wrong and the workings of which only the doctor can understand. For the last fifty years or so obstetrics has represented itself as a science, in striking contrast to the comfort techniques, the herbal lore and 'old wives' tales' shared between women from time immemorial. The influence of mind on body, all the emotional dimensions of the birth experience, the meaning of that particular birth for a woman, any stresses in relationships between human beings and the quality of the interaction between the childbearing woman and her professional attendants, are all considered insignificant compared to the system of diagnosis, measurement and intervention.

This is not so new an idea. The case was presented forcibly to women readers of the *Century Illustrated Magazine* in the 1920s:[1]

'What would you do if your automobile broke down on a country road?'
'Try and fix it,' said the modern chauffeuse.
'And if you couldn't?'
'Have it hauled to the nearest garage.'
'Exactly. Where the trained mechanics and their necessary tools are,' agreed the doctor. 'It's the same with the hospital.'

The argument is still the same today. A woman's body is just a machine and only the obstetrician has the skill to service it.

Women themselves are no longer content with this model for health care. They are demanding a much more active role in looking after their own bodies and seek to understand how they work in health and disease. This is not just something that is happening in the women's movement but is evident too in the pages of almost every women's magazine. The contraceptive pill, the too-ready wholesale prescription of tranquillizers to housebound, anxious or depressed women, dehumanizing antenatal clinics and factory-style childbirth, all these are leading women from many different backgrounds and different social classes to want to know how their bodies function, how they can keep healthy, how to play an active part in childbirth without the need for obstetric intervention and also how they can resist unnecessary interference and have the chance of doing things in their own way and in their own time. They are aware that the right to do this has been taken away from a whole generation and there is a tremendous suppressed anger among women at all educational levels, among working-class women no less than among the middle-class women, who are often stigmatized by doctors as being of 'the vocal minority'.

This is why some of the newest and most exciting developments in childbirth have nothing at all to do with technology but are concerned with rediscovering ways in which natural, physiological processes can be supported. They are the outcome of pressure from women to retain responsibility for their own bodies in childbirth and of changing attitudes and a refreshing flexibility in maternity care. Some midwives and obstetricians – not many, but a brave and pioneering few – have handed over control to the woman herself.

One of the basic questions about health care is 'Who is in control? Who, ultimately, decides what is to be done? Who possesses power over the territory where this decision-making takes place?' The answer is that, at present, almost invariably it is the professionals who are in control, both of the woman's body and of the territory in which birth is conducted.

When a woman gives birth at home the territory is controlled by the family and the doctor and midwives are guests. In birth at home the mother is the central actor in the drama and everyone else is there to serve her and her baby. There is no management system by which she is processed or with which she has to cope.

But not all women want to have their babies at home or would feel safe there, and clearly many professionals feel that *no* women should deliver at home. Society directs women having babies into hospitals designed for the ill and dying and treats them as if they were suffering from a disease called 'pregnancy', which can only be terminated by delivery. And at the same time there is a complete handover of control. This issue of power is central to the whole interaction between childbearers and professional care-givers.

This is why the changes which are now taking place in some hospitals where a woman is helped to 'listen' to her own body and get 'in tune' with her uterus, where she has freedom to move around and change position as she wishes and make use of the hospital in the way *she* wants, without having her labour 'managed' professionally, are so important.

The birth room
Most women who comment on the physical surroundings say that they find the hospital 'forbidding', 'clinical' or even a frightening place to be. This is even more likely when the mother is in a large, modern unit than when in a smaller, older one. The problem of designing maternity hospitals which are attractive places to be in has not been solved. Even

when the foyer is charming and welcoming this effect has gone by the time the woman reaches the labour room.

I shall never forget visiting a hospital in an American city the lobby of which was of almost Mies van der Rohe style and luxury, with wall-to-wall carpeting, elegant wood and beautiful paintings, and then getting in an elevator to descend to the bowels of the institution where the labour and delivery wards were, consisting of windowless cubicles in long serried ranks with colourless hardboard partitions among the exposed and trailing pipes of the cellars. It was like being in the guts of some great monster. And this was the place for birth and the welcoming of new life into the world!

In their accounts of their birth experiences, women often said that they wanted something beautiful to focus on during contractions. Occasionally they took bunches of flowers into the hospital and kept them with them during labour. A few women took paintings or posters, but it was difficult to put them up. In one hospital which has flowered paper on the wall opposite the labour bed, several women remarked that the wallpaper helped make them feel more at home.

Mothers particularly enjoyed being able to see living, growing things when they were in labour, and some commented on the garden or trees they could see outside. Not enough consideration has been given to the natural surroundings for labour, and many hospitals have been built in which there are no windows in the delivery rooms and the woman quickly feels she is incarcerated in a hygienic box.

Many women remarked on bad lighting which shone straight in their eyes or was too harsh. Some hospitals turn off central lights, using a light on the woman's perineum for the delivery, and this seems to be more relaxing for the mother than strong central lighting. This mattered especially to those who wanted 'gentle birth' for their babies and who would have liked a dimmer switch on the delivery-room light or the use of candles so that the baby could be delivered in semi-darkness. Some hospitals have thick blinds which can be drawn for 'gentle birth'.

Some hospitals are now offering birth rooms on the model of 'birthing rooms' and 'birthing centres' first developed in the United States as a contrast to the usual environment provided and with a focus on family-centred care and gentle birth. Perhaps because the contrast between the obstetric and natural models for birth is much more accentuated in North America, the few birth rooms which have so far been made in the UK are often not so very different from what is provided in the ordinary labour and delivery rooms, apart, that is, from the patterned wallpaper, the curtains, pictures and the bed which looks more like a normal bed than a delivery table. Some hospitals are even offering so-called birth rooms which have a standard delivery table, or one only minimally adapted for natural birth. If you lift the pretty bedspread and look at what is underneath you see that it is basically an obstetric couch, with lithotomy stirrups and all the attachments.

The change of environment is appreciated by those women who have used them, however. Sometimes there is a rocking chair, a cassette player for music, a large delivery mirror so that the mother can see the top of the baby's head before it is born, plenty of cushions and other means of back support such as foam wedges, perhaps a birth chair or stool on the lines of the medieval birthing stool. One of the most important things is lighting. The woman should not have to look up at lights which, as one woman said, are bright enough 'to illuminate a football pitch'. Soft, indirect lighting should be possible, with a dimmer switch. There should be blinds or curtains, some kind of heater so that no one worries about the baby getting cold when in skin contact with its mother and facilities for making snacks and a cup of tea. Some of the rooms are carpeted, with somewhere a woman can pin up her own posters and a vase for flowers.

The important thing, however, is what people *do* in these rooms and the way they think about the act of birth, not the decorations. Professor Richard Beard says that what I call the 'patchwork quilt syndrome' is more than just that because it alters staff attitudes. I hope it does. Midwives and doctors who have confidence in natural birth and know how to help a woman have it deliver babies in the most institutionalized, white-tiled surroundings in such a way that the mother never notices the setting because she is involved in such a positive way with the people sharing the birth with her. It would be a pity if changes in our style of birthing were delayed because staff feel they do not have the right environment or equipment with which to offer gentle birth. It is the people who matter.

It is very difficult for the principles which apply in a good birth centre such as the New York Maternity Center or the Mount Zion Birth Center in San Francisco to be duplicated in a system where there is no continuity of care between antenatal, intra-partum and postnatal phases of the birth experience. One of the most depressing things in the NHS (and many women write about this) is the segmentation of birth into these three departments, the woman seeing different sets of people in each. The shift system during a woman's labour, being cared for by a team rather than by one or two individuals, also means that women are constantly having to come to terms with changing faces, people whose names they do not know and often too, other members of staff 'wandering' in and out. Birth is a concentrated task, and women find it very difficult to cope with what sometimes seems like hordes of gowned and masked figures staring at their lower ends or the machinery, or sometimes discussing the dance the night before or where they are going for their holidays.

In a birth centre in the United States or Australia the group of people who will be caring for a woman throughout her pregnancy, birth and the days after meet her early in pregnancy. They also get to know the father and often other members of the family too. And they have responsibility for providing birth education for the couple and any other members of the family who may be present. This is more like the UK system of community midwifery, where a small group of midwives have direct, personal responsibility for 'their' patients and follow them through the childbearing experience. It is extremely difficult to duplicate in large hospitals, except those in which the Domino scheme operates and a midwife goes in with her patient, delivers her there, and then returns home with her, providing postnatal care within the home setting.

The biggest obstacle to creating an environment which is emotionally supportive, not only for the woman but for each member of the family, is the fragmentation of care in British hospitals. Until this is changed there is no chance of providing the kind of care which women choosing birth centres are really seeking.

The people who help
The majority of women who wrote about their hospital experiences had nothing but praise and admiration for the midwives who had cared for them in labour. They often thought of them as friends, and some had kept in close touch since the birth of the baby. They spoke most warmly of their kindness, understanding and encouragement, and the way in which they made their husbands at ease and put the baby straight into the mother's arms.

There was less enthusiasm about doctors on the whole. Many seem to have formed no relationships with their patients, and in those hospitals where women saw many different doctors antenatally and even in labour it must have been very difficult for any relationship to be formed. It is, perhaps, not so much individuals who are innately 'cold', 'clinical' and 'robot-like', as some were described, as a system which is inadequate and needs changing so that there can be more continuity of care, more time to get to know expectant mothers and labouring women as people, not just patients, and greater flexibility for individual doctors to adapt to different women's needs.

Perhaps because doctors in some hospitals do not speak much to their patients, any words they do utter become imbued with significance sometimes out of all proportion. Some women went home from the antenatal clinic acutely anxious because of what was said.

Women also occasionally indicated that they liked being looked after by other women in pregnancy and labour, welcomed the care given by midwives for this reason and enjoyed having women obstetricians.

Care by midwives and by obstetricians, even within the same hospital, is often radically different. In some units midwives are 'holding the fort', asserting an old-style control of the patient against obstetricians who are seeking greater flexibility and are willing to hand over a good deal of the decision-making to mothers. In others, obstetricians are asserting an hierarchical authoritarianism while midwives are striving to give personal loving care and as much choice between alternatives as possible to women. In each case those who want change point to the training of those on the other side of the argument and say that rigid attitudes and lack of open-mindedness are inculcated in an outdated system of medical or midwifery education.

This lack of understanding and common purpose between members of staff working in the same unit tends to make women having babies even more confused – everything may depend on whoever happens to be on duty at the time. With the present system of fragmented care and lack of continuity between antenatal, perinatal and postnatal systems within the same hospital the expectant mother is left with no idea of whether she will be allowed to do what may have been discussed sympathetically in the antenatal clinic, whether notes made concerning her wishes will be respected in the delivery suite and on the postnatal ward and, sometimes, whether anyone will bother to read them at all.

This is where the overall spirit and atmosphere of a hospital, and the lead taken by consultants and senior nursing officers, is vitally important. In some hospitals regular meetings of obstetricians and midwives together take place to share ideas and plan change. In others meetings occur but tend to be confined to obstetricians *or* midwives. In still others, meetings are arranged by obstetricians to which midwives are invited, but anyone lower in rank than a nursing officer is unlikely to raise her voice.

Mothers' experiences may reflect the schisms which often exist between midwives and obstetricians. Where there is conflict and resentment between them it is mothers who probably suffer most of all. This is because in a bureaucratic institution much of an individual's energy is likely to be canalized into asserting and maintaining status *vis-à-vis* others just below and just above in the hierarchy. Sometimes, also, mothers get in the way by accident and are at the receiving end of apparently hostile behaviour which was never intended for them. Women having babies are only temporary members of this power structure as they pass through the hospital and become objects over which power is exercised and rights asserted.

On the whole British midwives are feeling under attack at present. Much of midwifery has been swallowed up in obstetrics. Machines have replaced midwifery skills. Obstetric intervention of a highly complex nature has a great deal more kudos than age-old, traditional midwifery practices. Electronic monitoring, fetal blood samples, ultrasound and biochemical tests have taken the place of clinical judgement. Some women having babies approach the midwife in trepidation, seeing a strong woman who exercises power over them and their babies. But however tough a midwife may seem, she rarely feels as powerful as she appears. Understanding of the stresses to which midwives are exposed and of what amounts to an obstetric takeover of childbirth could enable women to realize their common cause with midwives.

Continuity of care: midwives

One of the things that women find most distressing about the present system of care is that there is little or no continuity. This is partly because modern midwifery is task-centred rather than person-centred. In the antenatal clinic one member of staff takes the history, another weighs the woman, another checks her blood pressure, another her urine, another takes a blood test, someone else ushers her into the examination cubicle, someone else again chaperones the doctor during the examination and there may be other personnel giving advice on nutrition, baby feeding, and so on.

The 'nursing process' was developed in the United States to deal with this fragmentation of care.[2] It is being used increasingly in nursing but is only just being introduced in midwifery. The aim is care of the whole person. In the antenatal clinics, for example, one midwife is allocated to care for a woman and stays with her the whole time. When the woman books in for her next appointment arrangements are made for her to see 'her' midwife again. When this system was introduced experimentally in Queen Charlotte's, London, it was discovered that mothers felt more interest was taken in them as individuals, and that problems, especially when the mother was anxious, came to light earlier.[3] The midwives, on their part, felt more involved in the care of each woman and midwifery tutors found that the much fuller histories recorded were extremely useful in teaching. The result is that midwives got to know their mothers much better and visited them also in the labour and postnatal wards. In the same hospital they allocated student midwives to mothers on the antenatal wards with whom they continued a relationship on the post-natal wards, and students said they much preferred the feeling of responsibility engendered by working with specific people rather than just being assigned tasks. In labour, too, women appreciated the greater personal interest they had from midwives whom they came to know, and after childbirth they liked having a particular person with whom they could discuss any problems. The student midwives became much more sensitively aware of the mothers' emotional and other needs and also recorded observations about the mothers in their care more accurately.

It might seem strange that conveyor-belt midwifery ever came to be accepted as normal. The idea behind it seems to be that if you break down large operations into a number of small tasks and divide them between different staff members they can be completed more speedily. Such a system did not take into account the dull repetitiveness of always doing the same task and having little chance to get to know individuals and relate to them over a period of time. To change the system now involves a radical re-think and major administrative adjustments and at first means duplication of information and almost inevitably difficulties in re-educating midwives to use new methods.

Moving about in labour
Two items of equipment which have up till now been considered basic necessities in maternity units are being questioned; the bed and the delivery table.

Each is designed for the comfort of attendants rather than the mother and each, by its very design, implies that the labouring woman will adopt one or two of a few limited positions. Yet among all the technological innovations they may have been the least subject to careful scrutiny and up till now women have rarely been asked their preferences either in retrospect after delivery, or, which is probably more important, at various points as labour unfolds.

A small study of forty-eight women who had vaginal deliveries and sent detailed labour reports to me revealed that:

- Many birth attendants assumed that the woman would be in bed throughout most of labour.
- Women in bed felt they were expected to lie down or sit propped up, not move around.
- Pillows kept slipping and where foam wedges were employed they were often not high enough to give good back support.
- Women having back-ache labours were often in acute pain when lying or sitting, but were given little help or encouragement to kneel or get on all fours, and there were often no sufficiently big cushions (such as a bean bag) on which to crouch forward and rest between contractions.
- Beds were too high to get on and off with comfort and a stool was not always provided.

- Beds were too hard. This was commented on especially by women immobilized with an intravenous drip and/or a fetal monitor.
- Midwives and doctors palpating the uterus and doing vaginal examinations expected the woman to lie flat on her back for examination. This seemed to increase the pain women often experienced.
- Birth attendants assumed that the woman must deliver on the delivery table, or, occasionally, on the bed.
- All but five birth attendants in the study assumed that the woman would deliver on her back. These five offered the choice of delivery in the Simms position (lying on the left side).
- After a vaginal examination many women found it too exhausting to turn again into a more comfortable position and tended to remain supine; the move from bed to delivery table was traumatic for some women. They often became stuck between the two with a contraction while they were trying to scramble on the table.
- Even women who felt they had had enough pillows in the first stage of labour often felt they had insufficient in the second stage. When they were moved to a delivery table some were not permitted or did not think to take their pillows with them and were left with one or two pillows only.
- The delivery table made women anxious because it was too narrow and some felt suspended in space. They were concerned that they would fall off and, when the lower end of the table was removed, that they would push the baby out with no one ready to catch it. They became particularly anxious if the birth attendant turned away or was talking to anyone else and not concentrating on them.
- Some women said that a companion helped them by supporting their head and shoulders or by slipping a shoulder behind their backs to raise them further during the expulsive stage. But the partner was often very uncomfortable in this position and was reluctant to sit on the delivery table and no member of staff suggested that he should do so.
- In some hospitals midwives were accustomed to getting the mother to lie with her feet on the midwives' hips, in a simulated lithotomy position. If the assistant moved away this meant that the woman was lying with one foot supported and the other suspended in the air.
- Women were often told to put their hands on their thighs and pull head and shoulders up as they drew their legs back towards the trunk during pushing. Many found this very tiring and some felt under duress.
- Though most women described the baby being put on their abdomen after delivery, some wanted to watch the birth and others wished to help lift their babies out, but could not do so because they were lying too far back. Some asked if they could be more upright but said that birth

attendants refused to allow them to change position. Any activity on the part of the mother apparently conflicted with the manner in which they saw their own roles in doing the delivery.

The majority of the women would have preferred to get into any position they found comfortable at the time, in both the first and second stages of labour. But to do this they would have needed something other than the usual labour bed and delivery table and a pile of pillows. In few hospitals was anything else provided.

In historical terms the supine, lithotomy and semi-reclining positions for labour are innovations imposed by obstetricians. Medieval midwives were accustomed to delivering women on low, horseshoe-shaped birth stools or, for wealthier women who had fourposters, to have them sitting upright banked by large cushions. Until the introduction of hospital birth it was normal practice for women to walk around during labour and carry on working in the house or smallholding, often until the onset of the second stage. The postures adopted were all modifications of the squatting, kneeling and crouching postures commonly used in Third World countries today.[4] In these positions the uterus is not pressing on the inferior *vena cava* and thus reducing fetal oxygen supply, and gravity aids the delivery of both the baby and the placenta.[5]

Women tend to be more comfortable upright and walking about, at any rate until the active second stage. In the study by Flynn and Kelly at the Queen Elizabeth Hospital, Birmingham,[6] women encouraged to move around needed fewer pain-relieving drugs and were sometimes reluctant to get on the bed when they were told they could do so. Moreover, contractions were more effective in dilating the cervix, the first stage was consequently shorter and the babies had higher Apgar scores than those whose mothers lay in bed.

Yet even when staff are flexible about positions, women themselves are sometimes reluctant to experiment with different postures. Many have been conditioned into thinking that the correct position for birth is a semi-recumbent one. One study of mobility in labour seemed to demonstrate conclusively that women did not want to leave their beds. This is hardly surprising, as in that maternity unit many had already received large doses of pethidine so it would have been difficult for them to stand up, let alone walk about.

An upright posture produces greater pressure within the pelvis and allows the uterus to assume a globular shape during contractions. If you are leaning forward, as a woman usually does spontaneously, the head of the fetus is tipped forward away from your sacrum, so reducing back pain, and rotation is encouraged. Caldeyro-Barcia, with evidence from

electronic fetal monitoring, has drawn attention to the relation between
the supine position and fetal hypoxia and considers the conventional
birth position adopted in the West today to be dangerous.[7]

It is all very well deciding in advance that you would like to be out of bed
and walking around during labour, but when it comes to it there often
seems to be nowhere else to go in a hospital and you find yourself
wandering around the bed or aimlessly up and down the corridor. So it
can be a good idea to think ahead to some different kinds of postures and
movements which might be comfortable during labour, some of which
can be very effective in reducing or eliminating pain.

Active birth

Much of this teaching has grown out of yoga and one of those most active
in developing a range of movements which women practise in advance is
Janet Belaskas, author of *New Life*.[8] She stresses that your own feelings
during labour are your best guide.

In many hospitals you will find that midwives are happy for you to get
into different positions during the first and second stages, but when it
comes near to delivery a midwife who is not very confident often asks you
to get into a position in which she feels she can cope. Nevertheless, if you
are working well with your midwife, she will probably be willing to do the
delivery with you in a kneeling or squatting position.

You can, for example, kneel upright, knees well apart or with one leg
bent up so that you are in a half-kneeling, half-squatting position. Or the
midwife can deliver from behind with you kneeling leaning forward on
cushions with your knees well apart. The baby can then be passed to you
through your legs. Or you can turn over immediately the head is born and
lift the rest of your baby's body out yourself.

During the third stage of labour, for the delivery of the placenta, you
can either stand or squat during the contractions. In this way gravity
helps delivery of the placenta.

There is no need for hospitals to buy expensive equipment for women
to be able to move around in childbirth. Paint, perhaps a mural or two,
indirect lighting and a leaning bar on the wall similar to that used by
ballet dancers practising 'en pointe', would transform long colourless
corridors for use in the first stage. (Women who want to be out of bed
should not be reduced to pacing round and round the father's waiting-
room or crouching in front of the TV set.) Instead of special delivery chairs
and beds, hospitals could introduce the practice of getting the husband or
other labour partner up on the bed or delivery table behind the woman in
the second stage, supporting her with his body and, for those women

Figure 12 Positions for labour: first stage (Figures 12–15 are based on Janet and Arthur Belaskas, *New Life*, London, Sidgwick & Jackson, 1979).

STANDING

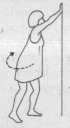 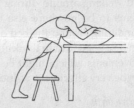

1. Walking and standing. Lean forward and rotate your hips during contraction.

2. Standing leaning forward with one foot on a stool. Rotate hips and lean forward for contractions.

SQUATTING

 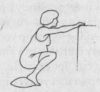

1. Squatting using a stool. Open your knees and lean forward slightly, keeping your back straight. Use this position during *or* in between contractions.

2. Squatting holding on. Squat frequently during or in between contractions. Place a firm cushion under your heels for extra support.

SITTING

1. Sitting backwards on a chair. Use a pillow so you can rest completely during contractions.

2. Sitting forwards on a chair. Knees apart and trunk leaning slightly forward with back straight.

3. Sitting on the floor.

KNEELING

*For all the kneeling positions, place something
soft under your knees – a foam pad or a soft pillow.*

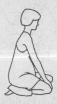

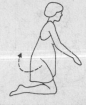

1. Kneeling on your heels (you may place a cushion between your buttocks and your feet). Keep your knees apart.

2. Kneeling upright, rotate your hips.

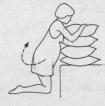

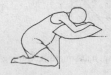

3. Kneeling leaning forward on a pile of cushions with trunk almost vertical. Rotate your hips.

4. Kneeling leaning forward on to cushion with trunk horizontal (only to be used for a fast labour).

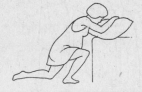

5. *(left)* Half kneeling, half squatting – rotate your hips or rock to and fro. Change legs from time to time. Keep your trunk almost vertical.

RECLINING

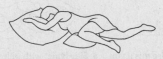

Side lying with pillows under trunk and upper knee. Use this position to rest or sleep.

Figure 13 Positions for labour: transition stage. This is the bridge between the first and second stages. Dilatation completing and bearing down beginning.

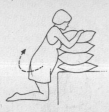

1. Kneeling upright with knees apart and trunk vertical.

2. Kneeling forward on to cushions and rotating hips. Keep your knees apart and your trunk almost vertical.

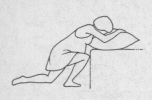

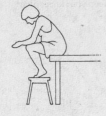

3. Half-kneeling, half-squatting, leaning forward.

4. Sitting leaning forward.

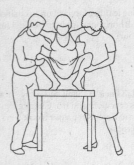

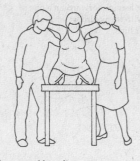

5. Supported squatting.

6. Supported kneeling.

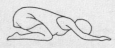

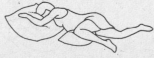

7. The knee–chest position. Use this if you have an anterior lip or if you feel like bearing down before you are fully dilated. Move your hips to assist dilatation.

8. Side lying, with pillows under your head, trunk and upper knee. Use this as a resting position only if necessary and change sides from time to time.

Change positions from time to time during a long transition.

who wish to, putting a sheet on the floor so that they can squat, supported by a partner behind, or one at each side.

Women today are seeking from doctors a much more flexible attitude to childbirth than in the past. Though many acquiesce to the medical view of birth as a clinical crisis in which the woman is a passive patient, others are questioning previously sacrosanct hospital practices and want to decide for themselves what kind of environment they would like for birth, what strategies are most effective for coping with contractions and how the baby is to be welcomed to life. Women and their care-givers could be collaborators in change. The important thing is to open up a dialogue, not as adversaries, but as partners.

Birth-beds, chairs and stools
Throughout medieval Europe women gave birth sitting on horseshoe-shaped birth stools. They delivered in a supported squatting position, feet firmly on the ground, with the midwife sitting or kneeling in front and other female helpers at either side. This was a physiologically correct posture, in which the pelvis is at its widest, the uterus can, without restriction, assume a globular shape during contractions, there is no pressure on major blood vessels in the lower part of the mother's body and gravity assists the descent of the baby through the birth canal.

It is also a position which reinforces the social nature of childbirth as an activity engaged in with the support of others working *with* and not simply *upon* the labouring woman's body. When a woman is upright, at the same level as her helpers, her role is very different from one in which she is only the passive body supine on the delivery table. It is a work posture not so very different from that in which she sat in front of her spinning wheel or milked a cow.

Throughout history while wise women (*sages femmes*) shared with labouring women the control of the territory in which birth took place and evolved the main comfort techniques and supportive actions which have been handed down in midwifery through the centuries, this upright, active posture was the norm. It changed only with the emergence of male midwives, the first obstetricians, in the seventeenth century.

In England the men called in to deal with cases of difficult delivery were the barber-surgeons. They had the instruments to cut up a dead fetus while still inside the mother's body so that her life might be saved, and they soon became the technical experts who were summoned in cases of protracted labour by those who could afford them.

In France the patronage of Louis XIV provided an impetus for the development of the new profession which was to become obstetrics. It is said that he gained enormous pleasure from watching the deliveries of his

Figure 14 Positions for labour: second stage. The birth of your baby. The baby comes down the birth canal, the head 'crowns' and your child is born.

SQUATTING

This is the most efficient position for the second stage as your pelvis will be at its most open and gravity will help your uterus to contract and the baby to descend.

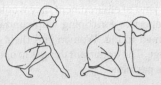

1. During contractions, squat forward on your feet using your hands for support. Rest by leaning forward on to your knees.

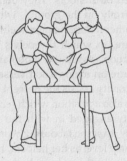

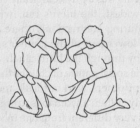

2. Squatting on the floor with two people supporting.

3. Squatting on a delivery table or bed, supported by two people.

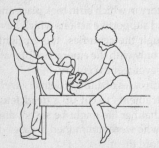

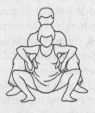

4. Supported squatting with one person. The supporting partner should stand straight with knees slightly bent, buttocks tight and pelvis carrying all the weight.

5. Supported squatting with one person sitting behind.

KNEELING

This is the next most open position and an easy position for the mother to give birth in. The kneeling position is especially recommended if your baby is lying in the posterior position or if you have had a previous Caesarean section.

Kneeling with body more upright is faster as the baby is coming *down* more.

To slow down lower your head to the knee–chest position, so the baby is coming more slowly.

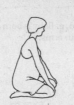

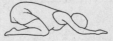

1. Kneeling and with your hands on the ground and trunk vertical.

2. Kneeling leaning forward on to cushions (trunk vertical).

3. Kneeling leaning forward, trunk horizontal. Use this if the second stage is *fast* to slow you down slightly.

4. Knee–chest position. Use this position to slow down a very *fast* second stage.

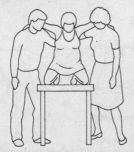

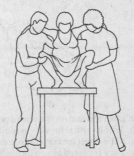

5. Supported kneeling.

6. Supported squatting.

Use positions 5 and 6 *(above)* if the second stage is very *slow* or if the baby is presenting in an unusual position, as these will open your pelvis to its maximum and assist the contractions and the descent of your baby.

Figure 15 Positions for labour: crowning and delivery.

KNEELING

1. Kneeling upright – this is the easiest way to deliver your own baby or can be used with the help of your midwife.

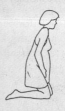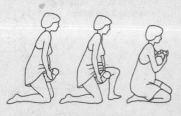

a. Kneeling upright with knees apart.

b. Half kneeling – half squatting.

c, d, e. Baby is born and lifted up into your arms.

2. Kneeling leaning forward.

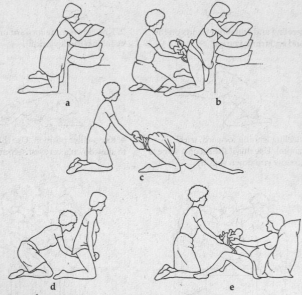

a

b

c

d

e

a. Lean forward on to a pile of cushions with knees apart.
b. Trunk vertical for slow second stage.
c. Knee–chest for very fast second stage to avoid tearing.
d. Baby is passed to you through your legs. You can also lift the baby out yourself.
e. Turn over, then baby is passed to you under one leg. It is also possible to turn over once the head is born and then lift the rest of the baby's body out.

mistresses from behind a curtain in the chamber. When the woman was on the labour stool he could not get a good view, so he arranged for a surgeon-accoucheur to deliver the baby with the labouring woman perched up on a high bed or platform. When it became known in court circles that the royal mistresses not only had a male accoucheur, but also adopted this new delivery position, the kind of care given by midwives and the use of the birth stool was soon thought to be outmoded and second-rate. The aristocracy all insisted on male accoucheurs and the supine position. In order to preserve modesty a sheet was often tied round the accoucheur's neck so that, though he could feel under the drapery, he could not see his patient's lower half.

Around 1600 a prominent barber-surgeon, Peter Chamberlen, invented the obstetric forceps. They were kept for one hundred years a closely guarded secret in the Chamberlen family. When the obstetrician entered everyone else was sent out of the room, the patient's eyes were often blindfolded so that she could not be a witness to this amazing new instrument, and an assistant might make a diversion (perhaps also drowning the woman's screams) by ringing bells and banging drums. The supine position became established as the only one in which it was feasible for obstetricians to do forceps deliveries and, since midwives were never allowed to use instruments, the distinction between the male doctor and the female midwife was still further intensified. The posture considered suitable for delivery was only one aspect of this, but a very important one.

Throughout the eighteenth century the strength of feeling against the presence of men during childbirth was such that some doctors put in an appearance dressed in cap and gown, masquerading as midwives.

The renowned Sir William Smellie wore a long dress under which he hid his instruments. He taught students using a model of a woman with a leather abdomen, an animal bladder stopped with a cork representing the uterus, and a wax doll for the baby. The living, active woman on her labour stool surrounded by female helpers was thus turned, in the eyes of the doctor, to a statue.

These first obstetricians had no experience of normal labour as they were rarely allowed to witness it; their only opportunity was to creep in on hands and knees and hide behind the bed. To this day the midwife has remained the expert in physiological childbirth, while the obstetrician is, *par excellence*, an interventionist. Obstetricians still get little chance to sit and observe normal labour, without interfering and with their hands in their pockets.

The more senior the obstetrician, the less likely he is to witness natural labour and delivery. By the very nature of his training and professional experience, he is the expert in pathological childbirth. This affects his whole view of what is happening in labour and delivery.

In the nineteenth century the lithotomy position, which was used for operations on gallstones, was first introduced into obstetrics. Thus a posture was adopted which further stressed the passive role of the labouring woman.

Whenever women were crowded together in maternity wards and staff carried bacteria from one to the other, puerperal fever was a very real threat after childbirth. In the Rotunda, Dublin, the first purpose-built maternity hospital in Europe, in one month of 1862 10 per cent of the women admitted died of puerperal sepsis. To combat it attempts were made to ensure a 'sterile area' around the birth outlet, though because of the juxtaposition of the vagina and the anus this is, in fact, virtually impossible to achieve. We have already seen how the shaving of the pubic hair and the use of enemas as part of the rituals of childbirth were used to help doctors and midwives feel more secure in the knowledge that they were doing everything possible to ensure 'clean' childbirth. To this was now added the draping of the whole area surrounding the birth outlet, including the legs. The woman lay as if under dustcovers with a slit in a sheet providing a window on to the genital area. All the obstetrician saw of his patient was a mountain of cotton cloth with a small gap through which a shaven vulva was exposed.

The legs were raised in lithotomy stirrups to which her ankles were attached by straps so that she was completely immobilized and in many North American hospitals her wrists were also handcuffed so that she could not move her arms at all. If she inquired about this she was told that it was to prevent her contaminating the doctor's 'sterile area'. A large part of her body had thus been effectively removed from her ownership. A process which started with the imposition of the supine position was now completed.

The average delivery table is a hard, narrow, cold shelf with pieces of metal jutting out at all angles and a lower section, extending from the woman's buttocks down to her feet, which can be removed entirely so that when she is about to deliver she is pushing into thin air, with nothing between the birth outlet and the tiled floor. There is often no structure at the head end to support pillows, so that even if she is offered them, they are likely to slip off as soon as she begins to push. Many women have felt trapped in pain on the delivery table as if on an exquisite instrument of torture.

Just as the worst excesses of 'obstetric' birth, together with the manacling of women and their reduction to inert lumps of flesh upon which the obstetrician operated, occurred in the United States, so also the first protests and the first attempts to discover equipment which could give physical support for women actively giving birth came from the United States. Niles and Michael Newton, a psychologist and obstetrician working together in Mississippi, invented a back rest which allowed the woman to sit propped up so that she could literally bear *down*. In France Pierre Vellay started using foam-rubber wedges, like enormous slices of cheese, for the woman to lean against in the first stage, and turn them round with the thick edge underneath her buttocks for the second stage and delivery. These were introduced into the UK by the National Childbirth Trust and for a long time, although they were used in antenatal classes, they were not acceptable in hospitals. Then some hospitals started ordering them, though they tended to use them only so that the woman could lie in an inclined position and did not usually think of sitting her up for the second stage, with plenty of pillows behind her, and her buttocks on the edge of the raised rubber wedge.

In the early seventies a hospital in Oxford first used a foam back-support – shaped very much like the back of an easy chair but with the lower part, behind the woman's lower spine, bulging outward – in both the first and second stages if the woman found it comfortable. At the same time they introduced polystyrene-granule-filled bean-bags for those women who wanted to get into other positions, who preferred, for example, to lean or crouch forward. The breakthrough had been made. The labouring woman had been got up off her back.

Meanwhile discussion had started in obstetric circles about the dangers of the supine position because of the reduced blood flow to the fetus. An obstetric chair was invented in Sweden which enabled the woman to sit up. It looks like a dentist's chair and has a block situated over either shoulder, to act as neck restrainers, so that she cannot easily move her head from side to side. But it was certainly an advance on lithotomy stirrups. Other chairs were developed in several other European countries. At about this time too, the 'prone trolley' was invented in Sydney, Australia. The idea behind it was that the woman with backache was more comfortable lying on her front, so that her back could be massaged, for example, and that the best thing to do with her abdomen was to cut out a hole through which it could be suspended. The argument went that this also removed any restriction on the contracting uterus. It was extremely uncomfortable when the woman was lying on a flat surface, so it was then curved upwards so that she was lying with her tummy hanging through the hole. It was not very popular with midwives and probably few mothers got a chance to use it, but it was, nevertheless, a genuine attempt to help those women who were having backache labours with posterior babies.

In the early eighties various firms started producing special birth chairs, the idea behind them being to offer mothers comfort but at the same time to provide obstetricians with completely equipped delivery tables if they should be needed. The Birth Eze, constructed of plastic and stainless steel, looks like something which has become detached from a forklift truck but does allow the mother to sit upright. In its original form it was extremely uncomfortable, with an upturned lip around the perineum which could be very painful. This has been remedied, but the back support is still unyielding and hard, pushing the mother into a position in which she cannot easily move her spine or pelvis. To sit in it for any length of time, even though not pregnant and not in labour, would produce backache. Its other disadvantage is that it is so narrow that the mother who is handed her baby after delivery, when the chair is designed to be tilted back so that the obstetrician can suture the perineum, often feels very insecure and fears that she is going to drop her child. Perhaps only a double bed can solve that particular problem!

Perhaps the most elegant of the new birth equipment is the Borning Bed, also designed in the United States by an obstetrician, providing 'family-centred' childbirth and aiming at getting a bed which was aesthetically satisfying, as well as being comfortable, flexible and easy for the obstetrician to work with. The mother can control her own position at the touch of a button, but one disadvantage is that the surface of the bed which provides back support is absolutely flat, whereas human bodies are curved.

The latest experimentation has been with the design of adaptations of the medieval birth stool, enabling the woman to get into a modified squatting position but, of course, forcing the attendants to get down on to the floor. Though many of the obstetricians and midwives were happy for the mother to adapt her position, they have not been willing to change their own positions in any way. Some have thought it a bad joke when they have to kneel on the floor to peer at the descending occiput with the aid of a flashlight. The original birth stool was backless, thus enabling the woman to rock her pelvis and change position with ease. Some of the birth stools designed nowadays have rigid backs. The best type may be the simplest. A low, horseshoe- or boomerang-shaped three-legged stool, small enough to be carried around with ease, allows the mother to tilt her pelvis and lean forward or backward without any hassle. It is stable if her partner sits behind on a higher stool or chair, legs apart, supporting her back and shoulders or if she has a large floor cushion behind her.

Figure 16 (opposite) The birth stool.

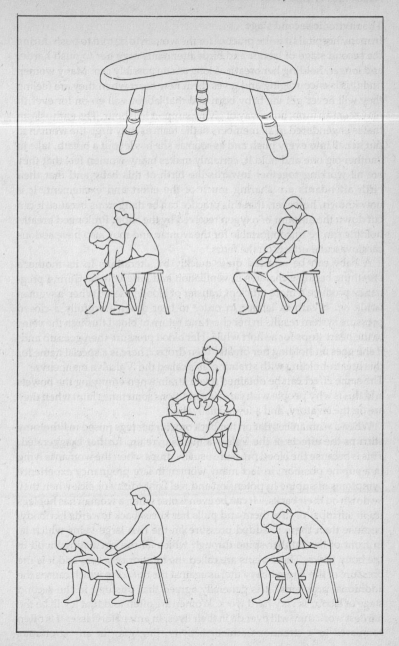

The rhythmic second stage

In many hospitals it is the practice for the woman to be told to push during the second stage of labour and birth attendants urge her to push harder and longer, holding her breath as long as she possibly can. Many women find this is encouraging and gives them new heart when they are feeling they will never get the baby born and that labour will go on for ever. It may seem an innocuous way of giving support in labour. The enthusiasm that is engendered in all members of the team as they urge the woman to put her all into every push and as soon as she has let out a breath, take in another big one and hold it, certainly makes many women feel that they are all working together towards the birth of this baby and that their birth attendants are sharing much of the effort and excitement. It is now known, however, that this practice can be dangerous because it can cut down the amount of oxygen received by the baby. Prolonged breath-holding can be uncomfortable for the woman and may also have serious cardiovascular effects on the fetus.[9]

A baby can be affected quite quickly by alterations in its mother's breathing because changes in ventilation and lung volume during pregnancy produce a more efficient transfer of blood gases.[10] When a woman holds her breath in labour in order to bear down forcefully a closed pressure system results in her chest and return of blood through the veins to the heart stops for a short while. Her blood pressure then goes up and, if she goes on holding her breath, then drops. There is a special name for this breath-holding with straining. It is called the 'Valsalva manoeuvre'.[11] The same effect can be obtained if you strain when emptying the bowels and this is why people with cardiac conditions sometimes faint when they are on the lavatory, and a few actually die.

When a woman lies flat on her back or with her legs raised in lithotomy stirrups the effects of the Valsalva manoeuvre are further exaggerated. This is because the blood pressure usually drops when the woman is lying in a supine position; in fact many women in late pregnancy experience symptoms of supine hypotension and feel faint, dizzy or sick when they lie down on their backs.[12] It can be even worse when a woman has her legs up in stirrups, or lifts them and pulls her knees back towards her body, because then there is added pressure on the two large veins which lie in front of the lumbar spine through which all the circulating blood in the body flows. These veins are called the inferior *vena cava* and it is the pressure of the large, heavy uterus against the *vena cava* which causes the additional problems. It is generally agreed that pushing in the second stage of labour is very hard work. Women are often told that it will be the hardest work they will ever do in their lives. In antenatal classes it is often compared to a strenuous athletic activity. Engaging in any strenuous activity while lying in an immobilized position is likely to produce cardiovascular stress.[13] Since blood cannot flow back to the heart the output of blood from the heart goes down.

Many woman have also received drugs for pain relief by the time they go in to the expulsive stage of labour. Some of these pain-relieving drugs – narcotics, such as pethidine or morphine, as well as sedatives – depress the respiratory centre of the mother's brain and the sensory and motor areas of her cerebral cortex and spinal cord, which can make the situation still worse.[14] Epidurals reduce sensory perception and motor activity and also produce lower blood pressure because there is a pooling of blood in the mother's abdomen and legs. This, too, may reduce the amount of oxygen-carrying blood going through to the baby.

You do not need to hold your breath in order to push effectively. You will probably want to hold your breath at the height of strong pushing contractions and will do this quite spontaneously, but there is no need to hold on to your breath deliberately. Unfortunately some women are urged to hold their breath still longer and try harder because the electronic fetal monitor has picked up ominous dips in the fetal heart which go on after a contraction has finished. The result is that the woman holds her breath longer in order to try to get the baby delivered quickly and this still further reduces the oxygen available to the fetus. In order to maintain a circulatory flow of oxygenated blood to the baby it is important to breathe again as soon as you can after having held your breath. Only hold your breath when you absolutely must. If you do this you will find that pushing is not nearly so exhausting, that you do not burst blood vessels in your face and eyes and that the whole second stage is gentler and more rhythmic. Your blood pressure is also likely to remain steady. It is usually when a woman can push no longer and gasps for air that her blood pressure shoots up above normal and drops again while she is pushing. These fluctuations in blood pressure can, as we have seen, be harmful for both her and her baby. When a woman pushes for not more than four seconds and then breathes out venous return is actually enhanced, the output of blood from the heart is maintained and fluctuations in blood pressure are avoided.[15] Keep as relaxed as you can in the second stage of labour and stress the breathing *out* rather than a gulping in of air. Follow your uterus and it will tell you when and if you need to hold your breath.

Leboyer

Some hospitals offer Leboyer or modified Leboyer deliveries, or say they will use 'Leboyer techniques' at delivery for mothers who request them. The first thing that should be pointed out is that Frederick Leboyer is the last person to approve of 'techniques'. He says that it is a matter of attitudes, of the spirit in which acts are performed rather than the acts themselves. 'The baby,' he asserts 'sees right into our hearts, knows the colour of your thoughts.' He is highly critical of a gimmicky approach to birth and though he has been caricatured as wanting flute music played at delivery or advising that the room should be pitch dark, he is not interested in such rituals and is much more concerned about how we *perceive* the newborn baby.[16]

Our own thoughts and emotions affect the baby at birth. Our anger, impatience or anxiety is, he believes, immediately communicated to the baby who 'feels everything'[17] and is like a mirror, reflecting ourselves. He says that 'it is up to us to see it doesn't cry'. This is a very confusing message, because if you are concerned to see that a baby does not cry you are likely to become very anxious when your baby *does* cry. And most babies *do* cry immediately after delivery.

Some parents feel they have failed because their baby cried loudly, even though they were doing all the things which they thought would comfort and soothe the child. It is almost as if the baby were passing judgement on them at the moment of birth.

Since then he has said that it is not a question of a baby never crying, but rather of the baby who goes *on* crying inconsolably.[18]

Leboyer teaches that the newborn baby is hypersensitive through skin, eyes and ears. When babies tumble into the world they are in a raw state, exposed in complete defencelessness to a barrage of stimuli. In our Western culture the baby is usually assailed with loud noises and bright lights and is handled in an efficient, business-like way as if it were a lump of meat being wrapped in a butcher's shop, not an exquisitively sensitive new human being. He seeks to make the transition between the soft, dim, warm world inside the uterus and the hard, noisy, cold one outside the mother's body as gentle and gradual as possible. Inside, the baby is contained, firmly held by walls of muscle. Outside the baby for the first time encounters space and such alien materials as rubber gloves, plastic, steel and cotton cloth.

One way he believes this can be done is by sinking the baby's body into deep, warm water and letting the child discover itself in an environment which is as near as possible to that from which it has just come. This is quite different from 'bathing a baby' to make it clean. An ordinary baby bath or a bowl is rarely deep enough, though a Perspex crib or a large thermal box of the kind used for picnics may be just right, and the latter will hold the water at a steady temperature. This is the part of Leboyer's teaching which is most often shelved in hospitals, because paediatricians and midwives are concerned that the baby will get chilled. It is true that the newborn baby has thermal control mechanisms which are not yet fully developed, and this is especially so for the low-birth-weight baby. The head is the largest part of a newborn baby and it is from this that there is the greatest heat loss. Some obstetricians have overcome this problem by having an overhead heater to keep the baby warm. Clinical research in the USA suggests that allowing a baby to lie, tummy down, on its mother's body after delivery is rather more efficient in getting rid of mucus in the respiratory tract than sucking out the baby, and that a baby retains body heat best when in skin-to-skin contact with its mother.[19]

The bath has come in for criticism for other reasons too. When midwives and mothers discuss it together they often wonder whether it is like a vote of 'no confidence' in the mother. Feminists question Leboyer's attitudes to women and ask whether he is not employing the well-known trick of coming in as an expert, even if a mystical, poetic, loving one, to take the place of the mother. Certainly his own writing does not give women confidence in themselves. During the birth he asserts that the mother is an 'enemy' to the child, standing between it and life. He calls her 'a monster' driving the baby through the birth passage: 'Not satisfied with crushing it, she twists it in a refinement of cruelty.'[20] A woman who is led to think that she is a torturer is hardly likely to trust herself to handle her baby with loving sureness.

For this reason some women decide that they would prefer to have the baby naked against their own skin for an extended period rather than use the bath. In some hospitals they are not allowed to do this because the baby will get chilled. The answer, of course, is to throw covers over both the mother and her baby. It seems a simple and obvious solution. Overhead heaters are often costly, but any sort of space heater which warms the area around the baby's head is suitable. Though in his film Leboyer himself baths the baby, there seems no reason why the mother should not do it if the bath is drawn up close to her or put between her legs on the delivery bed, or why both parents should not share doing it. Sometimes the father does it, and if so it should be near enough to the mother for her to be able to touch the baby.

The baby should be lowered into the water gently, your arm supporting the neck and holding the baby's hands in front of the chest so that a feeling of security is conveyed. When a baby, even one several weeks old, is suddenly dumped in a bath with arms and legs flailing it can be a terrifying experience for the child. If the mother or father then makes hasty or alarmed movements or communicates a lack of confidence through touch, the baby will scream, and go on and on screaming until taken out. It is understandable that anyone trying to give a baby a pleasant experience should react with anxiety when the baby makes it clear that she does not like it. This is why it is important to move slowly and firmly, talking soothingly to the baby as you do so. If the baby does not enjoy the bath at first, don't panic. Some babies have to learn to like a bath, even a Leboyer bath.

But the bath is only one aspect of what Leboyer teaches. The baby has come out of a smooth, slippery environment, and has been held by flesh. If wrapped in coarse cloth or bundled in a towel he thinks she may feel scorched. Warm skin is the only right substance with which to welcome a baby to life. This is why he delivers the baby up on to the mother's abdomen to lie against her warm flesh. After the strenuous activity of the second stage of labour the mother is usually very warm (even if she has an attack of shivering after) and this warmth is just right for the baby.

Leboyer also teaches that the baby should be allowed to uncurl gradually from the fetal position and that the pace should not be forced. This means that a baby should never be held upside down like a skinned rabbit. If it is put on its front against the mother's body the spine will slowly uncurl, though the baby usually assumes the familiar womb position whenever he falls asleep, and mothers who have had breech babies with extended legs or in some other less usual position often note that their babies adopt this position as they fall asleep over the first few weeks of life.

The mother spontaneously rests her hand on the baby's back. Quite often the father does so too. It is as if they are telling the baby through their touch that she is safe and has come home. The curve of the hands holding the baby are like the curved walls of the uterus which held her so recently. And then something else happens, often quite spontaneously. If the baby is lying against the mother's body in this way she starts to caress the child. It is a quite natural form of massage. Leboyer in his film shows a very deliberate, slow massage with the palm of his hands and some people try to copy this. But a mother who is in the kind of environment where she feels able to be herself and do whatever she feels like doing will often do this without thinking of it.

The room does not need to be in total darkness. It is enough for the blinds or curtains to be drawn or the lights dimmed. There is certainly no reason to think that the midwife or obstetrician should have to function in a black-out, and it is understandable that those who believe that this is what a Leboyer birth entails are anxious that if there is anything wrong with the baby's breathing or if he stays blue they might miss it. In a hospital outside Munich all babies are delivered into pink infra-red light. The matron of this hospital says it has the advantage of giving extra warmth and she very soon got used to assessing a baby's condition in this different kind of light.

Stillness and quietness are important. Though there is water in the baby's middle ear and sounds are probably muffled at first, newborn babies can be seen to startle at loud noises like the dropping of instruments into a dish or a shouted command. It seems odd that we should ever have thought in our culture that the average chit-chat and noise of machinery and instruments familiar in most operating theatres should have been appropriate for the birth of a new human being.

In some ways Leboyer's insight and the force of what he is saying are no novelties. Good midwives have known it all along, though they did not express it in his poetry. Far from being some extraordinary new technique, Leboyer-style birth means that the arrival of a new being into the world is greeted with respect and reverence, compassion and tenderness for a creature who has come on a long journey, and a careful watchfulness so that this particular baby's needs are responded to as he or she is helped through the transition into life.

In most obstetric units babies are routinely suctioned at delivery to clear the airways. A fine plastic catheter is pushed into the mouth and nostrils (and sometimes unnecessarily and dangerously far down the baby's throat) and suction used to draw out mucus. Yet a modern and reliable obstetric text-book states unequivocally 'Most babies are born in good condition and require nothing more than to be given to the mother.'[71] If the baby is already conscious and breathing some people think that aspiration of the mouth and naso-pharynx is an assault on the child. If you do not want your baby suctioned unless she is slow to breathe ask for her to be turned on to her front on your tummy, so that any mucus can naturally drain from the mouth and nose. When the baby's head is tilted slightly lower than the buttocks gravity will help this drainage. A lively baby with any mucus secretions will probably sneeze too, since there is a reflex response to irritation in the respiratory passage. (When the baby sneezes it does not mean she has caught a cold.) If the baby is flat on its back any mucus present tends to go down further towards the lungs. This is why the baby should always be delivered on to her front. It is a paradox that nowadays babies are often delivered and put lying on their backs *in order* to be suctioned. It should also be remembered that the baby who is suckled after delivery obtains colostrum, which breaks down mucus secretions through an enzymatic effect. So there is a strong case to be made for letting the vigorous newborn get his own breathing and control mechanisms working and for intervening only where careful observation indicates that it is needed.

There is a debate about whether the cord should be clamped and cut. Note that it is a question of when the *clamping* is performed, not the cutting. Leboyer believes that the cord should be clamped only after the

New Ways of Birth

blood from the placenta has gone through to the baby. Others say that letting the baby have this blood is likely to increase the burden of bilirubin (yellow pigment) to be excreted and that the cord should be clamped immediately in order to reduce the chance of jaundice. If avoiding jaundice was the primary concern in obstetrics, however, there would be no induction or acceleration of labour with oxytocin intravenous drips, no Valium given and no epidurals, all of which increase the chances of the baby developing jaundice.

There is concern among some obstetricians that unless the cord is clamped immediately some babies may become exsanguinated by blood draining back into the placenta. Studies have been done which suggest that if the cord clamping is to be delayed the baby should lie *below* the placenta. This problem has been solved by some obstetricians by delaying clamping of the cord, but having the mother sitting almost upright so that she can fondle her baby while it is lying over her thigh, in which position the placenta is situated above the baby.

While the cord is still pulsating it does not matter that the baby has not breathed yet. One argument for delaying clamping is that it gives the baby a literal 'breathing space'. On the other hand if a baby needs resuscitation with sophisticated equipment and with drugs it may be that she cannot be given this treatment until the cord has been cut and she can be conveyed to the resuscitation table. There are no nerve endings in the cord, the exterior surface of which is composed of a gelatinous substance called 'Wharton's jelly', so neither mother nor baby feels the cutting.

Modified Leboyer

Many hospitals which claim they offer 'Leboyer' births do nothing of the kind. What they are providing is a sop to the mother. They may not see it this way but the attitude is that it is sufficient if she is kept happy and reassured.

This happens in those hospitals which deliver the baby with hushed voices and lights lowered, put the child on the mother's body, and then take the infant away into a brightly lit room to be checked over by the paediatrician, measured, weighed and wiped, before being returned to her. An important aspect of a Leboyer birth is that anything done to the baby is done not only in the same room, but whenever possible with her in skin contact with the mother. Instead of the baby going to the paediatrician, the paediatrician should come to the baby.

There has been a great change in hospital attitudes towards breast-feeding and it is now generally accepted that a mother can, and even should, put her baby to the breast while still on the delivery table.

But in some units she is told that she cannot suckle her baby until the third stage has been completed or until she has been stitched. In such units hospital routines take precedence over the important meeting of mother and baby. The baby who is suckled after delivery obtains colostrum, the precursor to milk, which helps to dissolve any mucus secretions in the respiratory tract, contains antibodies against a wide range of diseases and gives protection against allergies such as eczema. It is another way in which natural processes are subtly adapted to the baby's needs and why interfering with what is going on between the mother and baby can disrupt a delicate balance which is as yet incompletely understood.

The checking over of the baby can itself be an assault if done insensitively and roughly. In some hospitals a tube is passed down the throat into the oesophagus to check for oesophageal atresia (a blockage in the digestive tract). If a midwife or doctor is carefully observing when the baby has her first feed there is no valid reason why this should be done. A finger is introduced into the baby's mouth and pressed against the upper palate to make sure that there is no cleft palate. This can be done so gently that the baby likes it and even starts to suck on the finger.

The paediatrician checks for a dislocated hip by holding the legs and extending them and bringing them together again. When done firmly and slowly the baby does not object to this. He also feels over the head to see if there are swellings and does an abdominal examination, but neither of these need make the baby at all uncomfortable.

It is sometimes claimed that a paper which appeared in the *New England Journal of Medicine* giving results of research carried out at McMaster University, Hamilton, Ontario, 'disproves' Leboyer.[22] Babies delivered with Leboyer-style births were subsequently compared with those who had delivered in the usual way in that unit. The Leboyer babies showed no benefits. Those who accept these findings as indicating that Leboyer is wrong have failed to ask what the usual treatment of babies is in that hospital. The obstetrician concerned, Murray Enkin, offers 'family-centred care'. He believes that babies belong to their mothers and fathers, and that women should be able to choose the kind of birth they want. *All* babies in his unit are treated with loving-kindness and are handed to their mothers, the difference in the babies in the control group being only that the cord was not left to stop pulsating, they were given to their mothers wrapped up and the mothers suckled their babies rather later.

One interesting thing the Canadian researchers did discover was that when women were told in advance that they were going to be in the Leboyer group they had easier labours. This simple piece of information seems to have done something for the *mothers*. It may be that preparing for a Leboyer birth already affects the feelings a pregnant woman has about her baby coming to birth and about her body in its birth-giving.

Odent
Dr Michel Odent, director of the maternity unit in the Centre Hospitalier General of Pithiviers in France, believes that women need an environment which allows them to get below the conscious level of action in childbirth. He feels it is important to 'regress' to a state of pre-cultural learning, in which they can get in tune with their bodies and lose self-consciousness. When a woman lets go and allows the primitive brain to take over, she knows exactly what to do without learning any exercises or being given instructions.

He points out that many mammals seek semi-darkness during labour, and that women, too, need a sanctuary, a safe, quiet place where the light is dim and there are no intrusions. A darkened room, silence, warmth and the continuous, loving support of a midwife who says little but stays in close physical contact with the woman in labour are all important elements in the setting for a truly natural birth. Odent believes that the presence of a male doctor can be a negative influence on labour and that the emotional, and even the physical, link through touch, between a woman and her midwife is vitally important.

When a woman is able to do whatever she feels like she usually gets into positions in which she has gravity to help rather than hinder her. She tends to move around in labour, adopting different postures, often ones in which the angle of the pelvis is asymmetrical. He teaches that this is much safer than having her lie down, and he, too, points out that the heavy uterus is likely to compress the mother's aorta and inferior *vena cava* and impair uterine and placental blood flow and the venous flow back to her heart, resulting in hypotension and increasing the risk of haemorrhage. In ancient times and in peasant societies today women adopt upright positions. They stand, sit, kneel or squat. We have to break with three centuries of culture in which the mother has been supine. In French, the very word for giving birth, *accoucher*, is based on the assumption that the woman is lying down – *accoucheé*.

Odent has nothing in his natural birth room which suggests to a woman a posture she *ought* to adopt, no bed or delivery table, no medical equipment and nothing which would not be found in an ordinary living-room. The dominant colours are brown and orange; there is a low wooden platform covered with brightly coloured cushions and, probably most important of all, there is no clock.

A warm pool is available in case the woman would like to get into water and many women, especially those having a painful backache labour, enjoy being immersed in water in a subdued light. Once a woman is in water, even if she was having a difficult labour, she usually finds it easier to relax and may go into a dreamy state. Being in water changes the patterns of the brain and induces a predominance of alpha rhythms.

A woman often chooses to kneel, crouch or be on all fours with her abdomen suspended. This is a good position in which to get rotation of the fetal head to the anterior and also helps her change her level of awareness. It is the posture adopted in religions all over the world for prayer, involving a change of consciousness and surrender of the conscious, critical brain.

Odent believes it is important that a woman should feel free to make any noises she wants. Women in his hospital do not have to be quiet and often shout just as the baby's head is crowning and then again as it is being delivered. This shouting helps release of the perineal muscles so that the woman actively opens her body to give birth. For some women it is a shout close to ecstasy.

For the second stage of labour they often choose a standing position, bending their knees to squat, shoulders supported by an assistant standing behind. During expulsion this produces the maximum degree of pressure within the pelvis, the woman uses least muscular effort to help the baby down the birth canal and there is optimal release of the perineal muscles. The squatting position is especially safe for a breech presentation because it reduces delay between delivery of the baby's body and that of the head. It is this delay, created by the supine position, which can be dangerous when the baby is being born bottom first. He says the squatting position is also very useful for the delivery of the second twin and is the most efficient position for the expulsion of the placenta, which simply drops out.

The supported squat is a position which prevents severe perineal tears. When a woman is lying on her back a tear tends to occur at the base of the vagina, near the anus. But when she is upright a tear occurs only in the superficial skin and does not involve the vaginal *mucosa* (the lining of the vagina).

In the upright position a woman also tends to have a more active relationship with her newborn baby than if she is lying flat and it is simply dumped on her body. It is very difficult to have eye contact with a baby when lying flat or almost flat and still more difficult if the baby is placed up on your chest.

The baby can smell the mother when held close and there is evidence to suggest that smell is important in establishing breast-feeding.[23] Mothers and babies do not, Odent believes, have to be *taught* how to breast-feed if they are able to start out together from the very first moments exchanging signals with each other. Odent also stresses the importance of waiting for the baby to show signs of rooting and seeking the nipple and not trying to fix it on to the breast before it is ready. The mother's vertical position is also important physiologically in the third stage of labour, since it avoids the constriction of the *vena cava* which can occur when she is lying down after delivery, a contributory cause of postpartum haemorrhage. Skin contact with the baby reduces the risk of haemorrhage too, since it produces a rush of oxytocin which contracts the uterus. The placenta then drops out by gravity and there is minimal bleeding. If a woman is horizontal she often bleeds, and continues to bleed, until the placenta has been delivered.

In Western culture femininity has been associated with passivity for a long time. Odent believes that obstetric practices should be changed so that women can become active birth-givers. Attendants should learn to wait and watch and provide a loving and supportive environment in which the woman can 'listen to her archaic brain' and her emotions can be freely expressed. He remarks that the practice of the father giving the baby the Leboyer bath may result from the conventional supine birth position which tends to make the mother passive. When parents want to give their baby the Leboyer bath he finds now that the mother and father usually like to do it together.[24]

Michel Odent's perinatal mortality rate at the hospital in Pithiviers is between 8 and 10 per thousand and his Caesarean section rate approximately 6 per cent. There is a 6 per cent episiotomy rate. He does no inductions, no amniotomies and no forceps deliveries.[25]

Section III

The Days After Birth

The night after delivery

This was an ordeal for many women who wrote about their experiences – they longed to have their babies with them, but found that hospital rules meant that babies had to spend their first one, two or three nights in the nursery. Women often wrote vividly about their thoughts during this night, when many had little or no sleep. This appeared to be the case particularly with those who had not had pethidine, who frequently felt wide awake and exhilarated. It seemed that during these hours they relived the experience they had gone through and yearned to have the baby to see and touch. Many felt that not having the baby with them was a deprivation and some specifically mentioned that it would not have been like this if they had had their babies at home, and that therefore they were determined to have a home birth next time.

Some women missed their partners during this night and felt they wanted to have them close to share the experience and to talk it through. Some mentioned that their men had felt 'lost' or 'miserable' when they had gone home leaving them and their babies in the care of the hospital. Few hospitals yet make provision for a husband, wife and baby to be able to stay together, unless the baby is handicapped or has been stillborn, but this is something we ought to be thinking about for the future.

Postnatal care

Most women who wrote about their experience wanted hospitals to be as much as possible like home and to do what they wanted *when* they wanted in a relaxed, informal atmosphere and feel they were among friends. Or if not home for some women, then the smoothly run atmosphere of a really good hotel where staff were ready to provide help and care when guests wanted it, rather than when the administration considered it necessary.

In spite of economies in the Health Service and the difficulties of running any institution when the management is unable to afford to replace outworn equipment or modernize existing facilities, the atmosphere of the postnatal wards is clearly dependent on the people running them rather than on the physical conditions. Although women in the older hospitals complained about too few showers, baths and lavatories, no bidets, and on a few occasions even dirty bathrooms, and long queues to use these facilities, relationships with the staff were far more important. This was the key to everything about postnatal care which was liked or disliked.

Women often said that they had too little rest in hospital and some discharged themselves so that they could get more rest at home. A fair number mentioned that they took some time recovering from the rush and bustle of hospital. But, and this is significant, it was hardly ever rest from *the baby* that they wanted, but rest from hospital routines which meant that sleep or cuddling or feeding-time with the baby was interrupted or, in a few hospitals, that the husband's or other children's visits were rushed.

In many hospitals women said that sedatives were given routinely at night postnatally. Some women became very anxious that if they had sedatives they would not wake to feed their babies, and were distressed at having to take them. If sedation is the rule, ask to discuss it with the paediatrician.

Most women wanted to be able to have their babies with them whenever they wished, day and night, but – and there is obviously a problem here – they disliked other women in the ward having their babies with them if they were crying. Some found that the answer was to have a private room or to ask for an amenity bed. Other women welcomed the Domino scheme whereby they went into hospital with their own community midwife and returned home after eight hours or so. But this did not apply to those who were booked for consultant care, and they often found themselves 'stuck' in hospital for periods longer than they wanted. Some women thought that depression they experienced during the first ten days after the birth was attributable to this, and said that a depressive crisis had cleared up as soon as they got home again.

There were also women who thoroughly enjoyed their hospital stay and were sorry to leave. For some hospital was a 'sanctuary' into which they withdrew, and for others it provided the comradeship of other women who were all going through the same kind of experience. On the other hand, the jokes that were shared, the gossip and laughter were too much for some, who compared the atmosphere to a 'school dorm', which they felt was inappropriate to the particular adjustment to the new baby that they were having to make.

Different women will want different things. If an expectant mother is doubtful about whether she will want to be with a number of other women (although modern hospitals tend to have wards not larger than four to six beds) or cope with hospital routines, it is probably better for her to seek an amenity bed or to plan in advance for early discharge if everything is going well. It is best to do this well ahead since then the community midwife can be booked, and she will visit the home to take over care of mother and baby for the first ten days at least after the birth. If decisions are left to the last moment there may be delay while arrangements are made so that there is no gap between discharge from hospital and the midwife coming.

Feeding the baby

There have been dramatic changes in hospital attitudes to breast-feeding over the last five years and it is now generally agreed that women should be encouraged to breast-feed their babies for the first months of life and that feeding whenever the baby wants it is better than a strict schedule. In most hospitals midwives and nurses give enthusiastic support to the breast-feeding mother. This is largely the result of two government reports, the Oppé Report of 1974[1] and its revised version published in 1980. The official committee, under the chairmanship of Professor Oppé, came out unequivocally with the conclusion that breast is best, and recommended that all health authorities should promote breast-feeding and ensure that women get help and advice. The more recent publication stressed that fathers should be included in antenatal health education about infant feeding and stated that babies do not need to be given glucose water or any other fluid under normal conditions.

Yet in many hospitals babies are still being given additional fluids, especially during the night, with the intention of letting the mother sleep, sometimes even if she is awake and listening for her baby. In some hospitals paediatricians insist on babies being given water before they go to the breast in order to rule out oesophageal atresia (obstruction in the upper digestive tract). There is no evidence that observing a feed with water is safer than observing one when the baby is getting colostrum. Colostrum has many advantages: it lines the baby's gut with a kind of protective paint which guards the baby against bacterial, viral, gut and respiratory infections;[2] it also prevents large molecules of cow's milk protein reaching the intestinal tissues and producing an immune response in a baby who is receiving any artificial milk. The practice of giving water first should, therefore, be open to question and you should make it clear if you want your baby to have breast milk only.

In spite of the Oppé Report, many babies are still receiving sterile water in hospital. This is quite pointless. It is also more expensive than giving a baby who is thirsty plain water. If extra fluids are required because the ward is kept at such a high temperature that the babies are becoming dehydrated or if they are ordered because the baby is jaundiced, it seems reasonable to give plain, boiled water. (It should not be water which has been artificially softened or boiled repeatedly, which has a high sodium content.)

Enthusiasm for breast-feeding sometimes means that mothers who wish to bottle-feed cannot admit to this and some feel bludgeoned into trying to breast-feed when they do not want to. Some mothers who wrote said that they wished to bottle-feed but felt guilty that they had chosen to do this, and thought that staff attitudes caused this. One mother said she was handed her baby for a feed and the nurse said, 'Poor little baby, your mother doesn't want to feed you herself. You're only getting a bottle.'

Sometimes breast-feeding mothers remarked on lack of support for bottle-feeding mothers from staff. On the other hand, some members of staff who were concerned that a mother would not have enough milk for her baby expressed pleasure when it was decided to put a baby on the bottle. When this was the case, nurses noticeably relaxed when the bottle was given, and sometimes said, 'It'll be all right now,' or words to that effect.

The really important thing, according to the mothers, seems to be that they should have genuine choice and feel free to feed the baby as they wish without disapproval.

The middle-class mother is at an advantage here and is more likely to be able to say what she wants. But she is also the one who tends to breast-feed. Some working-class mothers feel under artificial constraint in hospital and start breast-feeding there with the intention of putting the baby on the bottle as soon as they get home. While there are undoubted advantages in starting a baby off with breast milk, even if only for a week or two, it would be more realistic for hospital staff to accept that there is going to be an early transition from breast-feeding to bottle and show the mother how she can cope with this; this is especially important for women who are returning to work outside the home. It would also be useful to have full discussion about combining paid employment with partial breast-feeding for those mothers who wish to do so. Caribbean immigrant mothers are expert at this and can give a good lesson on how it is done.

Enthusiasm for breast-feeding does not necessarily mean that expert help is forthcoming. In many hospitals women say that though nursery nurses and other members of staff were keen on breast-feeding, they did not know how to give practical help. Different nurses tried different ways of doing things and a major criticism coming from mothers is that they are subjected to conflicting advice. One nurse comes up and positions the mother with the baby's head in the crook of her arm; another comes and moves the baby's head so that she can control it with her hand; yet another arrives and suggests that the baby's legs would be best tucked under her arm; then a fourth puts in an appearance and places the baby on a pillow. Some mothers say that they have to keep a look-out to see who is approaching and quickly switch the baby round to the 'correct' position. This makes an athletic, quick-change exercise of even the simplest feed and it is surprising that mothers persist under these conditions.

Suggesting different ways of doing things, trying out new methods, searching for 'the trick' which will get that baby on and sucking, is understandable if we see it as a side-effect of the nurse's own anxiety. It is not merely that in many hospitals there is no coordinated policy about how to help mothers with feeding, but that the professional's anxiety is expressed in the offer of advice – the more anxious she gets, the more she adds to this advice. If we envisage this happening with many different members of staff, both those on duty at the same time and those coming on with different shifts, we can see that the mother is subjected to a veritable barrage of instructions. In her research on the relation between care given at the time of birth and later problems encountered in the mothering role, Jean Ball[3] discovered that women who were given a great deal of conflicting advice in the early postpartum days were those who rated themselves low in a scale of ability to cope as mothers six weeks later.

Most mothers probably do not need advice. What they do need is 'a facilitating environment'. This means peace and quiet, a chance to relax and enjoy the baby, to do things in their own time and their own way, and one or two supportive persons available who let them know that they are doing well and who give warmth and friendship.

In some hospitals rules about feeding are still too numerous to be described, as Jo Garcia points out, writing on the Community Health Council[4] surveys on maternity care. Though well-intentioned, the regulations invariably make the early days of feeding more complicated and intrude between a mother and her baby. One of these rules is that a mother feed her baby in the nursery at night, the idea behind this probably being that she will not then disturb other mothers who are sleeping. Women describe sitting on hard, straight-backed chairs set in a row, with lights glaring, and sometimes with pop music playing non-stop on the radio as well. It is no wonder they find it difficult to enjoy the experience. Sometimes mothers even found that there was a queue for the chairs.

Another frequent rule is that mothers must fill in the length of the baby's sucking time on a chart. This occurs where the hospital has moved on from scheduled to 'demand'-feeding, but nurses have such little confidence that it can work that it is considered necessary to record the length of each feed or nibble. Mothers often seem to make these times up. If they are not to sit with one eye on the clock they *have* to, and experienced mothers, aware of hospital 'norms', realize they are expected to feed for 3 minutes on each side the first day, then 5, 7 and 10 minutes on the second, third and fourth days, and not more than 10 minutes each side after that. First-time mothers, however, may not know what is considered normal and have the added difficulty of often not being sure when a baby is sucking and swallowing or simply enjoying suckling without swallowing.

A study was done in a London teaching hospital to find out if limited sucking time reduced the incidence of sore and cracked nipples.[5] On two postnatal wards mothers were told to limit sucking time and on two others they were encouraged to feed as long as the baby wanted. Interviews on the fourth day after delivery, some time between the sixth and eighth day and at six weeks revealed that there were highly significant differences between the two groups. There were no significant differences in the numbers of women who had nipple problems or engorgement, but many more women were still breast-feeding in the free suckling group. So it seems that if you want to succeed with breast-feeding sucking should not be timed.

In spite of valiant efforts in many hospitals – and in some a considerable measure of success – many women who wrote about their hospital stay found that postnatal wards did not provide a flexible environment in which to care for a newborn baby. It was difficult to get enough rest, sleep undisturbed between feeds, behave spontaneously with their babies, sit comfortably, get into and out of bed without difficulty, get a bath or shower when they wanted one, and often simply to get sufficient clean linen, sanitary pads and baby clothing.

In hospital after hospital mothers complain about excessive heat. The temperature is high because a newborn baby has just emerged from a tropical climate inside its mother's body. Some newborn babies, especially pre-term ones, chill rapidly when exposed to cold air. But these babies tend also to overheat when they are in an atmosphere that is too hot. Although a very high ward temperature may make most babies merely uncomfortable, it may introduce special risks for the baby who is not suckling well, who can become dehydrated.

The worst problem of all for many women was the constant stream of staff requiring information or wanting to do something to them, which made their stay exhausting, and for some women, disorienting. Some mothers sent detailed diaries of events during the twenty-four hours; it was clear from these that one would have to be very fit to be able to cope and that for some women the never-ceasing activity at a time when they were at their most vulnerable constituted a form of torture.

Closeness to the baby

The work of Klaus and Kennell[6] has focused attention on the early postpartum minutes and hours in the bonding of mother and child, and much research is taking place in different countries on the environment offered for birth and postpartum care in relation to the parents' reaction to their child, their ability to feel that it really belongs to them, and the factors which release maternal care responses.

De Chateau,[7] working in Sweden, has suggested that hospital practices have to change now that the sensitive period for attachment between mother and baby is more fully understood. He studied the differences in interaction between first-time mothers and their babies on the third day after delivery and again when the babies were three months old. In one group the mothers had ten to fifteen minutes of skin contact with their babies during the first half hour after delivery. In the control group the mothers were not allowed to touch their babies in the first half hour. The observers recording the interaction were not told to which group the mother had been assigned. At thirty-six hours they found that mothers who had been able to touch them at birth were holding their babies more often than the others, and that there were surprising differences in their behaviour, especially with boys: they were twice as likely to smile at their sons as the mothers who did not touch their babies, and six or seven times as likely to hold them with their arms right round the babies' bodies. There remained differences at three months. The mothers who had touched their babies spent more time face to face with and kissing their babies and less time cleaning them than the other mothers, and their babies smiled and laughed more and cried less than the others; here again the differences were more marked for boys than girls.

Research in other countries too points to the importance of early and extended contact between mother and baby for the subsequent relationship between mother and child and for success in breast-feeding, and indicates how the bonding process that normally takes place between all mammals and their young can be supported or interfered with by hospital practices.

Some mothers can never love their babies, and the results can be disastrous not only for that mother and child but for the whole family. Separation of mother and baby obviously does not in itself create baby batterers. But some women are especially vulnerable because they are under intolerable pressure from an unhappy marriage, for other social or economic reasons, or because they themselves were deprived of love in their own childhood, and when separated from their babies in the immediate postpartum period may later reject or be very hostile towards them. Many more mothers take care of their babies well enough but suffer a sense of loss or of ill-ease, and find difficulty in relating to them because they seem to 'belong to' the hospital and they cannot trust themselves to be adequate mothers or to act spontaneously towards them.

We must remember, too, that non-accidental injury of babies is often done by the father. So it is not just a question of bonding between mother and baby, but also of giving the man a chance to grow into fatherhood. The environment offered by the hospital, and everything the staff do and say, can either contribute to that development or seem to diminish the man as a person, a husband and father with responsibilities towards his wife and child.

Whether or not the baby is with the mother and she is given emotional support to get to know her baby may, therefore, be highly relevant to the subsequent emotional well-being of the family as a whole. Rooming-in of mother and baby, and freedom for the father, too, to handle and share in its care, is not just the cream on the top of the cake, a luxurious extra which the hospital can provide when all physical needs are met – it is a vital part of an environment which facilitates the unfolding of care-taking responses and the ability of a couple to grow from being just two adults having a baby to being parents.

There are wide variations in hospital practices concerning the care of the newborn and the rules which the newly delivered mother encounters once she is moved to the postpartum ward, either with or without her baby. It is probably worth asking about the practice in each hospital and, if possible, having a look at the postnatal wards and talking to mothers who are there. Even if babies are in cots at the bottom or side of mothers' beds, it cannot be inferred that mothers are allowed to pick them up whenever they want to or cuddle them freely. On the other hand, if some babies are in a nursery attached to the ward, there may still be a liberal regime in which mothers can decide themselves when they want some time without the baby. Some women find uninterrupted contact with the baby just too much to take in the early postpartum days; this may be partly because they have had a long, difficult and tiring labour which has left them feeling exhausted or emotionally drained, but perhaps even more frequently it is because, for a first-time mother especially, taking on full responsibility for a tiny baby is a mammoth task, demanding a great deal of confidence. We might see a good part of the task of staff on postnatal wards as being to help that self-confidence develop by letting the woman take her own time to get to know her baby, and by providing a friendly, supportive environment in which she can begin to discover herself as a mother and the baby as the unique human being it is.

Klaus and Kennell make some practical recommendations about

hospital care which can help attachment develop between the parents and their baby. These include:

- Childbirth education classes which prepare the mother and father for an active role in the birth.
- A companion for the woman in labour, who gives emotional support.
- Delaying giving any medication in the baby's eyes (which is not given so often in Britain as in the USA where Klaus and Kennell's work was done) till after the first hour.
- Privacy for the couple to be with their baby in the first hour after delivery and to get to know each other in a warm room with skin-to-skin contact.
- Rooming-in of mother and baby for at least five hours a day.
- Responsibility for care of the baby being given to the mother, with help ready in the background.
- Opportunities for those in the new family to have extended contact with each other.
- Praise and encouragement for the parents from hospital staff.

Some women believe that if for any reason they are separated from the baby there are bound to be long-term consequences. This is not so. It would be odd if it were, when one thinks of the intense love that a mother can have for her adopted child. Studies which show long-term emotional deprivation as a consequence of separation between mother and baby after birth are those which have been done among disadvantaged women. Both were undertaken in the United States, one among black, single women who were extremely poor and themselves came from deprived homes,[8] the other among low-income women.

Both of these showed long-term 'disorders in parenting' lasting two years or beyond. Many mothers who have had babies in special care units, sometimes for prolonged periods of time, can testify that this has not ruined the bond between them and their babies and that they love a baby who has been separated from them just as much as other children in the family. It seems that the women and babies who are most likely to suffer from separation are those who for one reason or another are *already* vulnerable and that poverty and social deprivation are powerful determinants in emotional handicaps between parents and children.

Babies in wards at night
Hospitals are not really designed for mothers and new babies to be together. It seemed that the only choice between having the baby in the nursery at night was to have it with you in the company of other mothers' babies too, some of whom would be certain to cry. This meant very

disturbed nights for many mothers. There is no answer to this unless maternity hospitals are radically redesigned so that all have single rooms. A compromise was to take the baby who was restless to a nursery attached to the ward, but there were two snags to this: the nursery was not sound-proofed, so that mothers at one end of the ward heard everybody else's and their own babies crying, and sometimes there were insufficient night staff, so nurses wheeled babies to a central nursing station where they could keep an eye on them.

On the postnatal ward of one hospital mothers are encouraged to take their babies into bed with them to sleep, and there is peace and quiet at night. A photographer, who was taking pictures of these mothers and babies nestling in bed together one night, told me that although he and the paediatrician were walking round the ward and taking photographs, not a single mother woke, they were all sleeping so soundly. In the morning several mothers asked, 'Didn't you say a photographer was coming?' Perhaps mothers and babies can sleep more deeply when they are in skin-to-skin contact during these first days after delivery. This is a risky thing to do if the mother is heavily drugged however. Since some hospitals routinely hand out sleeping pills to all women on postpartum wards, if the baby is to be in bed with the mother such a practice would certainly have to change. Some writers also, who were concerned about overuse of drugs in our society, objected to this on the grounds that drugs should not be used unnecessarily.

Special care baby units

Enormous changes have been made over the last few years in special care baby units. Women often speak of the welcome they get, consideration, help with getting breast-feeding started and encouragement to help in the care of their own babies. In most units both parents are given a warm welcome and can go in at any time they like, day or night. In some the father, too, can help look after his baby. In nearly every unit women say they are given full and honest information, in terms they can understand, and feel that nothing is being kept back or watered down for their benefit. Some units have mother and baby rooms where a woman can stay close to her baby and get to know her for at least the day or so before they both go home. One hospital has the mothers right in the unit so that they are never separated from their babies.

The full significance of the research on bonding is appreciated by all staff working in SCBUs and in some hospitals a mother gets a much better chance of feeling the baby belongs to her and not the hospital if the child is in the SCBU than if she is on an ordinary postnatal ward!

Women who wrote about these units valued being intimately involved with their babies' welfare and being themselves an integral part of a group of people all working together for the sake of the baby. They often said that they never felt they were put into the position of being 'visitors' to the unit and they appreciated it whenever there was free access to the paediatrician (which was not the case in all units) so that they were up-to-date about the baby's condition from day to day. They also often referred to ways in which nurses, by calling the baby by name, talking to him or her, and treating the baby as a person, not just a sick patient, helped them with their often conflicting feelings about the baby. It is not enough simply to allow the mother or father freedom to come and go as they please. Many have to cope with very negative feelings about the baby, who, spread-eagled like a frog in a plastic box, with all sorts of instruments attached, may not look like a baby at all. Where staff understand these emotions, and accept them, and the waves of guilt which a mother may feel about having a pre-term low-birth-weight or handicapped baby, parents are helped to come to terms with these powerful feelings and start to fall in love with their baby.

Day and night in the hospital
When a woman is admitted in labour or is moved to the postpartum ward at night the care she gets may be very different from that she would get in daytime.

Though I am discussing these differences here mainly in the context of the time following birth, they can also have some disturbing consequences on what happens to a woman during labour, as we shall see.

Care at night appears often to be dramatically reduced and to produce difficulties, especially for breast-feeding mothers who want to feed their babies when they wake. A completely different system for feeding may be instituted when the night shift comes on (frequently made up largely of agency nurses, who may be unaware of or not interested in that hospital's ethos about maternity care or the methods of the day sister on that particular ward). The result can be conflict, with mothers and babies at the receiving end, and even when there is no direct hostility, such an uncoordinated system always seems to result in muddle and confusion.

Another effect of this is that discipline may be so slack at night that women find it difficult to get to sleep because of other patients or staff chattering and walking around and babies who are left to cry. In these hospitals writers frequently reported that they left hospital exhausted, longing for a rest and a good night's sleep.

Mothers were very critical of agency nurses, as were some midwives and obstetricians who wrote, but staff shortages meant that they had to be used. On the other hand it was precisely these agency nurses who sometimes let a chink of daylight and a relaxed atmosphere into a rigid hospital system where babies were fed by the clock, and mothers looked forward to the night when they could cuddle their babies. In one hospital where there was not much help with breast-feeding from harassed, overworked staff, one nervous first-time mother appreciated an agency nurse who sat with her on and off through a large part of the first night when her milk came in, helping her to get her baby to 'fix' and suck well, and got off to a flying start with breast-feeding because of the loving attention this nurse gave. So there were obviously individual agency nurses for whose help women were very grateful.

In some hospitals apparently women were not supposed to be in labour at night if they could help it, or not, at any rate, in advanced labour. Labour was supposed to take place in the right place, the labour ward, and at the right time, which seemed to correspond roughly with office hours. In one hospital, for example, a woman on the antenatal ward, with rapidly escalating contractions every four minutes, said she was told to go back to sleep and stop imagining things. The night sister appears to have recognized that she was in labour however, because when she handed over to the day staff she gave a message to the sister, who immediately examined her and moved her to the labour ward, and then at rapid speed to the delivery room as she was starting the second stage. In some hospitals, too, if a woman was admitted during the night she tended to be given sedation, her husband was told to go home, and she was put in a darkened room and told to sleep, unless she was recognized as already in strong labour. This meant that some women were deprived of their partners' support and of help from staff when they most needed it, and they either passed some hours in anxiety and pain until the hospital 'started up' again, or were subjected to a sudden dash to the delivery room in the early hours of the morning while being told to stop pushing, and consequently their husbands missed the birth of the child.

Certain methods of managing labour, notably acceleration with an oxytocin drip and the use of epidural anaesthesia, often seemed to depend on the time of day labour started, and a woman who was labouring during the night was unlikely to be accelerated or to have an epidural. On the other hand, if she started labour one day, laboured gently through the night, and was still in the first stage when general activity started in the morning and doctors' rounds were done, in some hospitals she was very likely to be put on a drip. That is, it seemed that the management of labour related to *the social divisions of time* rather than to the overall length and progress of that specific labour. The impression was that a few women who could have done with some stimulus to their labours did not get it because it was night-time, and that a much larger proportion of women were automatically accelerated after a weary night when they were given inadequate support and their morale had dropped, and that in these cases acceleration may have been used in place of other more directly human means of support.

It was unfortunate that a woman in labour at night was sometimes not allowed to get out of bed, or was occasionally enjoined to be quiet and not disturb other patients, when she longed to change position or move about. It is possible that her own spontaneous urge to get on all fours, rock her pelvis or stand up might have produced more effective contractions and that, here again, the oxytocin drip was introduced in place of, rather than in addition to, other simpler methods of stimulating labour. This applied also to daytime care but appeared to be a more frequently encountered difficulty at night.

In some hospitals night was artificially foreshortened by rigid routines which meant that mothers were woken for feeding their babies but did not get morning tea till half an hour after they had finished, and in one hospital did not receive breakfast till an hour after that. Or mothers were all woken at 5 or 6 a.m. or another specific time, regardless of the fact that some at least of those who were feeding their babies when they cried had already given one or two night feeds and their babies were still sleeping.

While flexibility obviously causes problems for ward organization, lack of it makes life particularly difficult for the new mother who may be short of sleep anyway, and was one of the reasons why some women discharged themselves from hospital early – to get some rest at home.

It is probably staff recognition of this problem that led to the wholesale distribution of sleeping pills at night-time, which one mother said were 'dished out like Smarties'. Perhaps it is because nurses are so used to giving medication to ill people that they sometimes could not understand why a new mother should refuse sedatives each night, and failed to sympathize with women who were concerned that they would not hear their babies cry and might not wake to feed them, or that drugs would contaminate their milk. This seems one of the areas where there needs to be some consultation between paediatricians, night staff and mothers.

When a baby dies

Judith Lumley, an Australian obstetrician, says, 'The birth of a dead fetus is not something which precedes and prevents a relationship between the mother and her child, but something which disrupts an existing relationship.'[9] This is why the advice to 'have another one' as soon as possible is invariably wrong.

A few letters came from women whose babies had died. There were not many of them, but they had a special view of hospital care and helpful suggestions to make.

These mothers wanted their husbands with them, both when they were told that the baby was dead if this occurred in pregnancy, and also if they were told during labour or delivery. When it seemed certain that the baby had died before birth hospital staff did not always think of getting hold of the husband so that he could be there to give support to his wife, and as a result sometimes women had to face lengthy tests and then a long journey home alone. Husbands were also sent out when epidurals were given, again a time when the mother bearing a stillborn baby would have welcomed her partner's support.

After delivery women were sometimes put where they could hear other women and their babies, and some found this very distressing. Sometimes the woman was kept heavily drugged and this made her feel groggy and ill without doing anything to help her cope emotionally. One woman said that 'the full effects of the ordeal did not reach me until I came home'. Women sometimes found themselves lying doped in rooms by themselves, without their husbands, and said they were more or less ignored by hospital staff: 'The doctors and nurses seemed to be apprehensive about seeing me or talking to me.' Not all staff members were informed of what had happened: 'A cleaning lady asked me where my baby was.'

When women went back to the hospital postnatally to hear the results of the postmortem it was unfortunate that sometimes they encountered a doctor whom they had never met before and who appeared to know nothing about the case, so that they had to sit for some time while he read through the case notes and the postmortem report. On at least one occasion the obstetrician did not even know that the baby had died and 'looked briefly through my notes and to my horror said, "Oh well, you've only come for your postnatal then." We had to wait an agonizing 15 minutes while he went through the case history, notes and reports . . . We were astounded that something as important as this should be treated so lightly by the hospital.'

Some obstetricians seem to have little understanding of the desperate need that some bereaved women have for someone to sit with them, share in what they are going through, listen patiently and allow them to weep: 'I remember feeling as if my right arm had been cut off and buried in the ground,' said one woman who failed to get adequate emotional support from any member of staff in a large London teaching hospital.

Sometimes women suspected that nurses were embarrassed by the mother's grief and avoided her for this reason. If doctors and midwives do not feel that they personally have sufficient time or the necessary skills or personality to do this it looks as if those hospitals which deal with complicated births should have people on their staff who are specially able to 'share the grief-work'. These same people may be able to help members of staff cope with their feelings of failure and guilt when a baby dies. This is already being done in some large hospitals and is a hopeful development.

Visiting

Free visiting on the wards almost invariably proved too tiring, especially when it meant listening to other people's visitors as well as one's own. A solution appears to be for free visiting to be possible in some place outside the ward, and where such arrangements were made they were welcomed.

Women liked having a special time when husbands only (or one person with whom it was arranged in advance) could visit. Many hospitals have evening visiting for partners only, and this seemed to work well, especially if the father could cuddle the baby and help care for it and be there during the evening feed. There was a general feeling that it would be best for this to be *every* evening, not just a few evenings in the week.

Women who already had other children often worried about them when they were not allowed to visit. They liked special visiting times for other children, and wanted them to be able to get to know and handle the baby too.

Although on the whole women welcomed restricting general visiting, they liked the visits of husbands and other children to be very flexible and generous, and in those hospitals where a husband could come in any time he was free there seemed to be a specially relaxed, warm, welcoming atmosphere.

Food

There were frequent complaints about food, usually that there was too much 'stodge' and not enough salads and fruit. There is an idea in some hospitals that fruit is bad for breast-feeding mothers because it tends to give the babies 'wind', and there were even occasions when grapes, which are supposed to be the worst offender, were denied women after visitors had brought them in. It might be a good idea if hospital dieticians and paediatricians discussed with staff on postnatal wards suitable diets and dietary supplements for breast-feeding women.

Many mothers were constipated after childbirth, or at least there was general concern that they should empty their bowels within a couple of days. (If a woman has had suturing of the perineum it is important that she should not have hard stools or the repair can be damaged.) In some hospitals all had to have laxatives. In a few the emphasis was on fresh vegetables and fruit and roughage.

Women sometimes remarked on the inadequate meals offered to women who were on special diets. Vegetarians often had a difficult time. Asian women sometimes found the food so unfamiliar that they ate practically nothing, although in some hospitals special curries are provided. Kosher food was also sometimes very poor.

In some cases the food was scanty, and breast-feeding mothers in particular found it inadequate. (Breast-feeding means that a woman usually requires about an extra 1,000 calories in the twenty-four hours.)

Many hospitals now have an odd system whereby one orders food two days in advance. (Try doing *that* in a hotel!) For the first two days after delivery the mother has food ordered by the woman who was previously in her bed. Many who wrote about this thought the system should be changed.

Planning Ahead for Birth

Communication

Many conflicts between the providers of health care and women having babies have been attributed to failures in communication. Obstetricians often assert that if only more effective ways of communicating with women could be found, mothers would accept the style of care provided without demur. Some accuse the media of whipping up resistance to standard hospital practices and types of intervention, and the 'middle-class vocal minority' of making other women dissatisfied. They sometimes say that the answer to all this is better communication by the medical profession. They may go on to say that any treatment or investigation should be explained, so that patients comprehend what is being done to them and why, the inference being that once such explanations are given all will be well. They are, of course, confusing persuasion with communication. It is a fallacy that communication is to do with telling people something and giving out information. True communication is two-way. It involves dialogue.

But even if communication were perfect, people might still not agree. There is every sign that there are genuine differences of opinion between many doctors and childbearing women about the environment and style of birth and the degree of intervention which is desirable. This is essentially a conflict about *who is in control:* whether all labours should be 'managed' by obstetricians or whether the woman should be helped to control her own labour.

Many midwives today also feel threatened by losing control both to obstetricians and patients. Under attack from both quarters, some side with the obstetrician against the encroachment of 'consumers' and see themselves as defending professional standards against a horde of uninformed and demanding women. Margaret Myles, the doyenne of British midwives, expresses an attitude which is shared by some other midwives today when she writes:[1]

To the expectant mother, labour is a very personal experience which engenders the presumption that she ought to participate in professional decisions and dictate regarding her obstetric care. But she may have little understanding of the tremendous amount of knowledge and years of experience needed in the practice of competent obstetrics. If she knew more she would realize the wisdom of having faith in professional experts and allowing them to make decisions regarding her own and her baby's well-being and safety throughout labour.

155

This is a basic disagreement about power and cannot be solved by mere communication, however well intentioned.

The idea that talking together about birth will solve all the problems also ignores the fact that doctors and others taking care of patients have greater power than the women who are merely visitors in the hospital. Even cleaners and tea-ladies have more power in the system than the patients. This power is often exercised benignly. But in the last resort it can be employed decisively. This is particularly the case when women are partially drugged or naked from the waist down, immobilized, connected to equipment and recording instruments and perhaps also in pain. Communication between doctors and women having babies is not between equals.

Learning to be assertive
Something not often taught in childbirth education classes, least of all those in hospitals, is how to state what you want, say 'No, thank you' and assert your rights as a human being. You need to be able to do this in the alien setting of a hospital confronted by professionals whom you do not know and who are acting as official representatives of an often imposing institution, and in spite of heavy cultural conditioning which leads almost everyone nowadays to assume that birth is a medical process.

As Mary Chamberlain says[2]

Many women, as part of their conditioning as women, have internalized masculine expectations of themselves, especially in health matters where the line between medical and social judgement has become thin and confused, and where access to knowledge is controlled by the doctor in an essentially unequal relationship. Patients in our society are required to be passive, and so are women: women as patients carry a double burden of expected behaviour.

The insistence which many antenatal teachers put on adapting gracefully, on getting on good terms with those caring for you and your baby, and, though they do not say it, on 'how to make friends and influence people', is now being challenged by couples who believe that this approach to birth education has resulted in conformism and in the passive acceptance of unnecessary obstetric intervention. John Hargreaves, writing in the London Birth Centre's Newsletter[3] is critical of the NCT's type of antenatal teaching because, he says:

The NCT is very careful *not* to set standards: drugs and every form of intervention are fine if that's what the mother wants. (But by refusing to set a standard advocating natural birth, the NCT is in fact accepting the status quo, rather than helping parents break through both cultural conditioning and medical pressure for unnatural labour.) Fathers are often peripheral, being invited to one out of eight classes. Labour is seen as inevitably painful, though the 'funny breathing' routines may distract you enough to get through some of it, so that you can delay the use of drugs which so many accept will be necessary eventually. Parents are often not prepared for coping with the hospital routines and with one wrong step on the conveyor belt they have no idea how to get off, so that what they thought was an innocuous routine – such as amniotomy – leads eventually to oxytocin, epidural, forceps, the intensive care unit for depressed breathing, and postnatal depression.

If our culture of birth is to change, *we* have to change it. That means never smiling and politely saying 'Yes' when we mean 'No'. Women are taught as little girls that to be attractive and desirable is to be pleasant and if a man seems to *want* us to smile and agree with him, we tend to do so because that is how we have been brought up. That is our 'feminine' view of ourselves. So we smile when a lout whistles or smacks his lips in the street, even if inside, we feel sick, just as we smile back at the male doctor who is telling us something for our own good in a kindly, condescending manner.

You do not *have* to agree with your obstetrician, even though he appears to have superior knowledge. It is *your* body and *your* baby. You can say you want to discuss the matter with your partner or someone else before deciding, that you need further information and time to think through the advice he is giving you. You can refuse to be stampeded.

Women often need to learn how to express anger and how to be assertive. We are taught to placate, to be tactful, not to annoy anybody, rather than to express the anger we feel. We try to cope with what society expects of us, bottling up inner rage and frustration until it bursts out when we least expect it, often against those closest to us, and in situations in which it is strategically inappropriate and self-defeating. When this happens in relations between women and doctors the emotionally over-wrought woman is then seen as requiring psychiatric help. She has been neatly categorized and, so far as the doctor is concerned, the problem is dismissed and the confrontation won.

There are some things you can do to prepare yourself to be confidently assertive during labour. The first is to get together a group of couples expecting babies and others who have recently had babies to talk together about the birth experience. If you can find people who have been and are planning to go to the same hospital that you are going to this will be very useful. Groups like this sometimes form quite spontaneously in antenatal classes and couples get together informally in each others' homes to discuss such subjects. But if you are not yet attending classes get in touch with your childbirth educator and ask if you can be put in contact with some other people. Some of these groups consist of women alone, but it is always useful to have with you the support person you intend to have with you during labour, whether male or female. Your general practitioner may also be able to put you in touch with other expectant parents and with people who have recently had babies. If you are attending the hospital for antenatal care you can probably meet other women during the long waits in the clinic. So it is usually easy to build up a mutual support group of this kind.

Some of the questions you may want to discuss are:

- How do we feel about going into hospital?
- What are our goals and our priorities in the birth experience?
- How can we ensure the best chance of reaching them?
- If anyone in the group has been cared for by doctors or midwives others are likely to meet, how easy was it to work with them?
- How can we avoid being manipulated?
- To reach our goals, what strategies work best?
- How can we ensure intervention takes place only when really necessary?
- What decisions do we want to be able to make ourselves during labour?
- How can we ensure that we make clear our concern and retain the right to make these decisions?

Another thing you can do is to use role play to rehearse how you might cope with difficulties in social relationships. Remember that labour is dramatic, especially once you have reached the end of the first stage and that, however much you are enjoying it, you will be under *stress*. The physical and emotional release which you need in order to let your body work freely involves an inner stillness, concentration, a psychological state which is probably best described by the Quaker phrase 'being centred down'; feeling that you have to argue about or discuss things in the middle of contractions, or to fight for your rights, is bound to interfere with this. So you need to work out ways of dealing with well-meant intrusions and questions and with irrelevant occurrences so that you can keep this harmony with yourself. Your support person is obviously very important in this. In fact, in the thick of labour, it is only when you have a strong support person that you feel that you can surrender conscious control.

The next exercise is best done in a group too, since you will need two or three people who know the kind of thing that goes on in hospital to take part in your play-acting. You will need your support person there too.

Start by discussing together the techniques which you plan to use for handling contractions. Then go on to discuss how this other person can best help you. Rehearse these together.

The next thing to do is to work out together a way of simulating uterine contractions. This will not be anything like real labour, of course, but it can be useful to develop a technique of rehearsing contractions with – and this is the important thing – somebody other than yourself deciding when they begin and finish, the interval between them and how strong each is to be. This could be provided simply by a verbal stimulus with your partner saying 'a contraction is starting now – it is getting stronger – and stronger – stronger still – now it's really tight – and now it is beginning to fade away a little – getting fainter – and now it's going – contraction finished'. But this is usually not the best way to do it, if only because when you are actually in labour you will feel tremendous sensations of pressure, tightening and stretching, and it is very difficult to represent these intense physical sensations in words. So here are some other ways of doing it:

Your partner takes a little bit of flesh from your inside thigh (not over a varicose vein) and pinches it, lifting it up off your leg. He starts gently and gradually presses tighter and tighter. You change your breathing to cope with the contraction as it gets stronger and use whatever other means you have decided on to handle the contractions. After forty seconds or so he releases the pressure and lets the contraction gradually fade away. With this technique it is a good idea to start very gently at first so that you feel you can cope with the sensations. But as you get more expert it is useful to be able to cope with pain, real pain.

If you don't like the pinching on your inner thigh you may prefer pressure at the back of your ankle. It works well, but does not have the advantage of being in approximately the same area as where you will experience tense sensations in labour.

Some people prefer a Chinese burn on the forearm.

Or your partner can do much the same, pressing firmly with his hands on either side of your rib cage.

Some couples hate doing this because the support person cannot bear to cause any pain. So you may want to talk about this together. It is a marvellous morale booster to know that you can cope with pain before you go into labour. You may also find that you want to alter some of the techniques of breathing, relaxation and so on you already know when you find that some are more effective than others in handling pain.

Another way is to use the stress and intensity of very powerful sound. Your partner produces waves of sound 'contractions', using a cassette tape-recorder and gradually turning up the music very loud, holding it at its loudest for half a minute or so, and then turning it down again. Unless you live in a very isolated area you will probably want to wear earphones for this!

A method which has been used to test coping strategies for pain is to immerse the hand in ice-cold water. Some people choose this method. The disadvantage here, though, is that your hand is either in or out of the water, whereas with contractions there is usually a gradual build up and a gradual fade away.

Once you have got into the swing of handling contractions, you can now go on to work out ways of coping with interruptions, people asking you questions, staff coming in and out and talking together, intrusive sounds such as bells ringing or a voice suddenly heard on an intercom and the invasion of body space which occurs when attendants come close and handle a part of your body, do a vaginal examination, for example, listen to the fetal heart, palpate your abdomen or roll you over into another position. You will need another one or two friends to act the part of hospital staff. It is important that they should take this seriously. Your task is to continue to concentrate on what you are doing and not allow yourself to be 'thrown' by any interruption or intervention. Your partner's role is to continue giving you support and also to communicate to the attendant that you are busy with a contraction so that no intervention takes place without your permission.

In many hospitals you will never be faced with this kind of problem, but even in the best there are sometimes one or two members of staff who, perhaps completely unaware of their negative effect on you, risk breaking your concentration and interfering with the way you are working with your body in labour.

One of the things you may discover is that making eye contact with this person and at the same time raising your hand with a gesture which says 'not yet!' is an effective way of communicating even while you are in the middle of a contraction. Knowing you can do this without breaking your concentration can do a great deal for your confidence.

These are some of the things the friends who are acting the part of doctors, midwives and medical students might say:

'Are you having a contraction now?'

'Have your waters gone yet?'

'Just roll over, dear, and I'll give you something to help the pain.'

'Do you want a boy or a girl?'

'Where are you going for your holidays?'

'You'll get dehydrated if you go on breathing like that.'

Or two people might have a discussion in front of you about the dance they went to last night or about the activities of somebody else in the hospital. An obviously disturbing conversation, to which some women in labour are subjected, is for two nurses to discuss the last difficult case they attended or a very complicated labour occurring in the next room.

You will probably find this hilarious the first few times you try it, but it is worth continuing till you are quite sure that you can keep your cool and that your partner goes on working with you without being distracted by anything that is going on around you. It is *your* labour and you can keep it that way.

Patients' rights

If you ask the doctor to tell you something, you have the right to a full and truthful answer. If you do not ask, however, the implication is that maybe you do not want to know. It is therefore up to *you* to ask.

You have the right to be told about any possible risk to you and your baby as the result of a treatment proposed by the doctor.

Your consent must be sought before starting any procedure or giving you any drug which could have side-effects on you or your baby. You can, if you wish, refuse to give your consent.

If you are given any drug you have the right to be told what it is. During pregnancy, in labour, after the baby is born and while you are breast-feeding, you may wish to ask about possible effects of that drug on you and your baby. The doctor has a duty to give you full and factual information if you ask for it.

Before any intervention takes place during pregnancy and labour you can ask to be told the likely effects on you and your baby of the procedure which is proposed. This includes such practices as the use of ultrasound, induction and acceleration of labour, amniotomy and the use of electronic fetal scalp electrodes. You have the right to choose not to accept any of these procedures. Examining or treating you without consent is a form of assault.

If you are told that a procedure is about to be performed and do not question it, it is taken for granted that you have agreed to it.

In Britain you do not have the right to see your case records, which are the property of the National Health Service, though if they are given to you to hand on the another member of the hospital staff you can, of course, read them.

If you discharge yourself from hospital against doctors' advice you may be asked to sign a statement saying that you accept responsibility for anything that may happen to you and your baby. You cannot be kept in hospital against your will.

If you do not wish to be observed or treated by medical students you can simply say so and your wishes must be respected.

A father, or other support person, has no inherent right to be present during labour and delivery. This is a matter for negotiation between you and your attendants.

Research

There are international rules governing medical research. They grew out of the Nurenberg war trials and the shocked reaction to experiments carried out by doctors in concentration camps.

A patient must be told when she is part of a research project. The implications of what it is proposed to do, and any probable short- and long-term effects on her and her baby, must be made clear in a way that she can understand. No research should be done unless she has given her informed consent. At any point she can withdraw from the research series.

If any special investigations are done during your pregnancy or labour, you can ask if this is part of a research project and if so, whether it can be explained to you. In many cases the research is interesting and being involved with it means that your pregnancy is specially watched. Sometimes it involves extra visits to the clinic or special tests which you may not wish to have, or the use of drugs in labour, for example, which you would prefer not to receive. You can then withdraw from the research.

It is unethical for a woman to be asked to engage in a research project when she is under stress. This is why it is wrong to do so when she is actually in strong labour. In a well-known London teaching hospital a woman was asked, late in the first stage of labour, to help research and was given an injection. When her baby was about to be born she saw a paediatrician standing by the delivery table and asked why she was present. The paediatrician said, 'Oh you have had Valium and your baby may need help breathing.' This woman was quite happy with the situation. Another woman might not be.

Similarly, no tests should be done on your baby after birth unless you are informed and give your consent. This includes psychological tests.

Making an informed choice

One view of childbirth is that it is a medical event about which doctors make all the decisions. Another view is that it can be an important experience in the life of a woman and in the unfolding of a family, and that therefore a woman should choose herself the setting for birth, the kind of care she prefers and, if all goes well, the details of what happens.

A birth educator and writer in the United States, Penny Simkin, developed the first Birth Plan to enable women to make their choices clear.[4] The aim of the *Birth Plan* (see p. 168) is to think through the kind of birth you would like to have and state your preferences, both if everything is straightforward and also if you encounter one of the variations in labour which means that you need help from an obstetrician. I have called the latter a *Contingency Plan*.

It is important to be flexible, to adapt to whatever happens. You cannot, obviously, legally bind doctors and midwives to do what you want. But working together on a Birth Plan is a valuable opportunity for discussing your hopes and anxieties, and for cooperating with the people caring for you and your baby to make birth not just something that happens *to* you, but a creative act which you have patterned by your own forethought and preferences.

You do not need to 'leave it to the experts'. It is *your* body, *your* life and *your* baby. It is your right and your responsibility to choose between alternatives.

In some parts of the United Kingdom there is very little choice, but in cities and in many suburban areas you may be able to choose between hospitals, between a consultant or a GP unit, and between hospital or home. If you are not certain about policies in any hospital, write to or ring the senior nursing officer with your questions. The kind of response you get will give you some idea of attitudes as well as policy.

Your GP may undertake obstetric care himself or he may refer you to a GP colleague who is on the 'obstetric list' or to a consultant 'firm' at the hospital. Even if your GP does obstetrics you can choose to go to another GP for maternity care. It may seem like a vote of 'no confidence', but you are perfectly entitled to do this and can return to your GP after you have had the baby. You may choose to do this if you want a home birth and your usual family doctor does not do home births.

It is a good idea to discuss with your GP the kind of birth you hope for *before* you are referred for consultant care. This may make a difference in the referral, for some consultants are known to be keen on epidurals, or induction or 'active management', some are particularly good at surgery or managing diabetes, for instance, and some encourage natural birth. Once you have booked in with a consultant it can be embarrassing for the GP to ask for a change, though you have a right to change your consultant at any time if you wish.

Whatever kind of doctor you choose you will need to discuss your birth plans with him or her at the booking clinic and again late in the pregnancy. Before discussing your plans with the doctor it may help to talk with women in your local NCT branch and the nearest antenatal teacher, or discuss their experiences with other women who have had babies in the same place recently.

A Birth Plan can only be drawn up when you have given yourself time to find out about the different alternatives available, and is best done when you already know what is offered in your locality. It obviously can't be done in a vacuum without reference to the usual views and accepted practices of birth attendants in the hospital or community services. Though it would be pleasant to pick and choose what you might like, it will remain a daydream unless you are able to *negotiate* with the people caring for you so that the dream is carried forward into reality. To have a birth plan without such careful negotiation is a bit like deciding on a menu without reference to what the cook has in the kitchen, since some of the things for which you are asking may be strange and new to some doctors and midwives. It can also be rather like asking the cook to prepare an *omelette norvégienne* for the very first time. If it is not something you know you can do it is an alarming undertaking, especially in front of an eager audience. It is understandable that some professionals would rather go on doing what they have always done and exercising skills in which they feel competent.

When professionals come over as heavy-handed and authoritarian this is sometimes not a simple matter of wielding power but can be an expression of their own doubts about their ability to do something new. Doctors who have nearly always done deliveries with episiotomies, for example, may be very unsure as to whether they have the necessary skill to deliver without an episiotomy and fear that an enormous tear will be produced. Similarly when doctors and midwives are accustomed to having women lying flat for delivery they find it disturbing to have a patient who insists on kneeling or standing. It means that they do not know how to position themselves for the delivery or which hand to use for what.

Professionals accustomed to a good deal of intervention may feel completely at sea when they do not have machines to help them. Not using electronic fetal monitoring, for example, can make an obstetrician very anxious because he feels that he simply does not know what is going on. It is hard for doctors who rarely witness completely natural births to believe that labour can progress normally without them doing anything at all.

A Birth Plan is not something you devise just for your own emotional satisfaction – though it can be important in this way also – but an expression of your thinking about the environment in which you want your baby to be born and the manner in which he or she will be welcomed. It is one way in which you start caring for your baby even before birth. Doctors and nurses offer professional skills and sometimes it seems as if they have accepted complete responsibility not only for you but also for your baby. In a sense this is what professional responsibility is all about. But nobody cares for your baby more than you do, and you can choose to accept responsibility *yourself*, together with the task of making informed choices between the alternatives available.

Working out a Birth Plan provides a basis on which you can discuss your preferences with the doctor or midwife, or, if you have no idea who is going to attend you in labour or deliver the baby, with representatives of the institution concerned. The fragmentation of care resulting from a system in which one set of staff mans the antenatal clinic, another set takes over the labour and delivery and yet another runs the postnatal wards in the hospital makes discussion much more difficult but not impossible. The shift system also complicates things. You may have agreed on a course of action with the doctor and midwife attending you, only to find that they go off duty and other staff come on. In these situations it can be specially helpful to have something in writing in your records.

It is probably a good idea to discuss your ideas initially very early in pregnancy because this will influence your choices about the place of birth and the people attending you. When you are about seven months pregnant the time has come to have another discussion and to ask the doctor to insert your Plan in the case notes so that whoever attends you in labour knows what you want and what has been agreed between you and your doctor. These agreements are not, of course, legally binding.

Some questions women ask
It may help you to decide what questions to ask if you know the kind of questions other women ask their doctors during pregnancy. If you share ideas in a childbirth education class you will probably find that other people in the group have sought and got information from the hospital where you intend to have your baby, and it can be useful to pool experiences in this way. But if you cannot get to classes, or attend a class where these discussions do not often happen, here is a list of some of the questions which people in my own classes have asked. Obviously it is not exhaustive, but it may give you some idea of the range of subjects to discuss.

- Will my husband be able to be with me right through labour and delivery?
- My partner isn't able to be with me, but I would very much like another support person throughout. Can this be arranged?
- My partner doesn't feel very confident about being with me and helping me during labour because he has been abroad most of the time, but he is willing to be there if we have another support person with me who has attended childbirth education classes with me. Is it possible to arrange this?
- Since it looks as if I shall probably have a Caesarean section will it be

possible for the baby's father to be with me during the operation?

- I'd like a woman friend with me to help me during labour and I hope that she will be able to be with me throughout. Can I be sure that she will be welcomed?
- I would like my friend with me when I have the Caesarean section. She has been to classes with me and has read about Caesarean birth. Can I be sure that this will be easily arranged at the time?
- If everything is straightforward shall I be able to walk around during labour?
- Shall I be able to have a bath/take a shower during labour?
- If I want to eat and drink during the first stage of labour shall I be able to?
- Shall I be able to choose whatever is the most comfortable position to give birth?
- Shall I be able to sit up/be on my side/squat?
- I would prefer not to be shaved. Will this be possible?
- I don't want to have an enema. Can I be assured that I shall not be compelled to have one?
- Is it routine for women to have their waters broken when they are admitted or later on during labour?
- What percentage of women are induced in this hospital?
- Could you tell me the percentage of women whose labours are stimulated?
- What percentage of women have electronic fetal monitoring?
- I would prefer not to have an intravenous drip if labour is straightforward. Can I be assured that I shall be allowed to labour without a drip?
- Could you please tell me the percentage of women in your care who had episiotomies?
- Could you tell me the percentage of women in this hospital who have forceps deliveries?
- I should prefer to have no drugs for pain relief unless I myself ask for them. Can I be sure this will be easy to arrange?
- Could you tell me the percentage of women who have regional anaesthesia?
- With Caesarean births, what percentage of women have epidural anaesthesia and what percentage general anaesthesia?
- What was the Caesarean section rate in the hospital last year?
- How much time can we be sure of having to cuddle the baby after delivery?
- Is it possible to ask for extra time?

- If I need a Caesarean section shall we both have the chance to hold the baby after the baby is born if all is well?
- If the baby is born by Caesarean section can I ask for extra time to cuddle the baby?
- If I have a Caesarean section will my baby automatically go to the nursery?
- If I have a forceps delivery will my baby automatically have to go to the nursery?
- How long is my baby likely to have to stay in the nursery for observation?
- Can I go with my baby to the nursery?
- Can I stay with him or her as long as I like?
- Will my baby be able to be with me right through the twenty-four hours?
- Is there breast-feeding on demand?
- Does that include the night?
- Are babies routinely given water after feeds?
- What percentage of women choose to breast-feed in the hospital?
- How long is fathers' visiting time each day?
- Can my older children visit every day?
- Will my husband be able to cuddle the baby when I am on the postpartum ward and can he help with things like baths and changing?
- Will my other child be able to cuddle the baby?
- I should like to leave the hospital a few hours after having the baby if all is well. Will it be possible to arrange to go home within about eight hours?
- Can I arrange twelve-hour/twenty-four-hour discharge please?

When you have had full discussion on these subjects and have come to some consensus it can be useful to have a single sheet of paper which constitutes your personal Birth Plan and which can then be put into your case records. It might look something like the example on p. 168:

Planning Ahead for Birth

An example of a Birth Plan in hospital records

MARY BROWN	
Antenatal classes attended:	National Childbirth Trust
Teacher:	Marilyn Smith, 12 Sisley Way, Brighton. Phone 73216
Tour of hospital:	12 May
Companion during labour:	Roger Brown
Preparation preferences:	enema no shave no
Preferred ways of coping with contractions:	Breathing, relaxation, keeping mobile, changing position as needed, massage if liked.
Pain-relieving drugs discussed:	Entonox if requested; would prefer 75 mg if pethidine requested; if epidural, to be timed to wear off for second stage.
Delivery:	Would like quiet room/dimmed light/to lift baby out herself. Baby straight on mother's body and extended skin contact. Father to cut cord after it stops pulsating.
Care of baby:	Completely by mother. Father to visit any time and help.
Feeding:	Breast, no formula to be given. Demand-feeding, including at night. No top-ups. No dextrose.
Postnatal plans:	Twelve-hour discharge if all well. Husband has time off work to help. Contact already made with community midwife.

Some birth alternatives

The following options will not all be available in every hospital or for every home birth, but when you ask questions you will probably discover that there are more available than you realized. Doctors and hospital administrators often say that they did not know their patients wanted certain things because they had not asked.

168

Here are some subjects which you may want to think about in advance and discuss.

Please do not assume that everything in one column is good and everything in the other bad. You can choose things from each column and mix as you wish.

The medical pattern	*The physiological pattern*
The place of birth: hospital consultant unit	The place of birth: home or hospital GP unit
Induction of labour	Spontaneous start to labour
Enema/suppositories	No bowel preparation
Shave	No shave
Amniotomy	Spontaneous rupture of membranes
Companion allowed except for certain procedures	Companion welcome throughout
Electronic fetal monitoring	Monitoring by the midwife
Nil by mouth	Eating and drinking or not as mother prefers
Intravenous drip	No intravenous drip
In bed in first stage	Up and about in first stage
Analgesia/anaesthesia e.g. pethidine, epidural	Breathing rhythms; focused concentration; relaxation; help from birth companion
Drugs/intervention ordered when doctor considers advisable	Any drips/interventions result of discussion and mother's own decision
Catheterization	Emptying own bladder
Timed second stage	Untimed second stage
Commanded pushing	Spontaneous pushing
Deliberate breath-holding	No deliberate breath-holding
Passive position	Upright position/position of choice
Episiotomy	Breathing the baby out – tear/intact perineum
Mother not touching – 'sterile field'	Mother touching the baby's head before and at delivery Mother lifting the baby out herself

169

The medical pattern – contd	The physiological pattern – contd
Conventional delivery of baby	Leboyer or Odent-style birth
Delayed contact with baby or separation from baby	Immediate skin contact with baby and extended time for both partners with baby after delivery
By-the-clock mothering	Baby with mother as long as and whenever she wishes
Bottle-feeding	Breast-feeding

Birth variations

Stimulated labour (i) If induction, prostaglandin pessary and/or intravenous oxytocin and/or amniotomy. (ii) If prostaglandin pessary, with immediate/delayed/no amniotomy; with/without intravenous oxytocin. (iii) If intravenous oxytocin in/out of bed; lying down/upright. Choices of pain-relieving drugs: type, dosage.

Epidural Any delays in getting one? Topped up by anaesthetist only/also by midwife. Aiming at anaesthesia for second stage/to wear off for second stage.

Electronic fetal monitoring Continuous/for 20 minutes or so on admission (strip monitoring); external/internal; mother in bed/out of bed/walking around (possible only with telemetry).

Caesarean birth Epidural or general anaesthesia; partner present or absent; baby touched/held immediately or not/by mother and/or father; baby kept with or separated from mother.

Forceps delivery/vacuum extraction Type of anaesthesia; delivery performed completely by obstetrician or mother lifting baby out after assistance.

Some hospitals are now beginning to adopt the concept of a Birth Plan agreed on by the obstetrician and the pregnant woman. One such hospital, the McMaster University Medical Centre in Hamilton, Ontario, has a well established system and each pregnant woman is given a copy of a document about patients' rights. In this hospital these rights are:

1. To be seen fully clothed before being examined.
2. To be seen on time or to be given an approximation of the waiting time.
3. To be treated respectfully and in privacy.
4. To have any tests explained to you before they are done.
5. To have the results of tests explained to you in language you understand.
6. To know the name and dosage of any medication, and also any side-effects.

7. During an examination to see what is happening if you wish.
8. To make your own decisions. Your doctor can only make recommendations. In cases of important decisions you have the right to seek a second opinion.
9. To read fully all consents – you should never sign under duress.
10. To change doctors if necessary, and have your information sent to your next doctor. In order to effect change, it may be helpful to tell your doctor why you are leaving.

In this hospital the patient plan, agreed on by the obstetrician and expectant mother during the pregnancy, is produced as soon as the woman goes into the hospital in labour and the nurse discusses with her how she would like her labour to be so that everybody in the team knows what is planned.

British midwives are now getting interested in full patient participation in decision-making and in working out together with the woman the agreed goals for care. Many are excited by new ideas of *active* birth and are keen to help women have the kind of birth experience they seek.

Postscript

There are choices open to us in the care that we give our bodies and the things we allow to be done to them by doctors and nurses. Decisions can be *shared* decisions, in which professionals give us information and a selection of alternatives in care, and then *we* make the choice.

Birth is intimately linked with a woman's feelings about and sense of her own body, her relations with others, her role as a woman, and the meaning of her personal identity. This is one reason why the way we bear our babies is so important.

Birth, like death, is a great universal experience. It can either be a disruption in the flow of human existence, a fragment which has little or nothing to do with the passionate longing which created the baby, or it can be lived with beauty and dignity and labour be itself a celebration of joy.

Section V

The Hospitals

The idea behind 'The New Good Birth Guide' Directory

When a woman is having a baby it is often very difficult to find out anything about the maternity hospitals in her area. Especially if it is her first baby, when she may not even know the questions to ask or, if she has recently moved to a different town, she may have only the vaguest idea of what lies behind those imposing doors, and this very uncertainty can lead to unnecessary worry in pregnancy.

Women need information so that they can choose between alternatives. After all, if women can use birth control effectively so that they plan how many children to have and *when* to have them, it seems reasonable for them to have some choice about *where* and *how* they have their babies.

One thing that can be done is to ask one's own doctor about possible hospitals, and it is a good idea to do this. But the matters which most interest the woman having a baby may not be things her general practitioner knows about. He or she is busy, and maternity care is just one aspect of the work he does, if he takes it on at all. (An increasing number of general practitioners do not, but send the woman straight off to the antenatal clinic at the hospital.)

The expectant mother can also ask to speak to one of the labour ward sisters, the supervising midwife, or the consultant, and can request an appointment when her partner can be there too. Or she can simply phone, with a carefully thought out list of questions beside the phone, and ask about hospital policy on the things that matter to her. Some women are concerned that they will be thought 'anxious' or even 'neurotic' if they do this. But it is a sensible way to find out.

The expectant mother can also ask round among other mothers at playgroups and seek information through friends, but this is pretty haphazard. Moreover, different women may want different things, and the kind of care that pleases one may be unsuitable for another.

If the expectant mother is interested in preparation for childbirth she can ask her antenatal teacher, but since women are usually booked into hospitals long before they start classes, what she learns about the hospital may come rather late in the day.

The idea behind this guide was to find out women's own experiences of large and small maternity units all over the country, to hear in their words what they appreciated, what they did not like, and how, if at all, they thought things could be improved, and to collect these together in such a way that expectant mothers could have *a basis on which to find out more.*

The Directory of Hospitals starting on page 193 can be useful even if your local hospital is not there. Some hospitals do not appear in these pages because too few women wrote about them. If you do not find your local hospital here it does *not* mean that it is too awful to be included but that I should welcome information on it. The thing to do is to look at what is happening in other hospitals close by, and then if you want to learn about your nearest hospital write to the senior nursing officer with questions you would like answered or ask if you can meet someone on the staff to have a talk together about the hospital. If the hospital has antenatal classes, the people who run them will usually give you information.

Things are changing rapidly in the Health Service. Do not take anything in these pages as 'gospel'. If you are keen to feed your baby on demand, for instance, and you read that your nearest hospital does not really approve of it, get in touch with somebody in a position of authority at the hospital and say you hope to feed this way and ask if you can be assured that it will be possible. Even if the system has not changed already, you may be the person who has the opportunity of changing it. This means being sure of what you would like, and being able to explain your reasons with clarity.

This is another point of the Directory – that women cannot know what they want until they know what is possible. An expectant mother may not realize that some hospitals are happy for mothers to give birth squatting, and for them to deliver off the delivery table or have special kinds of support behind them, so she does not know that this is a reasonable thing to ask for.

I hope that readers glancing through these pages will get an idea of the wide range of behaviour that is possible in labour and the variety of things hospital staff can do to make women more comfortable and to give them emotional support and guidance.

Midwives and doctors, too, often do not know what is being done in other hospitals. In an isolated maternity unit it might be considered rather weird for the mother to have her naked baby against her own naked body for an extended time after delivery, while the baby is still attached to the placenta, and staff may worry about the baby getting chilled. But this is being done in many hospitals. Mothers usually like it, and paediatricians approve of the way in which it helps the relationship of mother and baby from the very first moments. The problem of the baby getting cold is solved by having a heating lamp over mother and baby or throwing a blanket over them both.

I have had letters from midwives about the first edition of *The Good Birth Guide* (published in 1979) saying 'this will help us know what women want'. It is good to know that maternity staff are keen to give women in childbirth whatever will make them feel happiest within the limits of medical safety. It is easy when one is in a big hospital to feel that one is just part of a machine, and not to ask for things because everything seems to run so smoothly, on well-oiled wheels, that personal requests would interfere with the organization. It is clear from the letters I have received that many midwives are concerned to adapt to the wishes of each woman. When women know this, they may be less hesitant about asking for what they would like. So I do hope that hospital staff and administrations will find this Directory as interesting as mothers will.

There is difficulty in keeping up to date about hospitals. As with the *Good Food Guide*, staff will have changed, new things will be tried, so although this guide can give an idea of what a hospital was like when the women who write about their experiences had their babies it may well not be like that now. Odent-style births, for example, are being tried out in many different places, usually first by individual doctors and midwives who want to see what happens and who have a mother who especially wants to do it that way. Then perhaps everyone finds that they enjoy this kind of birth enormously and the idea catches on, and mothers are asked whether they would like the lights dimmed, what kind of music they would like on the cassette tape-recorder and encouraged to stand and deliver.

The constant change-over of staff means that it would be unwise and very unfair to write about individuals as if they were permanent parts of the system. On the other hand, the personality of each individual the woman meets during antenatal care, her labour and her postpartum stay must affect what she thinks about the hospital. There have been many reports of hospitals which obviously have a good system and forward-looking policies where the words or actions of one individual have spoiled things for the mother. I decided that it was probably best to overlook the latter, unless a number of mothers mentioned the same problem, when I have included the comment. These incidents may reflect a lack of interest by the management in the style of personal contact between staff and parents. On the other hand, when a mother has felt very positively about members of staff, or even one, I thought it would be a good idea to include it even if only because it makes *everyone* feel more positive.

How the Directory was written
Accounts came from women in response to radio and TV programmes, articles in magazines and newspapers and to my books about birth. A number of readers of the first edition of *The Good Birth Guide* filled in the form at the back of the book similar to the one on page 445. They often added further material.

Very few of the accounts that came were merely angry or destructive. A great many praised hospitals and members of staff. When women had criticisms to make it usually seemed that they were trying to be fair, and they often added, 'it was because they were so busy', or even suggested that it could not have been easy working in that particular hospital. Some women were so grateful to have a baby that they did not really analyse what had gone on in the hospital or ask if it could be improved in any way. It is all very well saying 'Fantastic!' but it does not tell much about the care given. I have put in the 'fantastics' and 'wonderfuls' and was glad to be able to add many details about these exceptional hospitals, but included even for these hospitals practices which some women questioned and procedures they felt were unnecessary.

Some happy letters were received about every hospital in this book. The writer often finished off with: 'I would go to X Hospital to have my next baby' or something like 'All in all, I am very satisfied with the care I received there.' They often had constructive criticisms to make too and even when they were delighted with one aspect of care suggested that improvements might be made in some other aspect. Their suggestions are also included.

A letter was sent to the senior nursing officer of each hospital asking about any changes in the last few years which might interest expectant mothers and for statistics relating to induction, acceleration of labour, forceps deliveries, Caesarean sections and episiotomies.

The replies from the senior nursing officers varied widely, ranging from curt refusals to give any information at all to very generous four or five pages of single-spaced A4. Occasionally the SNO handed the task over to a consultant obstetrician; one consultant said that since these were matters of a technical nature he did not wish them to be the subject of public comment, so was unwilling to let me have any information. Very often I was told that the requests I was asking about had never been made by their women patients. This occurred frequently with Leboyer-style deliveries, rooming-in of mother and baby during the postpartum stay including at night, and the father having an opportunity to cuddle, change and bath the baby himself. The replies usually went on to state that if such requests should be forthcoming in the future the hospital staff would be glad to make arrangements for these things to be done. Perhaps it is a bit like a shop; the assistant says, 'We don't have any demand for that, madam,' but if enough people ask, and go on asking politely, the management realizes that there *is* a demand after all and sees what it can do about it.

My impression is that women often do not ask for what they would like, and feel rather intimidated by the organization of the hospital, however kind and helpful the doctors and nurses. Or perhaps they ask, but they ask whoever happens to be on duty, who may be a junior or a student midwife or an auxiliary, and who may deal with the request in the way she thinks will make least fuss. It is important to discuss the things that matter most to you with a consultant or registrar or with the senior nursing officer or the sister, people who are able to take responsibility for allowing changes.

As a general rule only those hospitals are included about which I have received information from at least twenty-four women, except in the case of GP units, for which I used twelve accounts as the baseline for inclusion, and a scattering of the larger hospitals about which I received very detailed reports, but from not more than twenty women.

Where no information has been received from hospitals about their policies the entry is marked MO – mothers only. Where I had insufficient accounts from mothers about any particular hospital but had an official letter from the hospital about its policies I have marked it HO – hospital only.

Where material is most likely to be out of date I have inserted the date the information was received, e.g. (1979).

Readers should understand that the information is not based on a statistical sample of mothers and that the women most likely to write in about their experience are probably those who either had a very good one or a very bad one. Though this makes for lively material, your own experience of the same place might be somewhere in between!

Medical details are included only where they relate to *choices* and to *emotional* aspects of birth. There was some borderline material as, for example, when a baby contacted an eye infection from wearing goggles under phototherapy which had been worn by other babies, which I trusted would be by now outdated since the hospital staff would have been alerted to this problem. So this kind of thing is not included.

I have included specific instances of failures in communication and very happy or unhappy experiences only when there was sufficient corroboration from other women's reports of the same hospital to conclude that this woman's experience was not unique.

Any hospital is bound to have changed since the material was written up. When I did the first edition of this book I was concerned that it would become outdated very soon. This has not been the case. Though in some well-defined areas, such as infant feeding, there have been radical changes, some hospitals are slow to modify practices or to try out new ideas coming from mothers till they have been through half a dozen committees! Nevertheless, the best way to use this book is as a basis for discovering more.

It is important not to read only the entries for hospitals in your own area. If you do this you will get no idea of the range of possibilities and what is done in other hospitals.

I have omitted the phrase 'breast-feeding encouraged' from this new edition of the *Good Birth Guide* because it is now official policy to encourage all mothers to breast-feed and staff are encouraging it in just about every hospital. I have concentrated attention instead on how skilled staff on postnatal wards are at giving help.

The suggestions at the end of each entry are those made by writers themselves about that particular hospital. Where no suggestions are included, writers had not responded to the request to make constructive suggestions for change.

In the first edition of the *Guide* every phrase that added any information from SNOs was included with meticulous care. In the present edition so much information has come from some hospitals that exigencies of space have forced me to sift the material and I have often omitted data about buildings and numbers of beds, for example, in favour of information which suggests more about the atmosphere and human relations in a hospital.

The reader may be surprised that some hospitals which sound rather good do not have a star. I must admit that I have not felt able to quote all the things writers described and there were some instances of unsympathetic care and even, occasionally, of callousness which might alarm readers without achieving any positive results. It may be that such things happened to only one woman in any hospital, but the fact that they *could* happen meant that I felt one had to reserve judgement about that particular hospital, and certainly not give it unqualified praise.

Some hospitals sent me sheafs of grateful letters from satisfied parents. Though I realize they would be unlikely to send letters from those who were less satisfied with the care they received, I have, wherever possible, incorporated the positive comments made by these couples into the material on the hospital. Both consultants and senior nursing officers at some other hospitals, however, in particular those which had stars in the last edition, have told me that unless I am frank about criticism, staff tend to get smug about being in a good hospital and changes for the better are delayed. If this is really the case I hope that SNOs in these hospitals will start sending me letters from dissatisfied parents.

Different kinds of hospitals

Regional hospitals are those which serve a large area, and in some cases women must travel forty miles or more to attend them. In these hospitals patients are under the care of consultants. A woman may never see the consultant with whom she is booked, but may see senior registrars, junior registrars and housemen.

Teaching hospitals are associated with universities and here again women are under the care of consultants, but may not see them. A good deal of research goes on in teaching hospitals, and medical students may also observe and care for women under supervision. A woman has the right to ask not to be observed or attended by medical students if she wishes.

General practitioner hospitals are for straightforward obstetrics, and are not intended for women classified as 'high risk'. Women often like the friendly informality of a GP unit. If the doctor thinks it is all right to have your baby in a GP unit, you might also consider birth at home if that is what you would really like.

Both regional and teaching hospitals often have general practitioner units attached. GP units also exist which are not an integral part of the big hospital, and some are simple cottage hospitals. In GP units the woman is cared for by a community midwife and general practitioner, although the GP may not be present for the birth. In those GP units which are part of larger hospitals specialized care can be obtained quickly should labour not be straightforward. In distant GP units women may have to be moved in an ambulance during labour to a consultant unit if labour is complicated.

Catchment areas
Can I have a baby in another area and yet get National Health Service care? Yes, you can.

The concept of 'catchment' areas is based on administrative convenience, as it is obviously simpler for hospitals to accept patients mainly from the immediately surrounding district. This is why a GP tends to send the majority of all his or her patients to one hospital. But there are no rules about this, and the Department of Health and Social Security say that flexibility and choice are an important part of the system.

'There is,' the Department states, 'no *statutory* basis for catchment areas.' That is, it is not a matter of law. General practitioners in the country sometimes decide to refer a patient to a consultant who is known to be very good at dealing with a particular kind of case and who is in London; so referrals outside regions, as well as outside smaller areas, are common. If the general practitioner can do this, the woman is also free to choose to move to a hospital in another town, provided, of course, that the consultant will accept her under his care. Sometimes consultants have more patients than they can cope with and do not want to take on anyone

Continued on p. 186

The Hospitals

A statistical comparison of some teaching hospitals (all have a large percentage of high-risk patients) in percentages

	Induced	Accelerated with oxytocin	Epidural	Electronic monitoring
Liverpool	22	—	—	—
Queen Charlotte's London	19 (most with prostaglandin)	—	73 primiparae 46 multiparae (50% Caesareans with epidurals)	—
London Hospital, Mile End	12	8	—	—
Greenwich	(22) but may not all have syntocin 13 (incl. 3% prostaglandin)	5	—	—
St Mary's, Paddington	9	—	26	—
Hammersmith	(20–27) 18 (with ARM)	—	—	—
UCH London	20	20	29	—
John Radcliffe, Oxford, consultant and GP units	25 (60% of which prostaglandin only)	19	28	—

A statistical comparison of district hospitals in percentages

	Induced	Accelerated with oxytocin	Epidural	Electronic monitoring
N. Devon, Barnstaple	—	—	33 approx.	
Pilgrim, Boston, Lincs.	14	30	—	—
Royal Victoria, Bournemouth	—	—	—	—
Southmead, Bristol	14	—	—	—
Burton-upon-Trent, Staffs.	23	—	—	—
Fairfield, Bury, Lancs.	—	—	—	—
Cheltenham	—	—	—	—
Royal W, Sussex, Chichester	20	23	—	—

Episiotomy	Vacuum	Forceps	Caesarean	Breast-feeding on discharge
45 (25 with normal delivery)	—	20	15	—
—		26*	13	—
25	—	7	10	—
35	3	13	15	—
70 primiparae 40 multiparae	—	15	13 (3 elective, 10 in labour)	—
42	—	15	13	—
—		18*	—	—
48	—	17	10 (5 elective, 5 in labour)	—

* Vacuum and forceps together.

Episiotomy	Vacuum	Forceps	Caesarean	Breast-feeding on discharge
—	—	—	—	80 approx.
—	1	10	10	58 52 at 10th day 47 at 28th day
—	—	10	6	—
—	—	10*		—
—	—	10	6	—
—	—	25*		—
30	—	—	—	75 approx.
47	—	6	7	—

A statistical comparison of district hospitals in percentages – contd

	Induced	Accelerated with oxytocin	Epidural	Electronic monitoring
Coventry	12	—	—	—
Enfield District	(25–30) 29	—	—	—
Royal Devon, Exeter	23	—	—	—
Northgate, Great Yarmouth	—	—	—	—
N. Herts, Hitchin	10	10	—	—
Royal Lancaster	—	—	—	—
Newham, Forest Lane, London	7	2	12	—
British Hosp. for Mothers and Babies, Woolwich, London	30	—	—	—
Luton and Dunstable	—	—	—	—
Northampton including GP unit and home births	18	—	20	65
Poole General	—	—	—	—
Freedom Fields, Plymouth	18 surgical, 33 ARM in labour	—	13	—
Odstock, Salisbury	20 (75%+ with prostaglandin)	—	20	
Northern General, Sheffield	20 approx.	—	—	—
Copthorne, Shrewsbury	(33) 20	—	—	
Queen Mary's, Sidcup, Kent	20	—	6	—
Princess Margaret, Swindon	20	—	—	—
Musgrove Park, Taunton	(30) 16 (60% primiparae, 10% multiparae)	—	—	
Manygates, Wakefield	—	—	—	—
Schrodell's, Watford	(over 55)	—	75	—
Queen Elizabeth, Welwyn	—	—	—	—

Episiotomy	Vacuum	Forceps	Caesarean	Breast-feeding on discharge
2	—	13	9	—
48	—	14	13	—
—	—	16	13	—
—	—	28*		—
—	2	15	10	—
—	1 approx.	8	14	—
1	—	10	7	85
—	—	10	10	—
—	—	9	7	—
—	—	10	12	—
—	—	15	6	—
—	—	14	9	—
—	—	—	—	—
—	—	—	—	—
3 approx.	10	11	9	—
4	—	18	7	90
—	—	—	—	—
—	—	10	15	—
—	—	8	7	—
primigravidae multigravidae	—	—	—	65
—	—	—	—	65

A statistical comparison of district hospitals in percentages – contd

	Induced	Accelerated with oxytocin	Epidural	Electronic monitoring
WALES AND SCOTLAND				
Glyn Garfield, Glamorgan	18	—	—	—
Eastern General, Edinburgh	22	—	15	—
Western General, Edinburgh	22	—	—	—
Glasgow Royal	35–8	14	44	—
Paisley	(30) 30	—	—	—

Continued from p. 181

new; and it is understandable that they must retain the right to say that, in certain circumstances, they have to give priority to women within the hospital's catchment area.

In the past, when there was heavy pressure on maternity beds, with too many women seeking places in hospitals, this may have happened quite often, but now, with the drop in births, few hospitals are under this kind of pressure.

The thing to do if you want to have your baby in a particular hospital or with a particular consultant is to talk to your general practitioner, and he or she will then write to the doctor concerned. A word of warning here though: it is not a good idea to move a long distance if it means you have to stay (before the birth) in a hotel or boarding-house, or with friends or relatives you do not really get on with, or if you have to travel a long way wondering whether you are going to deliver on the roadside.

Episiotomy	Vacuum	Forceps	Caesarean	Breast-feeding on discharge
—	—	11	11	—
—	—	14	13	—
72	—	14	13	—
—	—	—	25	15
—	—	—	—	43

Forceps and Caesarean together.

1. Scotland

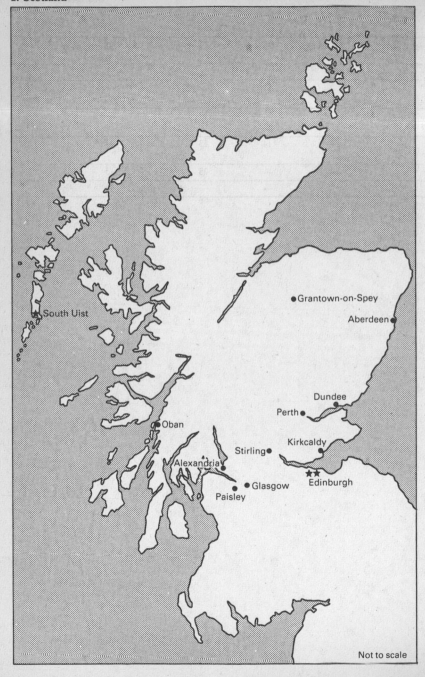

- Grantown-on-Spey
- Aberdeen
- South Uist
- Dundee
- Perth
- Oban
- Kirkcaldy
- Stirling
- Alexandria
- Edinburgh
- Paisley
- Glasgow

Not to scale

2. North-West England and North Wales

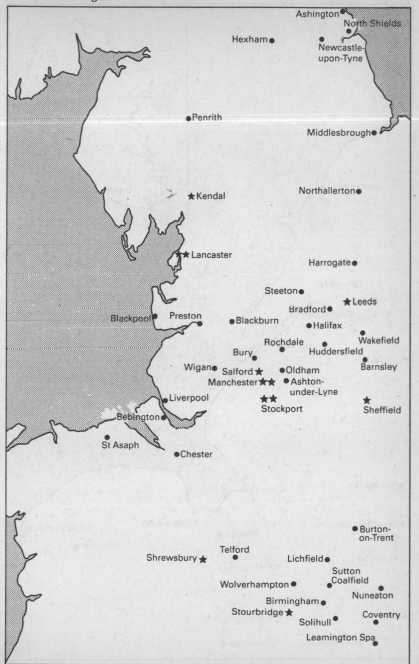

Ashington

North Shields

Hexham

Newcastle-upon-Tyne

Penrith

Middlesbrough

Northallerton

★ Kendal

★ Lancaster

Harrogate

Steeton

Bradford ★ Leeds

Blackpool Preston Blackburn Halifax

Rochdale Wakefield

Bury Huddersfield

Wigan Oldham Barnsley

Salford ★

Manchester ★★ Ashton-under-Lyne

Liverpool ★★ Sheffield

Stockport

Bebington

St Asaph

Chester

Burton-on-Trent

Shrewsbury ★ Telford Lichfield

Sutton Coalfield

Wolverhampton Nuneaton

Birmingham

Stourbridge ★ Coventry

Solihull

Leamington Spa

3. Eastern England

Ireland (inset)

Drogheda ●

● Galway   Dublin ●

Cork ●

Not to scale

Scarborough ●

Beverley ●

Hull ●

Grimsby ●

● Doncaster

● Nottingham

● Loughborough

● Leicester

● Rugby

● Northampton

Wisbech ●

● King's Lynn

Great Yarmouth ●

Norwich ★★

● Peterborough

★★ Huntingdon

Cambridge ●

4. West of England and South Wales

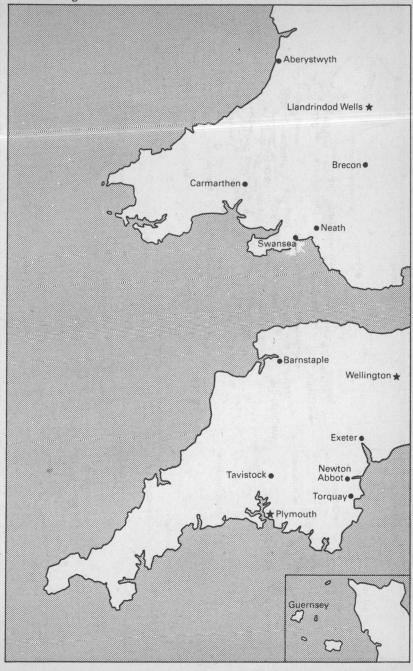

5. South of England

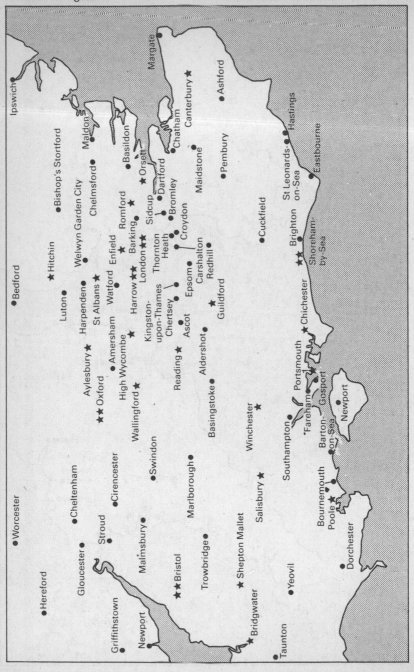

Ipswich

Margate

Canterbury ★

Ashford

Maldon

Hastings

Bishop's Stortford

Basildon

Chatham

Eastbourne

St Leonards-on-Sea

Orsett

Chelmsford

Dartford

Maidstone

Welwyn Garden City

Sidcup

Bromley

Pembury

Hitchin

Romford

Croydon

Enfield

Barking

London ★★

Thornton Heath

Cuckfield

Bedford

Watford

Harrow

Brighton

Shoreham-by-Sea

Luton

St Albans

Kingston-upon-Thames

Carshalton

Redhill

Harpenden

Epsom

Amersham

Chertsey

Guildford

Aylesbury ★

High Wycombe

Ascot

Aldershot

Chichester ★

Oxford ★★

Wallingford ★

Reading

Basingstoke

Portsmouth

Gosport

Fareham

Newport

Winchester ★

Swindon

Southampton

Barton-on-Sea

Worcester

Cheltenham

Cirencester

Marlborough

Salisbury ★

Stroud

Malmsbury

Bournemouth

Poole ★

Gloucester

Bristol ★★

Trowbridge

Shepton Mallet ★

Dorchester

Hereford

Yeovil

Newport

Bridgwater ★

Griffithstown

Taunton

The Directory of Hospitals

Northern Ireland
Information which has come in about Northern Ireland has been scanty – not
enough, unfortunately, to be able to include details of hospitals. I should be
very glad to receive more reports about maternity units there.

England

Louise Margaret, Aldershot, Hants   MO

Old building. Well staffed. Well equipped.

Antenatal Long waits, up to an hour. Doctors take time to talk. A lot of
queuing. Scans often done. Helpful nurses. All questions answered honestly
and in full. 'Nothing was too much trouble' . . . 'I never felt rushed'.

Labour Shave/enema. Electronic fetal monitoring used. Woman is free to have
pain-killers or not as she wishes. Partner allowed in but may be asked to leave
for internal examinations and stitching. Episiotomies not routinely done.

Postnatal Baby is with mother from second day. Nurses helpful with feeding.
'The physio makes you do all the exercises. It is like being at school.' Talks on
health care, teeth care, baby bathing, making up feeds, nappies. 'Far too hot.'

Suggestions Reorganization of antenatal care. Turn heating down.

**Maternity Unit, Amersham General Hospital,
Amersham, Bucks**   MO

Old building. GP unit. Own midwife from GP practice cares for woman in
labour. Complications require flying squad from Wycombe.

Antenatal Busy clinic. Usually long wait, 'never less than an hour'. No drinks
available. Staff 'always friendly', 'greet you warmly', some 'imprinted with
old, rigid schemes and less likely to chat in relaxed, equal way'.

Postnatal Two large postnatal wards. 'Peaceful.' Many women transferred
here at 1–2 days from Wycombe. Seem to be 'more staff than patients', under-
occupied. 'Very sweet nurses.' Have room down corridor and 'you have to
seek them out'. Day staff helpful but tend to treat you as a 'patient' rather
than a person. Night staff sometimes 'aggressive', 'do not smile', 'talk more
about you than discuss things with you'. Silly rules: not to change baby in
ward 'which entailed trundling baby in cot to nursery', 'very wearying
process'. Felt 'taken over by the system' here. 'Found myself worrying
whether I was doing the right thing.' No rooming-in. 'Felt tremendous
pressure to give baby a bottle and when I said definitely no, a tin of Wysol
(non-allergic) milk was produced and waved at me while I breast-fed.'
   Women advise early discharge to go home and do your own thing.

Suggestions Rooming-in. Dispense with minor rules and be more flexible. Stop
topping up and develop up-to-date relaxed attitudes to breast-feeding.

194

Heatherwood, Ascot, Bucks MO

Antenatal Clinic overcrowded, long waits, queues at reception with urine samples, but ample space and seating in waiting-rooms and refreshments usually available in out-patients if not in maternity wing. Doctors and nurses 'sympathetic', 'cheerful', 'thorough'. Opportunity to see round labour suite and postnatal wards – ask sister. Toys for children. Some writers said communication with GP doing shared care was not good.

Antenatal classes – rooms too hot, seating uncomfortable, women with other children say times clash with times for fetching children from school. No facilities for toddlers.

Labour No shave/enema. 'Shower not properly cleaned after last occupant.' Husband may be sent to waiting room during admission procedures but 'well-sited kitchen for sustenance of dads during labour' and they are offered coffee. Doctor's wife comments, 'Though there was a generally accepted framework of procedures, it was constantly adapted to my needs as an individual, and time was taken to find out what they were.' Fetal heart monitors used: 'They explained when they strapped it on that the baby's heart beat might disappear if the baby moved so I shouldn't worry if that happened.' In early labour 'when they found that everything was going steadily, a sister took the strap off' and encouraged women to move around. One woman for whom pethidine was suggested to bring down blood pressure said she was very affected by pain-killers and did not want to be drowsy, was asked if she would have ½ mg of Omnipon instead: 'I felt it was *my* labour and they were there to help.' Some women have delivered in standing and squatting positions. Doctors described as 'kind' and 'are making a conscious effort to communicate'. Mothers say 'baby is popped on tummy' while stitched, then checked. Then given to father: 'A huge pot of tea and we were left with the baby for ¾ hour . . . he was able to cuddle and I to suckle at leisure.' Birth chair available.

Postnatal Ward 'lovely', 'new and shining'. Very hot. Baby goes to nursery first night, rooms in by day. After first two nights all breast-feeding mothers have to go to nursery to feed 'with bright lights on, screaming babies and a queue for chairs . . . not pleasant!'; 'I was nagged to give the baby complements of SMA because she was not gaining enough and she was test-weighed once,' writes mother with family history of allergies. Several writers described 'standard practice' in 1980 of giving SMA to all babies, whether breast- or bottle-fed first couple of nights, but mothers who put notice on cot such as 'Mother willing to breast-feed any time', 'NO SMA', found that request was willingly complied with. Nursing shifts have different ideas about breast-feeding. One shift believes 'on demand' means every 3 hours and not more than every 2 hours. Writers describe sucking strictly limited to 2 minutes a side first day, 5 minutes second, 7 minutes third, 10 minutes fourth: 'They are fierce about sucking time.' Mothers have to fill in chart about length of sucking: 'I used to say I had given her lots of little sucks and not own up to 15 minutes each side'; 'We had to fill in input/output chart every time we changed a nappy.' Truthful mothers get 'rebukes' from nurses 'for feeding too often or too long'. Antiseptic spray given out to all breast-feeding mothers. Glucose and water handed out at every feed but 'as long as babies are not jaundiced and don't cry no pressure to give it to them'. Nurses helpful and very kind: 'Nurse spent 1½ hours kneeling on floor helping me hold her on breast and encouraging me'; 'Every feed that day a nurse sat with me and helped.' Fathers very involved in caring for baby, though some mothers wished they were given more help to understand what to do. Lack of privacy, and writers said cases were discussed, also family planning methods and sterilization operations, in front of other people. One woman was operated on for haemorrhoids and repair of episiotomy under local anaesthetic on ward during visiting hours. Sleeping pills 'not pushed'. Flexible, friendly atmosphere.

Food good for institution but 'sparse'; brought in hot cupboard by 'two extremely friendly Scots girls'. Mother who is caterer advises: 'Think before you choose dish which might be favourite at home, but spoiled if cooked in vast quantities or too long at wrong temperature.' Shepherd's pie cooked beautifully. Visitors offered cups of tea. One woman 'skulking round a corner with husband and glass of champagne' was amazed to be wished 'Cheers!' by passing nurse.

Of 106 women in one month of 1980, 74 had normal deliveries, 20 forceps, 12 Caesarean births, 60 had pethidine, 59 gas and oxygen, 28 epidurals (including 15 forceps and 3 Caesarean).

Suggestions Reorganize so that woman in labour sees at least one midwife she met in antenatal clinic. Help nurses help breast-feeding mothers so that advice does not change with every shift. More to eat for breast-feeding mothers. Reduce length of general visiting but keep long visiting for fathers.

William Harvey, Ashford, Kent   M O

Large, new unit outside Ashford. Light spacious building with bright colours, 'route march' from main entrance to maternity section. Friendly atmosphere.

Antenatal 'Usually I didn't even have time to sit down'; 'longest wait was 15 minutes'. Women say they were treated as individuals. Usually saw same doctor. Doctors and nurses helpful. Plenty of opportunity to ask questions but voices have to be kept low as conversations heard in adjoining cubicle. Big playpen full of toys. Routine scans.

Antenatal ward efficiently run. Helpful staff. Extremely clean. Appetizing meals and drinks but day room full of smoking women. Toilet and bathroom facilities good. Some writers said doctors' opinions and advice differed and was confusing.

Labour Delivery rooms with bright curtains. Wedge-shaped bolsters and about three pillows provided. Staff 'friendly', 'efficient', discussed progress with women. Consent asked before administering pethidine but may be advised to have epidural. Midwives like women to deliver without episiotomy/stirrups/forceps, but when doctor takes over, midwifery-style birth is replaced by obstetric delivery. Father encouraged to be present. One man who looked at monitor to tell wife when contraction was coming was reprimanded by midwife and told equipment was for staff use only: 'A little knowledge is dangerous.'

Postnatal Views over grassed hospital grounds to open countryside beyond. Friendly, relaxed atmosphere. Baby can stay with mother at night, but this disturbs other mothers. Is usually in nursery first night. Breast-fed baby brought to mother for feeding at night. Helpful nurses, patient with breast-feeding difficulties. Dextrose administered liberally according to some writers. Inadequate bathing and toilet facilities. Physiotherapy class helpful. Ultrasound used for perineal pain. No phone in ward and women have to go to antenatal ward and have long wait.

Food good. Menus provided previous day. Plenty of variety and choice of size of portions.

Long visiting hours.

Can arrange 6-hour discharge.

Suggestions Postnatal wards less 'busy' to give chance to rest. Reduce length of general visiting but keep long visiting for fathers.

Ashington General, Westview, Ashington, Northumberland

Antenatal 'I felt I was a person, not just a pregnant woman.' 'Relaxed and informative mothercraft classes.' Scanning available. Can look round hospital at 28 weeks. Doctors say they prefer not to induce, but when induction is done prostaglandin pessaries are used prior to intravenous drip.

Labour Fathers encouraged and are informed about everything: 'They told my husband to time my contractions.' Electronic monitoring available but not used routinely. Pethidine offered. Woman may be encouraged to push with feet on midwives' hips. Episiotomy not done routinely.

Postnatal Staff friendly and helpful: 'Always someone on hand if I needed help or reassurance.' Baby is with mother except when she prefers nursery: 'I felt that the baby was mine from the beginning.' Baby given glucose solution first night, but otherwise mothers woken to breast-feed.

Meals 'very good', 'hot', 'kept back for you if you were feeding'.

Suggestions Babies not given glucose solution first night but put to breast.

Maternity Unit, Tameside General, Ashton-under-Lyne, Lancs   MO

Modern, well-equipped, efficient; also GP unit 'Not very different from consultant unit' and excellent midwives unit, underused, 'home from home'.

Antenatal Outer waiting-room 'smoke-filled'. Women say they see different doctors each time. Staff 'pleasant', 'willing to answer questions but you have to ask them'. 'No advice on breast-feeding,' said one mother, who expressed worries. Long waits, up to 3 hours sometimes, conveyor-belt feeling. Older children welcomed. Staff explain to children what they are doing. Opportunity to see wards, labour and delivery rooms and SCBU in advance. Writers say fewer inductions done now than previously, but many had labour accelerated. One woman whose baby was due 20 December says she was told by doctor 'Induction done routinely 10 days past EDD.' He was undecided whether to book her for clinic on 27th or induction; prostaglandins used for softening cervix overnight before induction and may be sufficient without drip.

Labour Partial shave/enema. Partner asked to leave for this but can stay if you ask. Partner can be present for forceps delivery and stitching. Women say they were encouraged to stay at home until they felt they needed to be in hospital. Plenty of pillows available in first-stage rooms, not enough in second stage. Upright position advised for first stage. Most women who wrote had had pethidine, which seems to have been given in rather high doses. Several writers felt it very important to have labour companion with you. One woman described how she was taken to labour room 'and left with gas and air machine' feeling 'completely drunk' from pethidine: 'The feeling of isolation was awful.' Doctors seemed to have active, interventionist role, taking over tasks done by midwives in other units, e.g. one writer said she was not given VE when admitted at 7.30 a.m. but told duty doctor would perform this on his rounds at 9 a.m. Writers also describe some disagreement between doctors and midwives over augmentation of labour with oxytocin: 'Sister objected, said contractions were strong and regular.' 'Spartan' delivery room 'all white, bright, quiet'. Baby can be delivered up on to mother's abdomen and put to breast immediately after cord cut, but she may have to ask. One writer says she was only offered 'quick look' before baby was cleaned up. 'Sister asked my husband if he had taken all photos he wanted before she cut cord.' Midwife helps put baby to breast. It may not be suggested that father holds baby but he can go ahead and do so. Baby is wheeled to ward with mother.

Postnatal Baby is beside bed except on first night when goes to nursery. Paediatrician 'explains everything' during examination of baby. Breast-feeding now on demand and can breast-feed during visiting times. May be offered dextrose and topping-up bottles but 'nobody argues with a firm, well-informed, sensible mother'. Some nurses insist on giving artificial milk first 2 nights and on rigid 3–4 hour feeding, 'but after 2 days I fed 2½ hourly and nothing was said'. 'Staff don't have to know what time you fed.' Wards modern, babies in see-through cots nicknamed 'goldfish bowls'. Fathers allowed to handle baby only after asking permission, washing hands and donning gown, though in fact staff may not be around you during visiting time and fathers touch babies then, but may get 'caught': 'Staff are almost neurotic about anyone picking up babies.' Help freely given with breast-feeding 'though quality depended on how vocal one could be with sister', and mothers praise care of babies though some feel that they did not get good enough care themselves: 'Only the baby is mothered'; 'often we had to go looking for staff if we had a problem'. Cheery atmosphere and help given freely with breast-feeding. 'Most staff acted as if you were their friend and were jovial and helpful', but staff shortages produced problems. Sleeping pills and pain-killers given routinely. No rubber rings for perineal pain. Showers and baths good, bidets 'heavenly'. 1–2 p.m. rest period. One major disadvantage: clattering tea-trolley which wakes everybody at 4.45 regardless, 'even if you have just finished a feed'. Bed has to be vacated while being made. One woman said day of discharge was 'luxurious' as bed not re-made till after she left. Breakfast not served till 8 a.m.

Visiting 3–4 p.m. Saturday and Sunday, 7–8 p.m. every night, but sibling visiting at weekends only for 1 hour, with advance permission from sister; otherwise mother has to be wheeled in bed to day room, baby is removed and women said they were made to feel 'an awful nuisance'. 'Someone special' visiting outside usual hours not refused; ask sister.

Food 'all pappy', 'suitable for psycho-geriatric ward and not enough of it'.

SCBU Both parents encouraged to visit baby at all times. Mother helped to express breast milk and then breast-feed. 'A nurse had to accompany mothers to SCBU – never too much trouble.'

Suggestions Less emphasis on induction and also on pethidine in labour. Father should never have to wait outside while woman examined or put on monitor. Improved communication between nursing staff about breast-feeding policy so that confusing and contradictory advice not given. Improved postnatal caring for mothers. Stop waking them before 5 a.m. When problems with baby keep mother better informed. Nursing auxiliaries should be taught about bonding, demand-feeding and rooming-in. Provide extended visiting for fathers. Children should be allowed to visit every day.

Royal Buckinghamshire, Buckingham Road, Aylesbury, Bucks

Old building. Modern GP unit on second floor. Cheerful, relaxed atmosphere; clean; friendly staff. Special care unit serves Milton Keynes hospital. Mothers allowed in SCBU any time.

Antenatal 'Dreary' 1930s clinic next to hospital also houses physiotherapy: 'very impersonal'; 'fleeting'; 'several women have appointment at same time'. 'Old men shuffle by while you sit with your specimen bottle.' Nurses and doctors 'gentle', 'reassuring'; 'The more you are interested in yourself and your baby the more they will be.' Enjoyable antenatal classes cover every aspect of baby care. Many writers had induced labours; one woman simply told 'in the baby's interest'.

Labour Shave/enema. Partner allowed throughout labour. Pethidine offered but 'not pushed'. Electronic monitoring used selectively. Plenty of supporting

199

pillows. Woman who asked for Leboyer delivery told not possible but baby given to mother cord still attached. Can be put to breast after weighing. Father can go to nursery and spend time with baby.

Postnatal Chintzy, comfortable wards. Baby in nursery at night but with mother all day. Loving care of nursery nurses remarked on: 'Very patient with breast-feeding mothers'; 'When they said "I'll be back in 2 minutes" they always were.' Mother free to cuddle her baby whenever she wants. But 'auxiliary nurses would not let me go to my screaming baby at night. Said he would "Get spoiled"'; handled babies 'roughly'.

Food criticized: 'baked beans, overcooked, stodgy vegetables . . . then the nurse gives you a laxative', though some writers enjoyed food. One writer said there was one bath between twelve women. Writers liked bidets.

Visiting 2 hours in afternoon, 2 hours in evening; only father allowed to hold baby and must wear apron.

★ *GP unit* Women who had babies in GP unit had antenatal care from GP, with only about two visits to hospital. In labour own midwife takes one into unit. Woman is in room of her own, 'comfortable, relaxed environment'. Can walk about and labour without drugs of any sort: 'I only got on to the delivery table at the onset of the second stage'; Can have Leboyer-style delivery: 'very enjoyable and very peaceful'. Own midwife visits daily for postnatal care. Women can breast-feed at night and demand-feed, and baby can be in bed with mother when she wishes. Mothers say they are free to do what they want when they want.

Suggestions A separate room for feeding baby while ward being cleaned so that smoky visitors' room does not have to be used. Mothers should not be persuaded to give their babies milk complements.

Maternity Unit, Upney Lane, Barking, Essex

Pleasant atmosphere on ante- and postnatal wards. Staff friendly, helpful. Small garden where women sit in warm weather.

Antenatal Long waiting at first visit (3 hours) and last four visits; middle months can be in and out in 45 minutes. Staff 'rushed'. See different doctors each time; mostly pleasant and willing to explain things; after examination can sit down and talk; women who had glucose tolerance tests and scans said these were fully explained by doctor. NCT counsellors in clinic speak to women about breast-feeding as wait for scan. One woman suggests they need more time.

Labour A woman who was induced said 'Little consideration was given to my feelings.' Attempts at induction failed in the morning and everyone went away: 'I was left alone and not told anything till evening, when prostaglandin tablets given to soften cervix. Thus I was in a highly nervous state at the onset of labour.' She was 'moved to very dark side room alone, husband not called'.

Few night staff available, came in occasionally: 'I felt desolate.' Writers describe being given pethidine in high doses. Delusions reported by one. A woman in labour during the night says her husband was not called till 6 a.m. Partner may be sent out before delivery of placenta. (Why?) Is then allowed back and holds baby.

Postnatal 'Sister, nurses and student midwives all came to say congratulations.' Nurse helps put baby to breast. Baby stays with mother all day, can be with her or go to nursery first night, is then with mother all the time. Conflicting advice from day and night staff. Latter 'not very supportive as overworked'. On one ward at least inadequate help with breast-feeding; 'Sister who helps with breast-feeding worked mainly on other two wards' (1980). Nursery nurses and student midwives 'kind' and 'sympathetic'; 'helped keep a sense of humour and see things in proportion'.

Strict visiting rules enforced and afternoon visiting only Wednesdays and weekends.

SCBU Paediatricians and nurses 'kind', 'helpful'.

Suggestions Waiting times in antenatal clinic reduced *or* obstetricians give explanation for delays. Cooler postnatal wards. Extend visiting and make it more flexible.

Barnsley General, Barnsley, S Yorks MO

Antenatal Some doctors described as 'distant', 'silent'. Writers advise saying what you want: 'The system is not as immovable as it looks at first.' 'Patients more punctual than doctors and too many appointments are made for same time.' Women encouraged to ask questions. 'Something needs doing about junior doctors, often from different cultures, who have little or no knowledge of a woman's emotional needs in pregnancy.' Writers say they did not always have opportunity to discuss worries or get information, though those who attended parentcraft classes said they were encouraged to ask questions.

Labour 'It would have been nice to meet midwives working on the delivery side beforehand rather than be confronted by complete strangers when arriving in labour.' Most writers had had an oxytocin drip and augmented labours.

Postnatal Several writers felt they had insufficient support with breast-feeding.

Suggestions Domino scheme put in operation for mothers in area around Barnsley. More continuity of care. More skilled support with breast-feeding.

North Devon District, Raleigh Park, Barnstaple, N Devon   HO

Modern unit. Serves whole North Devon. 'Very warm and friendly.'

Antenatal Three obstetricians hold booking clinic each and follow-up clinic every week. Clinic staffed by midwives who are available to give advice.. Women interviewed and examined in single soundproof rooms. Appointment system works well most of the time although delays can occur if consultants are called away. Ultrasound scans performed, but there is 'no pressure to have any test'. Care shared with community midwives and GPs. Toys to amuse small children. Hospital tour and 'everything explained'.

Labour Delivery suite has sitting-room with TV. Partner is encouraged to stay with women in labour and during delivery. Women are free to move around in labour. A good epidural service is available and approximately a third have an epidural. Some writers say it is assumed they will need drugs for pain-relief. Each mother is under care of one particular midwife. Some women who live in Barnstaple or Bideford are cared for by their own GP. Fetal heart monitor is used on selected, 'high-risk' patients but not as routine. Baby is given straight away to mother to hold.

Postnatal 'Very pleasant'. Combined antenatal/postnatal wards – with views over green lawns. Babies stay by mothers by day and breast-feeding on demand is encouraged. At night babies sleep in small nurseries and mothers who wish are called to feed them. The breast-feeding rate has increased and is now over 80 per cent. Women who have been in wards before delivery are returned to same floor to ensure continuity of care. On average mothers are discharged home 2–7 days after delivery. SNO says, 'Many ask to stay in longer than they really need, for a rest!'

SCBU One in ten babies in special care. Mothers have choice of staying in and helping with care of babies or going home and visiting frequently. In all cases mothers encouraged to supply breast milk which can, if necessary, be pasteurized and stored for future use. Fathers, grandparents and siblings have free visiting.

Barton Hospital, Grove Road, Barton-on-Sea, New Milton, Hants   HO

Small GP unit threatened with closure but temporarily reprieved. Twenty-two miles from consultant unit at Southampton, ten miles from consultant unit at Boscombe.

Sister in charge writes: 'In holiday periods roads in either direction are very congested making journey to large hospitals slow and frightening experience for woman in labour. We based our case to remain open on right of women to have freedom of choice where they wish to have their babies, emotional difference to mother and her family in having her baby in small unit with relaxed atmosphere and individual care, and very real postnatal benefits we can offer to mother and baby and their whole family.'

Antenatal Sister in charge writes that at the moment midwives do not play any part in antenatal care but this is something they hope to remedy in near future, and that they are firm believers in value of antenatal care being carried out by midwives.

Labour Mothers are cared for by their own GPs and midwives. Normal deliveries only. There is no monitoring equipment and they do not use intravenous syntocinon. Sister in charge writes that they rely on clinical skills of experienced midwives and GPs are not necessarily present at deliveries. They try to respect mothers' own wishes with regard to relief of pain and support any method of relaxation and preparation for labour and delivery practised during pregnancy. They give pethidine and Entonox as needed and agreed by mother. Do not perform routine episiotomy but would do one if it was considered to be in best interest of mothers and/or babies. Episiotomy wounds or perineal tears are sutured by mother's own GP and she adds: 'We have found that these do not cause nearly as much pain as perineums sutured in consultant hospitals.' Mothers are encouraged to breast-feed as soon as possible after birth. They have facilities for giving positive pressure oxygen or for incubating babies asphyxiated at birth, but sister in charge says these are rarely needed. They welcome moral support and help given by fathers during labour and encourage them to share care of mother throughout.

Postnatal They are able to give individual care to mother and baby and have time to give personal support with feeding and care of baby. They encourage breast-feeding but there is no coercion 'and we respect the mother's own wishes if she decided to bottle-feed'. All babies demand-fed from birth and complements of artificial milk offered only 'in very rare circumstances'. Water and glucose also only given rarely because these interfere with establishment of breast-feeding. 'We have a follow-up clinic 2 months after birth and a high proportion of our mothers are still breast-feeding then.' Mothers have their babies with them as much as they wish. Most prefer babies in the nursery at night and sister wakes mother to breast-feed when baby wakes. After initial period of rest, mother taught how to care for her baby and, with support, will do this herself. Mother's other children welcome to visit her and baby and because there is homely, relaxed atmosphere this helps to make visits happy occasions. This hospital also cares for mothers and babies transferred from Southampton and Boscombe. Any mother welcome to stay till tenth postnatal day. 'We believe mothers with first babies need this time to gain confidence in feeding and caring for their babies and multigravidi benefit from the rest before going home to cope with the rest of the family.' Sister in charge writes, 'It is vital for us to increase our numbers' if they are to remain open.

Basildon Hospital, Nethermayne, Basildon, Essex

Hospital built in seventies. Consultant and GP units, and special care baby unit on ground floor. All nursing para-medical and hospital support staff wear name badges.

Antenatal Long waits though appointment system, sometimes 2 hours or more. Usually see different doctor each time: 'He just grunted twice.' In general staff helpful, though some doctors 'impersonal'/'brusque'. Rarely see consultant: 'I didn't even know what he looked like.' Scans done when doubts about dates, to confirm multiple pregnancy, no longer routinely as before. Relaxation and parentcraft classes, fathers encouraged to attend too; visit to maternity ward and labour suite; film, husbands welcomed. Several writers said they had been told by doctors that labour was induced if they went 1 week, or sometimes 2 weeks, over their dates. They were also told Caesarean section done for breech delivery at 38 weeks. Writers critical of 'conveyor-belt' system, queuing for routine tests – 'You are moved from queue to queue' – and of having to sit in cubicle waiting to see doctor: 'You mustn't keep the doctor waiting a second . . . but our time is of no value.' Shared care; many women have first visit at hospital, then to GP until thirty-second week. Midwives in clinic may examine woman rather than doctor. Hospital booklet stresses 'Should you at any time wish to seek advice . . . please do not hesitate to telephone us.' Also 'Please do not bring your children to clinic sessions unless absolutely necessary.' Very hard on women with older children and inadequate facilities for care. Notice up asking you to keep children under control. Inductions done with prostaglandin pessaries, ARM and syntocinon drips.

Labour Routine shave/enema. Staff shortage, 'but in spite of this they remained cheerful and reassuring'. Encouraged to use breathing taught in classes but no informed help with it. Pethidine offered; epidurals available but you have to decide in advance. Delivery room 'off-putting'. One husband said there were blood stains on floor and ceiling. Baby placed on mother's chest after delivery, but labelled first. (Is this necessary?)

Postnatal Hospital booklet states: 'Your well-being is our concern and so we should like you to keep as close to home, family and everyday happenings as possible.' Baby is at mother's bedside. Mothers' experiences variable: 'There were some staff who treated us like morons.' Consultant and midwife tutors do bedside teaching with groups of students; you may ask not to participate in this if you prefer. One writer described a nurse sitting with her 'for ages' when she was having feeding difficulties. Policy of demand-feeding; hospital booklet says, 'Some babies require a night feed', which is something of an understatement! Auxiliary nurses 'a bit bossy'; 'Made me feel like I was at school all over again.' Conflicting advice: 'By the time I got home I was thoroughly confused.' One writer says midwife who delivered her came up to postnatal ward to visit, which was appreciated. Some writers advised single room if you can get one, to get enough sleep. Smoking allowed in day room. Writers like best flexible attitude to husbands: 'It is taken for granted that husband will attend the birth.' They are allowed to pick up babies, in contrast to some other hospitals. One woman says doctor explained about induction to her husband and did not send him out when she was examined.

Basingstoke

Food 'quite nice'. Woman makes daily menu selection, though when first admitted gets someone else's choice. Breakfast 7.45 a.m., lunch 11.45 a.m., tea 2.45 p.m., supper 5.45 p.m.

Two visitors allowed every afternoon 3–4 p.m. Own children only by arrangement with ward sister. Hospital booklet says if there is difficulty with visiting time see ward sister. Some women asked if their parents could come in evening and were told 'no'; hard on working grandparents.

Suggestions Play area and toys for small children in antenatal clinic. Reorganization so that woman sees same doctor whenever possible. 'Doctor should ask how you are feeling or say hello, look at your face.' Half-hour visiting for grandparents every evening.

Hospital booklet asks for helpful suggestions to be made to the nursing officer to improve comfort and well-being of mothers and babies.

**Maternity Unit, Basingstoke District,
Aldermaston Road, Basingstoke, Hants** MO

Bleak, modern building outside, bright and friendly inside.

Antenatal 'Like conveyor belt'/'impersonal', but 'reception staff always willing to chat to anyone who seemed bored or miserable'. See different doctor every time. Different dates for birth given by GP and hospital worried some mothers. 'The consultant told me my condition was none of my business.' Of four mothers who asked for Leboyer delivery two were refused, two told that staff would cooperate as far as possible.

Midwife clinic for normal pregnancies; short waiting times; woman attends consultant clinic only once.

Classes available including two evening classes for fathers, birth film, tour of labour and postnatal wards and SCBU.

Labour Midwives 'supportive', 'friendly', 'attentive', 'kind'. Electronic fetal monitoring done; some women said monitors did not always work well. Some felt under pressure to have pain-relieving drugs, were given pethidine instead of gas and oxygen which they asked for, or given it during contraction and did not realize it had been done. Two women were given epidurals without understanding what was being done. But one writer said she did not want pethidine 'and midwife was delighted'. Women who had been to classes would appreciate more understanding from midwives of what they had learned. Fathers welcome, encouraged to do back-rubbing, though some had to go out for examinations/forceps delivery. Separate delivery rooms, so have to be moved. Depends on staff whether delivery room brightly lit. Baby is given mother to hold at once. Of 100 mothers delivering in five months of 1979: 3 had Caesarean births, 20 forceps delivery, 78 episiotomies (including those having forceps). The 58 who had spontaneous deliveries were not told why they needed episiotomies; only 11 women did not need stitching. Thirty-six of

205

these babies were in special care for periods of 12 hours or more (did they all need it?), 10 because there was a forceps delivery with complications, 10 simply because it was a forceps delivery, 3 because of Caesarean sections. In 9 cases mothers said they were not given reasons.

Postnatal Relaxed atmosphere on whole. Difficulties with ward routines. Some writers said it was hard to discover what they were and had to find out by trial and error or from other women: 'I was always being told off'; 'It was like being back at school'; 'I was treated like a moron'; 'I was shouted at.' Policy is to encourage contact between mother and baby but there are obstacles to be overcome. Some staff feed baby in nursery at night and do not always bring baby to mother for feed. Hospital leaflet states: 'Babies stay with their mothers day and night.' Writers said that if they got together and agreed to have their babies with them they could stay at night. Women are encouraged to put babies in cots between feeds. 'A nurse said "If he has not got wind put him down and leave him to cry," which he did for about an hour.' 'If you are caught cuddling your baby then you have to have a good excuse.' If the baby did not sleep the mother tended to be told that it was not getting enough breast milk and should be given bottle. Crying babies put in nursery. This meant that mother did not know how to cope when she got home: 'I didn't feel that he was really mine until I got home'; 'My husband wanted to hold him, but wasn't allowed.' Though policy of demand-feeding from birth, dextrose given out after feeds for first 24 hours and writers say support is inadequate. 'Staff have insufficient time and too few skills.' Instructions contradictory, e.g. on demand/scheduled feeding, topping up/no top-ups and if top-ups given whether water/dextrose/SMA. Jaundiced babies often given SMA as fluid supplement. Tablets to suppress milk sometimes given (despite dangers from oestrogens and risk of rebound engorgement). Ward routines often conflict with babies' needs. Some mothers did not feel free to feed baby and eat own meal later. Ward short-staffed and nurses busy. Women in single rooms may find it difficult to get advice and help. Conflicts between day and night shifts result in confusion for mothers. Wards have pleasant view, but women describe being wakened by other people's crying babies. Only two bathrooms for twenty-two-bedded unit but lots of lavatories with bidets. Some writers describe linen often in short supply; wet cot sheets arranged to let baby lie on dry patch or being dried on radiators. Fathers may only be allowed to hold baby for 5 minutes at end of visiting time.

Food good but 'not spectacular'; 'wide choice'; 'can order double helpings'. Menus every morning for following day. Vegetarian meals can be ordered. Tea 6 a.m., breakfast 7.30 a.m., coffee 10.30 a.m., lunch 11.45 a.m., tea 3.15 p.m., supper 6 p.m., evening drink 9.45 p.m. Rest time 2–3.15 p.m.

Writers appreciate fathers-only visiting 7.15–8.15 p.m. Own children may visit in day room, where people smoke, Wednesday and Sundays 2.30–3.30 p.m. Policy about visitors holding baby differs on different floors.

SCBU Staff praised for sympathetic help, but lack of liaison between wards and unit. Mothers trying to express milk for pre-term babies said they did not get encouragement from ward staff. Father can visit nursery but no other member of family.

Suggestions Better communication between day and night staff. Breast-feeding counsellor on postnatal wards. Longer visiting hours, especially for own children.

Clatterbridge, Bebington, Wirral, Merseyside   MO

Teaching hospital; well organized; post-war building.

Antenatal Doctors 'approachable'; 'treat you like intelligent human beings'. Consultants described as 'down to earth', 'reassuring'. Sister 'friendly'. Cheerful atmosphere throughout. Evening meetings to discuss anaesthesia/ baby care. Fathers' evening when couple shown round. Questions invited.

Labour Partner made to feel welcome. Midwife stays with her patient all the time and keeps her thoroughly informed. Woman can sit up to deliver. 'The baby was handed to my husband almost straight away.' One woman appreci-ated midwife explaining placenta. Couple cuddle baby for extended period of time. Mother can breast-feed on delivery table. Baby then taken away to be bathed and writers said babies did not go up to ward with them though brought soon after.

Postnatal Happy atmosphere, mother free to feed as she likes, is given every encouragement to breast-feed, and can be woken at night. 'We actually got rest.' Food adequate, with choice of menu.

Suggestions Mother should be able to have her baby with her without interrup-tion from birth on, if she wishes.

Bedford General, North Wing, Kimbolton Road, Bedford

Old building: 'all over the place', though maternity unit modernized 1981: 'The appearance of the buildings more than made up for by kindness and cheerfulness of staff.'

Antenatal Women having shared care attend clinic only at 8 and 34 weeks. Ultrasound scan done routinely; some writers said staff were not friendly, 'They wouldn't let me see the screen despite my asking. When she asked me to come back in 3 weeks' time to do it again I was sure there was something wrong' (there wasn't). Another woman said: 'Everything was explained and I was shown picture'; she asked if her husband could see it too but was told: 'No, strict rule.' Counselling service by midwife available at all clinics. Guided tour of unit.

Labour Pleasantly decorated rooms with wallpaper and toning curtains. SNO says perineal shaving no longer part of admission procedure, and enemas done only when necessary. Electronic fetal monitoring used. Epidurals available. Pethidine sometimes given without vaginal examination and therefore occasionally too late. One writer said she appreciated doctor telling her to get as comfortable as she could before he broke waters and to adopt any position she liked. He did it so gently that she did not realize it had been done. Father may be told to go outside before amniotomy. One woman having an induced labour which lasted only 3 hours from beginning to end said she was left alone for 30 minutes when contractions were strong. Another writer says 'cheerful' student midwife was great help chatting to her husband to relax him, helping with breathing and massaging her back: 'I found the staff were there when needed but they didn't hover or interfere.' Some women felt uncomfortable in position they were expected to adopt for second stage, 'lying flat on my back with my husband pushing my head forward and my legs against a nurse'. One who finished with a forceps delivery said she thought this position made pushing unnecessarily difficult. Another, also placed flat on her back, suggested she would be better sitting and was helped to a semi-sitting posture. Another said 'I wanted to sit up and they kept on telling me to lie down.' Several writers were asked whether they wanted episiotomies. Midwife may hold mother up to see baby's head and ask partner to support her so she can see rest of baby being born. Baby can be delivered on to abdomen and given straight to mother to cuddle and put to breast. Women described having 5-30 minutes cuddling baby. Unfortunately father is asked to leave after birth if it is night time: 'Very disappointing.' Women described long waits for doctor to sew episiotomy at night, sometimes without baby who was taken away to be bathed: 'The midwife was good company but I don't think I was really listening. All I wanted was my baby!'; 'We both agreed afterwards that we felt wide awake and desperately wanted each other to talk over our experience.' Two women wrote of inadequate pain-relief for suturing.

Postnatal 'Lovely atmosphere.' SNO says babies are with mothers at all times, unless mother decides otherwise. Writers said babies were usually sent to nursery at night and advised being firm if you want to keep baby with you. Mother does everything for baby herself. Plenty of help from all staff. Choice of feeding method respected and mothers did not feel under pressure: support for mothers whether breast- or bottle-feeding: 'The nicest thing was that the staff took time to help you'; 'Everyone asked my permission before touching or doing anything to my baby, which really made me feel that he was mine.' Policy of demand-feeding. Help good, with some exceptions. Formula was offered one mother who had sore nipples; top-ups suggested readily and one nurse actually squeezed a woman's breasts and told her she had no milk. One woman said nurse tried to push baby on to breast and she would have preferred to be left alone: 'Most staff are bossy and too set in their ways.' But most women praised staff. One writer, who appreciated never being treated as if ill, wrote, 'With few exceptions all the staff I came into contact with were happy, kind and fun. I felt that they were enjoying themselves, as I was. Nothing ever happened to me without it being fully explained first and my feelings seemed to matter to everyone.' But one writer said her hour-old baby was placed in cot by open window wrapped in blanket, so took her baby into bed with her: 'I was confronted by two nurses who argued that she should be in her cot . . . I was shouted at in front of a dozen mothers and reduced to tears.' Some women who had been sutured said rubber rings were not provided and wished hospital chairs were softer. No salt available. Several writers had great trouble with stitches afterwards. Double glazing and air-conditioning has now been installed to reduce extraneous noise. SNO says 'Length of stay is geared to individual patient . . . can go home to care of community midwife in 6 hours'.

SCBU Upstairs, and mother can only go up when someone says she may. Particularly hard on Caesarean mothers. One woman trying to breast-feed said 'only small, hard chair provided, very uncomfortable'.

Suggestions More kindness and gentleness with stitching. Some couples would have liked more time with each other and the baby alone after delivery. Mothers who wished their babies totally breast-fed should never find in morning that baby has not been brought to them and has been given bottle. It should not be a matter of a mother being 'allowed' to keep her baby with her at night, but rather her choice.

Beverley Westwood Maternity Unit, Beverley, Humberside

Small, friendly unit, clean, light and airy. Good continuity of care. Very much a midwives' hospital. Domino scheme practised.

Antenatal Women booked for shared care attend clinic only at 13 (or thereabouts) and 36 weeks. Routine ultrasound; opportunity to ask questions, though one writer who wanted doctor to talk with her husband says she was refused 'roughly'. Can look around in advance by appointment with SNO. Inductions apparently for only good medical reasons, i.e. placental insufficiency/very overdue.

Labour One writer thought reception 'cold and unfriendly'. Routine small disposable enema/mini-shave, carried out with consideration. Previously some husbands felt less than welcome (1978) but things have changed. Midwife waits until contraction over before talking or carrying out procedures. Midwives 'capable', 'efficient', 'sympathetic'; give information about baby's position freely without being asked. Woman is in single room, allowed only water in labour, but can walk round room. Atmosphere relaxed and friendly. Pethidine offered. Several women had large doses and were 'knocked out'. Another room for delivery. Amniotomy performed at about 7 cm from accounts. Midwives try to manage without episiotomy but may freeze perineum just in case. Baby wiped, wrapped and given to mother to hold. One mother says she was asked not to suckle baby until the placenta was expelled 'because it was a large one and they wanted it to come away cleanly'. (Since nipple stimulation helps separation of placenta it is not clear why she was asked to wait.) Father given baby to hold during third stage. After any stitching baby is brought to parents who have 'a few minutes alone'. Father then 'kicked out' and mother taken to postnatal ward.

Postnatal Friendly atmosphere. 'Grossly understaffed', though 'seem happy'. In 1978 mothers said they could not pick their babies up except at feeding times and babies were taken away when they cried – this no longer happens. Baby goes to nursery first night. 'When staff were busy with deliveries they were unfortunately left to scream until someone came.' Good support for breast-feeding, though 'you have to time feeds'. One writer says her husband was not allowed to touch or hold baby. Non-medical staff friendly and helpful.

Food good, 'especially salads, available at lunch and tea'.

Visiting 1 hour only in evenings in week, husbands only on weekend evenings, general visiting afternoons at weekends. Children welcome.

Suggestions Ban smoking on ward.

Birmingham Maternity, Edgbaston Road, Birmingham

Large, impersonal, though Chairman of Hospital Executive Committee says that 'care is individualized'. Good relations with NCT.

Antenatal All staff members described as 'kind' and 'sympathetic'. One woman who became depressed after an unhappy experience there with her first birth said she found registrar understanding: 'He suggested shared care with GP, answered every question fully' and talked with her husband. Labour care plan is discussed at clinic; 'increasing flexibility of attitude towards the needs of the individual'.

Labour Enemas have been discontinued. All first-time mothers who wrote had been offered epidurals. Caesarean sections done under epidural. Father may be asked to wait outside while woman is examined. Electronic monitoring may be used and telemetry available. Writers said staff questioned them during contractions, did not know how to help with breathing or relaxation, but were pleasant, always explained what they were doing and were 'chatty', 'friendly', 'help you feel at ease'. Some writers said they were told not to use breathing techniques learnt in antenatal classes for transition but gas and oxygen instead and partners were told to stop helping. Some women said they were urged to push harder and longer and threatened with forceps after next push if they did not do it well enough. There seem to be strict second-stage time-limits, but women have delivered in different positions, including squatting and on birth stool. Writers say episiotomy was more or less routine, that they were given no choice and would have liked some explanation when it was done. When forceps are used reason is explained by doctors. Several writers described strenuous pulling on cord with resulting need for manual removal, though 'I was given baby to hold and suckle straight away when cord broke . . . it was wonderful.' (Putting baby to breast helps the separation of placenta and could have been done before, not just after.) Mother can see and touch baby straight away and women write about this even following difficult deliveries, though baby is wrapped before being handed to mother. Several writers wrote that partners were able to go up to postpartum ward with them.

Postnatal Women care for own babies during day and after 'a few nights' are woken at night to feed but 'one night I woke up an hour after his usual feed time, went to the nursery and was told by staff nurse that my baby had woken up later than usual so she had fed him a bottle to save waking me up!' Otherwise feeding on demand is policy. Mothers query advice to 'give lots of water' to jaundiced babies: 'After struggling through a bottle of water he was simply not interested in a breast-feed before next scheduled water feed.' Nurses 'friendly', 'helpful', but some women could have done with more help. Not enough staff. Conflicting advice given. Woman with big baby was told she would have to give complementary bottle. 'Bidet was a real godsend and gave such blissful, soothing relief.'

SCBU Parents can visit any time. Women intending to breast-feed should make it clear this is what they want from start. One writer who went to *SCBU* 3 hours after delivery by Caesarean 'was amazed to find my baby had been fed cow's milk. I tried explaining I was going to breast-feed and didn't want him to have cow's milk because of eczema in family and was told by nursery nurse "It is all right because it is Cow'and Gate"!' Egnell pump available on ward to express milk. When baby is sucking is brought to ward for mother to feed.

Suggestions Staff should be taught more about physiology of breast-feeding. Mothers of jaundiced babies should be able to feed on demand and give water only in between breast-feeds. Fathers should be allowed to visit at any time, perhaps in day room.

Maternity Hospital, Bishop's Stortford, Herts   M O

Pleasant hospital.

Antenatal Helpful relaxation classes and 'it was nice to arrive and know other mums on the ward'. Fathers' evening.

Labour Most writers had labour accelerated. 'Drugs not pushed.' Woman is moved from labour to delivery room in wheelchair, no longer by trolley. Plenty of pillows on bed to get into good position. Writers said they were not allowed more than 1 hour in second stage, though some concessions can be made if woman asks. Deliveries normally done by midwives. It appears that midwives are not happy about Leboyer-style births and worry about missing breathing difficulties in baby if lights are low.

Postnatal 'Staff could not have been more helpful.' Most mothers breast-feed. Nurses 'have endless patience'. Woman in bed first day. Baby on 4-hourly feeds first 2 days and then demand-fed (1980). Anybody allowed in nursery 'if not overcrowded'. It is kept at very high temperature: 'All the babies developed heat rash.' Ask for heating to be turned down if this happens to your baby. Writers say staff are 'tremendous'. Verandah on which mothers can sunbathe in good weather.

Food 'bad': 'On one occasion the kitchen rang up to say don't eat the dinner.' Meals 'constipating . . . and we all had to resort to sister's magic potions'.

Suggestions Provide dimmer switch in delivery rooms so lights can be lowered for delivery.

Queen's Park Hospital, Blackburn, Lancs

MO

'Clinical', 'drab', and 'unfriendly'.

Antenatal Clinic has toys for children and plenty of room to play. Waiting at least 2 hours. Many men accompany their wives if they can afford time off work. 'Very keen on ultrasound scans' but 'staff can't be bothered to explain pictures'. Claustrophobic cubicles for waiting; may have to sit in one for over ½ hour. One woman who had recurrent bleeding says consultant, though very busy, visited her at home on request: 'A really dedicated chap.' Some nurses in antenatal clinic described as 'curt'.

Labour 'I was completely surprised at the friendliness and hospitality of the midwife when I arrived,' said a woman who had hated antenatal clinic. Membranes often ruptured on admission. Woman free to refuse pain-killing drugs, but if she asks for gas and oxygen may be brought pethidine. Partner made to feel welcome, but no refreshments available. (Bring coffee and sandwiches.) Babies wrapped before being given to mother: 'They showed and explained placenta to me.' Baby bathed and left with parents for time to get to know each other. Mother can carry baby with her on trolley going down to ward.

Postnatal Some women were not fed on going to postpartum ward and were hungry. Some had to wait before their babies were brought to them. Savlon sachets provided for bath, but several writers said 'bath was filthy'; 'rimmed with scum and muck with blood on the floor'; 'wished I'd brought some Vim as there was nothing to clean it with'. One woman who looked at bath but did not get into it had only been on postpartum ward 45 minutes 'when orderly came and told me to go and clean bath as left mucky . . . I fumed about Colditz'.

Suggestions Nurses in antenatal clinic could be friendlier. Partner should not be sent away while woman admitted, when she is examined and during stitching.

Victoria Hospital, Blackpool, Lancs

MO

Pleasant building; good layout, but large and impersonal.

Antenatal 'Easy-going' doctors friendly and concerned that women should be happy. 'Nobody explains where to go to undress, get blood tests' . . . 'Just got pointed in a direction and figured it all out.' Shared care possible and women described seeing GP throughout. Chance to be shown around wards. Many writers were induced. Some said they would have been much more relaxed if they had not had to go in night before: 'The worst night of my life.'

Labour Mini-shave but no enema. Midwives 'lovely', 'kind', 'encouraging', 'friendly', 'helpful'. But some women described pethidine given without discussion. Others were asked first and choice was theirs. Electronic fetal monitoring done. Women sometimes described difficult inductions, with oxytocin going in at fast rate: 'My husband had to ask midwife to switch drip off when contractions were lasting 3 minutes' (which they did, but it was a bit late for them to notice). Those writers who were not induced had labour accelerated: 'I was put on an oxytocin drip against my will' . . . 'left with a student who read the paper and ignored me' (1980) . . . 'The midwife came back 2 hours later and found me crying' (she was given more pethidine). Some writers who asked not to have oxytocin stimulation said it was done nevertheless. Partner can be present throughout and couple left in privacy if they wish it, but midwife comes promptly when rung. Episiotomies not done routinely. Baby given to mother after cord cut; put to breast for few minutes after delivery. Father can also hold baby. Baby is washed and weighed in delivery room. Time for couple and baby together. Partner may be sent out during stitching, which may be done by medical student. If suturing starts before anaesthetic has had time to take effect, writers advise shouting 'Stop!' If born during day baby is taken to ward with mother but at night goes to nursery, mother to ward and sleeping pills and pain-killers offered. Some writers said they had to wait long time for food after delivery: 'I was ravenous.'

Postnatal Baby can be with mother at night only after 4 days unless in single room when can be with her at all times. Woman only allowed up 12 hours after birth to bath. Everyone woken at 6 a.m. for tea, again at 7 a.m. and again at 8 a.m. with breakfast and make bed: 'Annoying after being up through night.' Policy of modified demand-feeding: 'Not less than 2 hours not more than 5.' Some mothers said little help given with breast-feeding. One mother said she greatly appreciated midwife who delivered her coming to ward before she went off duty to see baby: 'Seemed so pleased'. Writers remember things like 'the nurse who treated my baby as special and said how lovely she was' and being able to 'feed the baby and cuddle her and love her whenever I wanted to'. They particularly enjoyed being able to be together all the time and being left undisturbed to feed whenever the baby wanted it. All writers emphasized pleasure of being able to look after their babies without interference: 'I coped much better without someone watching me all the time.' Chart on baby's cot is filled in by mother recording nappy changes, feeding. Pleasant, enthusiastic physiotherapist 'reminiscent of school gym lessons'. All staff 'friendly', 'helpful', but 'changed round a lot'. Most writers said help always available if they wanted it and thought some mothers were reluctant to ask. 'Really sweet newspaper lady who brightened the day.' Plenty of bathrooms with bidets.

Visiting 8–9 p.m. only on weekdays. Saturdays and Sundays 2–3 p.m. and 8–9 p.m. Own children allowed Sunday afternoon only 'but not *two*. Strict about this.'

Food 'reasonable', 'average'. Menu chosen two days in advance. For first two days you get previous occupant's meals. Inadequate breakfasts and some women fill up with chocolates.

Can arrange day discharge. Some writers advise this as 'it is lovely to get home for a rest'.

Suggestions Paediatricians should examine baby in mother's presence and explain what is being checked. Since babies have to go home to cooler rooms, thermostat should be lowered. Women would like to be left to sleep when they get the chance. Longer visiting times for fathers and own children.

Royal Victoria, Shelley Road, Bournemouth, Dorset HO

Antenatal SNO writes that full range of antenatal screening tests is available. Shared care possible. Husbands welcome to attend antenatal classes.

Labour Induction when medically indicated. Monitoring apparatus used for all high-risk cases. Husbands present during labour and delivery – including forceps delivery. Forceps 10%; Caesarean 6%. Epidural analgesia available.

Postnatal Rooming-in; flexible approach to breast-feeding, with demand-feeding in many instances. Early transfer home to care of domiciliary midwife. When intensive nursing required babies are transferred to SCBU at Poole Maternity. Mothers usually transferred with babies.

Maternity Unit, Bradford Royal Infirmary, Smith Lane, Bradford, W Yorks

Busy, short-staffed hospital. 'Terrible' language problems for Asians.

Antenatal Rarely see same doctor twice, but 'all doctors give impression of genuine concern'; 'I was never treated like just another pregnant woman.' A great many scans seem to be done, some women think too many. Antenatal ward: 'understanding' staff. But 'Consultants do not bother to explain unless you show obvious knowledge.' Some women confused by medical terms which were not explained; some felt 'ignored'. Marked colour prejudice observed in some auxiliary staff.

Labour 'Lovely' delivery suite. Full shave; one woman asked for mini-shave but was refused. Enema. Waters may be broken with no explanation, even when requested. Continuous electronic fetal monitoring often used but several writers said it was not working properly. Pethidine offered: 'I had to have it even when I told them it was too late . . . I begged for examination before injection but was refused' (baby born 10 minutes after). Fathers welcome but may be sent out when doctor comes in. Midwives 'kind', 'gentle' and 'patient'. But one writer said she encountered midwives who were 'scathing of National

Childbirth Trust and said "Oh God, you're not going to sing 'Ten Green Bottles', are you?'''. Mothers allowed to cuddle and suckle baby after delivery but some separated for prolonged period afterwards. One did not see baby for 8 hours 'due to busy ward' and staff shortage.

Postnatal Several writers advise amenity bed if you can get one so that baby can stay with mother at night if she wishes. Some day staff 'a bit regimental'. Demand-feeding encouraged by most nurses but no feeding allowed at meal times and babies taken out for afternoon visiting. Water brought for baby at every feed, but no pressure to give it. Writers said staff gave babies bottle-feeds at night. Father can hold baby at evening visiting. Food 'appalling', 'not enough'.

Suggestions Improve antenatal clinic. Woman should be able to see same doctor more than once. Give more explanation of treatment. Children should be able to cuddle their new brother or sister, not just look at baby through door.

★ **Mary Stanley Nursing Home, Castle Street, Bridgwater, Somerset**

Small, friendly GP unit, 'very homely', run by midwives, rarely full. For normal deliveries and straightforward forceps deliveries only. If complications develop mother is transferred 12 miles to Musgrove Park, Taunton. Wards look on to beautiful gardens at back of hospital, though in middle of town.

Antenatal GPs do antenatal care at nursing home: 'Everything fully explained.' Older children welcomed. 'No them and us attitude.'

Labour If woman says she would prefer not to have drugs this is accepted by staff without question, a change from a few years ago. 'During early phases we were left with buzzer and pupil popping in about every 15 minutes for a chat on progress. Once things started moving sister joined pupil, but all the time they *talked* about what was happening and encouraged me all the way.' Writers said they were told to push as long and as hard as they could. Some queried wisdom of this. Woman can get into position she likes for delivery. One woman said student midwife told her she was going to do an episiotomy because it was part of her training. Baby can be put to breast immediately, with help from midwife. Father can hold baby 'and we took some photographs and the staff took some of us'.

Postnatal Though previous policy was to put baby in nursery for first few hours and every night, this has changed too. If she asks, mother can now keep baby with her first night. One writer said baby started to cry at night: 'the sister came in and said the easiest way was to have her in bed with me so she would be warm and I could feed her when she wanted, tucked her in bed beside me, with a pillow on the far side to make me feel safer and we spent the whole night like that, with her latched on my nipple, sucking whenever she wanted to'. Writers usually described 'warm', 'friendly', 'helpful' care especially with breast-feeding. Mothers encouraged to breast-feed on demand day and night, another great change from a few years back, when 4-hourly feeding was standard. One writer who had baby there 2 years before writes: 'Although the staff had been friendly before they were like friends this time.'

Food 'excellent', 'always hot and fresh and usually home-made'.

Forty-eight-hour discharge can be arranged. 'When I left several of the staff said that if I had any problems they were always there just on the end of the telephone.'

Suggestions Before midwife does episiotomy she should give mother reason and do one only with her consent.

Royal Sussex County, Eastern Road, Brighton, E Sussex   MO

Twelfth and thirteenth floors of 1970 tower block, perfect sea views; light and welcoming: 'smell and atmosphere is super'; 'I love the whole place.'

Antenatal Letters arriving in 1979 and 1980 gave overall impression that 'staff believed patients are either totally dumb and/or not to be trusted in anything they say and therefore are not worth listening to,' and women said they were expected to be 'passive' and that 'patronizing' advice was given. But most recent reports more positive and some writers say they are impressed with open attitudes of staff: 'I got straight answers with no flannel from anyone'; 'I was given credit for intelligence.' But things still not right: a nurse having her baby there said she felt treated like a 'stupid bovine'; 'I was left feeling like a moron'; 'I felt like a silly little girl if I asked questions'; 'Nobody patted me on the head, but came close to it.' All but one writer (28) mentioned that there were no easy openings for discussion and they came away with unanswered questions. Some women felt 'accused of being wrong in their dates', including one who had been keeping temperature chart and was sure. One writer said 'abrupt' midwife 'made it clear she thought I was lying' when she said she had taken Pill every day but conceived. On the whole writers felt that staff tried to be reassuring at all costs, and this failed miserably because women wanted information. One social worker was highly critical of way social workers are used. She was told she *must* see one 'simply because I was not married'. Shortage of space and chairs, and women wait in cramped, crowded conditions, frequently reporting hearing conversations between other patients and staff. See different doctor at most visits. 'The more senior doctors were, the more communicative.' Obvious staff 'hierarchy' noted. Doctors 'kind', 'charming', 'chauvinistic', 'self-assured', 'pleasant', and staff in general 'busy', 'efficient', 'kindly', but 'not interested'. Women having shared care with GP may visit hospital clinic only three times, booking clinic and in late pregnancy. One woman who was antenatal emergency said she was taken straight to labour ward even though labour not imminent: 'Nursing care did not seem so attentive as on antenatal ward because women who were in labour came first.' One woman was on drip and monitor for a whole day without being able to find out what was happening: 'Then nurse walked in and told me

I was going to have "a little prick". When pressed for information said it was something to help the baby's lungs mature. I felt I should have been consulted about this by doctors who prescribed it.'

Antenatal classes only for women in immediate vicinity. 'At one a midwife launched an attack on demand-feeding and the NCT. While the choice was ours, staff didn't like demand-feeding. It was nearly always young, inexperienced mothers who wanted to demand-feed. More experienced women had more sense.'

Labour Same room for whole of labour, but 'shabby' and 'depressing'. Routine partial shave, sometimes given in 'off-hand way', 'no explanation given beforehand'. 'I was always taught to tell patients what was about to happen,' nurse comments. Routine suppository, though some women refused it and 'no fuss made'. Partner may be asked to leave for prepping, vaginal examination, stitching. One father, who says he was 'fuming' at being told to leave during suturing, said doctor seemed 'pompous' and 'self-important', in contrast to 'informal, friendly attitude' of midwives. He may also be asked to leave when woman is washed afterwards: 'nurse was emphatic'. Some writers mention that partner did not have to wear gown, and some couples who asked not to be separated were allowed to remain together throughout. Some writers said membranes were ruptured at or soon after admission without informing them or asking for their consent. A good deal of technological intervention described, which distracted women and impeded mobility. One writer said that hearing fetal heart monitor was 'comforting'. Criticism of badly functioning monitors, 'The fetal heart kept stopping. Disconcerting, but only loose connection. But how could it be any use?' 'I was strapped up to machine which kept failing to operate and every time I had a contraction it didn't pick up baby's heartbeat. It was worrying to say the least.' Breech babies seem likely to be delivered by Caesarean section. Most writers describe plenty of attention given, but one woman with antepartum haemorrhage says she was put on monitor and 'left alone' for 2 hours. Midwives described very positively, however: 'delightful', 'motherly', 'informal', 'friendly', 'made suggestions rather than gave orders', 'always encouraging', 'keenly involved', 'showed great personal interest', 'most accommodating': 'I was made to feel an adult, responsible member of a team to ensure my baby's safe arrival.' Some women found staff did not realize supine position could lower mother's blood pressure dangerously: one was kept 15 minutes lying on her back while student doctor tried to rupture membranes and she fainted. Many writers wanted to walk about and think this would have helped labour. Midwives usually conduct labour and 'explain everything they are doing' and women having second babies say atmosphere much more relaxed than a few years back. Pethidine offered; epidurals available, including for Caesarean section. Writers describe lying flat on their backs in second stage and said there was little flexibility about delivery positions, but may be shown head crowning in mirror: 'I wish I had insisted on being more upright, which I feel sure would have helped.' Episiotomies not done routinely. Baby wiped and wrapped before being handed to mother. May be taken away to be cleaned while mother stitched and washed. Suturing done by doctors. Ask if you want to hold your baby during suturing. One woman says doctor complained about unpleasantness of suturing for *him* throughout: 'demoralizing!' Afterwards she was left alone with baby crying in crib but unable to reach him for ½ hour. Midwives may draw attention to baby's rooting and help to suckle on delivery bed. Some women who had general anaesthesia for Caesarean section would have liked husbands with them. After Caesarean baby is shown to father as soon as possible.

Postnatal On eleventh and twelfth floors overlooking Marina. Pleasant, friendly, 'personal' atmosphere. Baby with mother all the time unless she wishes it to go to nursery at night, or when she wants to rest. Most women breast-feed. Scheduled feeding has been abandoned both for breast- and bottle-fed babies. But some mothers say that not all members of staff understand what demand-feeding really is and some still have expectation that baby is fed every 4 hours. May be told not to feed more than every 3 hours: frequent mention of 'spoiling' the baby. No schedules for anything. No dextrose offered routinely; if mother wants it she goes and gets it. Staff willing to help, but mother must ask. It might be difficult for some first-time mothers to do so. Mother free to care for her own baby in her own way without interference: 'We were in charge of ourselves and our babies': 'Best just to get on with it and learn about your baby'; 'Do it *your* way.' This important because when advice is given it tends to be conflicting. One writer warns; 'The more anxious you are and the more you ask for advice the more conflicting advice you are given.' Mothers say best thing is universal attitude on part of nursing staff that mothers and babies should be together as soon as possible after delivery and stay that way. Mother can cuddle baby all day if she likes. 'No petty routines'; 'baby and I in bed together all night – marvellous!'; 'left blissfully alone to do just as I pleased'. Nurses 'kind', 'cheerful', 'helpful in spite of being overworked' but 'hierarchy pervades everything'. Some auxiliaries 'bossy'. Some women said baby was given artificial feed in nursery at night when they had given instructions that water only should be given, and were told they needed 'a good night's sleep'. On wards some women disliked lack of privacy but agreed it was good thing to talk to other women. Paediatricians praised: 'explain everything', but one woman with breast-feeding problems said she was told 'not to worry, cow's milk is not a poison'. Tend to be queues for bathrooms at some times, but plenty of hot water. Cleaning of floors, changing of sheets, supplies of baby items, salt for perineum inadequate. Some writers said no sanitary pads provided. But on whole pleasant place to be because 'some lovely people work in it'.

Food chosen from menu on previous day: 'terrible'; 'reminiscent of school'; 'cold and underseasoned'.

Visiting 4–6 p.m., 8–9 p.m. fathers only. Can arrange 48-hour discharge.

SCBU Some rather sad accounts of mothers shown their babies but not allowed to touch them; of older siblings left outside while father went in. One mother 'raised hell' for 3 hours until allowed to see baby, who was well enough to come on to ward as soon as she *did* go and see her. 'Administrative obstructionism?' she asks. A woman fetching baby after Caesarean section discovered that she had been given two artificial feeds without her permission. 'Sister insisted that she would be "jaundiced" otherwise.' But these are earlier accounts and from letters it is clear that in 1980 things started to change. Writers say that if a baby was in special care for short time and they were going to breast-feed, baby was given only dextrose, not artificial feeds.

Suggestions Improve antenatal clinic and 'move out some Hitlers working there'. Booklets should be more informative. More women doctors; more midwives. Some writers felt that some doctors should recognize that 'patients are people with right to control their own lives'. Evening antenatal clinics so fathers can attend, child care easier to arrange and ease overcrowding in day. Improve antenatal classes; should have more continuity, be led by one person. Fathers should be welcome at all times in labour and delivery. Women who cannot move because attached to drips and apparatus should never be left alone. Suturing should be done only with effective anaesthesia. Babies should be bathed, weighed and dressed in delivery room, not taken away. Suggestions boxes on postnatal wards. Open visiting for fathers, to help bonding of father and baby and give more emotional support to mother. Longer visiting for own children.

★★ Bristol Maternity, St Michael's Hill, Bristol, Avon

Large, modern, well-equipped hospital with personal touch. Writers say everyone 'helpful', 'friendly' and that hospital efficiently run: 'You are dealt with by trained people who don't treat you as idiots.'

Antenatal Shared between consultants and family practitioners. Sometimes long waits, often 2 hours, but clinic redecorated and carpeted throughout. Children's play area in main waiting area, with toys. Women praise consultants: 'one of kindest men I have ever met'; 'I could ask him anything, however trivial, and would always get a patient answer.' Low induction rate. Women are asked if they have special requests for labour. Antenatal wards 'boring'; 'day room full of chain-smoking women'.

Labour No shaves. 'Everything fully and kindly explained.' Partner can be with woman whole time. Delivery rooms wallpapered and redecorated. Pethidine offered. Some women described being encouraged to squat in second stage. Various writers wondered whether necessary to have so much encouragement to push, however. Episiotomy discussed before done and woman can make choice. Father can photograph birth if he likes. Writers describe quick, efficient suturing. Woman who had Caesarean section held baby as soon as she came round from general anaesthetic; 'My husband wheeled the incubator (baby stopped breathing for a short while) to ward with me and although I couldn't talk to him I was greatly comforted by his presence and glad he had seen baby so young.' Some fathers have been present at epidural Caesarean sections.

Postnatal Everything done to encourage good bonding. Father can help with feeding and changing of baby from start. Baby can be with mother all time if she asks, including first night. High percentage of women breast-feed, mother can feed baby whenever s/he is hungry, 'do what she likes' and take baby into bed with her. A woman who was in 'emotional turmoil' was grateful for expert psychological care. Auxiliaries very good. One of very few hospitals that has managed to create continuity of care. Each ward is 50 per cent antenatal and 50 per cent postnatal. Woman is moved back to same ward if she was in hospital before birth: 'I saw the same faces throughout.' Doctors involved in antenatal care and delivery and one's own GP may visit. Mothers can use own baby clothes. Paediatrician sees baby every day. Explains everything fully. Food good. Woman can choose when she is ready to go home and many leave after forty-eight hours.

Visiting 3–4 p.m., 7–8.30 p.m. Mondays and Wednesdays fathers-only night. Own children can visit. Women say nurses 'turn a blind eye' when fathers come at odd hours and stay late at night.

SCBU Women with babies in special care have room next to SCBU; also flatlet, redecorated and wallpapered for three mothers. Both parents help look after baby. Brothers and sisters encouraged to visit baby in special care. Low-birth-weight babies who do not need intensive care admitted to this ward with their mothers. Babies discharged from special care followed up at home by specially trained midwife as long as women require support.

Suggestions More bathrooms. Junior doctors should interfere less.

★ **Paulton Memorial, Salisbury Road, Paulton, Bristol, Avon**

GP unit: 'cosy', 'warm', 'friendly', 'relaxing atmosphere'. Midwives and auxiliary nurses work well together. Happy, efficient team: 'make every mum feel the birth of her child special'.

Antenatal Care from own GP. Hospital tour and talk from sister 'informative', 'reassuring'. Antenatal beds separated only by half wall from main ward and some women embarrassed to labour within earshot of other women and visitors.

Labour Mini-shave, enema seem routine. ARM often performed. Midwives 'kind', 'considerate', 'efficient'. Calm atmosphere. Partners welcome. Women encouraged to move around as much as they wish. SNO says 'pethidine is given only after consultation with the patient', though several writers seem to have had rather large doses and become drowsy and unable to work with their labours. Epidurals not available. Oxytocin acceleration of labour not done. Half-sitting position in second stage. Nearly all deliveries normal. Midwives keen to avoid episiotomies. Baby laid on mother's abdomen straight away, but cord cut immediately. Midwife helps mother put baby to breast on delivery bed and couple left alone with baby for while; 'a lovely experience'.

Postnatal Small ward. SNO says, 'In recent years the routine has become much more flexible.' Baby is in ward all day except for ward cleaning, but can go to nursery if mother wishes. Is in nursery at night. Baby may be given distilled water or dextrose at night till third day. Writers describe 4-hourly feeding but with some flexibility. No artificial feeds are given to breast-fed babies. Mother has to get up to breast-feed at night. Cares for baby after third day. Staff go out of way to encourage breast-feeding and are at hand to help. Sunny day room for sitting and meals. Food tasty, varied, ample portions. Soothing cassette tape played to crying babies 'with striking results'.

Visiting 2.30–4 p.m. and 7–8.30 p.m. First 40 minutes evening visiting for fathers only. Own children can visit. Forty-eight-hour discharge can be arranged but not if it is your first baby.

Suggestions More staff at busiest times. Babies should not be so often 'topped up' with dextrose/distilled water.

Southmead, Bristol, Avon

Pleasant grounds; gorgeous gardens, flowers and many green areas. Buildings fairly modern: 'lots of low, bungalow-type buildings', but general impression 'forbidding'. Very busy; most staff 'friendly', 'obliging', 'chatty', 'sympathetic'.

Antenatal Pleasant receptionists, relaxed atmosphere. One writer, who travelled 25 miles for scan, was told she could not have one because she had not drunk a pint of water and had emptied her bladder. She offered to drink something immediately, since her husband had taken time off work to be with her, but says this was refused: 'they made no attempt to fit me in, to the point of rudeness. I left in tears . . . My doctor later told me that at 24 weeks drinking water before a scan is unnecessary.' Staff 'kind' but overworked. Three-hour wait common; 'cattle-market approach'. Small play area for children. All queries answered and midwives will translate consultant scrawls on cooperation card if necessary. And writers say consultants always give time to answer questions. Women are encouraged to write down their plans for labour and these are put in their notes. Induction down to 14% (1981).

Labour Enemas no longer routine. Woman never left alone for more than 3–4 minutes. 'My husband was treated like a lord and helped with bedpans' (??). Electronic monitoring and telemetry used so women can move about. Epidurals available and Caesarean section done under epidural. Several writers describe snacks during labour; one mentions tea and home-made Easter biscuits. Hospital noisy. 'Windows were left open so that my mother could chat to me from outside.' Woman has to be moved to different room for delivery. Caesarean section rates remain low, about 10%. Nurses generally 'pleasant', 'helpful', 'give time to talk', have 'endless patience'. One writer who had a Caesarean section breast-fed 4 hours after delivery and 'due to patience and perseverance of two nurses who put my baby to the breast when I did not want to feed him or even speak to him, from then on we launched into a perfect feeding relationship'. All drugs and procedures fully explained. Woman who had Caesarean section said she was made to feel special even when she felt recovered, and staff had 'endless time' for her and baby. Sitting-room overlooks gardens, with sliding doors to patio; brightly decorated and carpeted. Wards so busy and noisy that it is difficult to sleep, but there are single rooms for those who want them.

One woman's day: 2.30 to 3.10 a.m. feed baby, 4.30 approx. back to sleep, 5.30 a.m. feed baby, cup of tea. 6.08 a.m. cup removed, bin emptied, 6.31 drugs trolley arrived, 6.49 given tablet, 7.26 water jug removed, 7.42 breakfast, 7.52 tea, 8.10 nursing auxiliaries asked if they may make bed, I say 'no thank you'. 8.13 bed made, 8.21 asked how I am, 8.48 weigh baby, 9.05 two nurses come, laugh and go away again, 9.49 fundus measured, temperature, etc., while feeding baby, 10.02 coffee, 10.46 offered paper. Cup removed, 11.51 post.

She said afternoons and evenings similar except that visiting and bathing also fitted in. She expressed breast milk and asked to sleep through night because she felt exhausted, but was woken to feed regardless. Some women worked out they were getting about 3 hours sleep in 24 hours and after 5 days like this became depressed. Several told to stay in hospital for rest said they 'could not stand it any longer' and had to get home for sleep. One said she left hospital 'exhausted physically and emotionally tense'. Choice of trayed meals.

Visiting 3–4.30 p.m., 7–8 p.m., but flexible. First ½ hour of evening visiting for father or nearest relative. Forty-eight-hour discharge possible.

SCBU Grandparents, parents and baby's brothers and sisters can visit at any time.

Suggestions Extend visiting times on antenatal wards. When forceps are used explanation should always be given beforehand and father should not be sent out. Redesign trolleys and cots so less noisy.

Maternity Unit, Farnborough Hospital, Bromley, Kent

Unimposing building but friendly staff. Cut off as far as public transport concerned.

Antenatal Long waits, but waiting-room with box of toys much enjoyed by children, and 'if you turn up between 9 and 10 a.m., even though appointment is later, you can be seen almost immediately before crowds start gathering'. Busiest time 10.30 on. Chaotic. 'Conveyor-belt treatment'. Mothers feel rushed. Woman is not introduced to doctor. One woman asked him his name, 'He was very abrupt with cynical attitude, always had students with him. Had to ask for explanations after he had made alarming comments.' Questions answered but not encouraged, though staff generally pleasant. Some women doctors: 'I felt more relaxed about asking questions.' Some women described induction when 10 days overdue, apparently for that reason alone, with prostaglandin to soften cervix prior to amniotomy and oxytocin drip. Full explanation of what this is and what may happen. Some writers advise having labour companion with you from start and one woman said she was 'left alone for most of 7 hours when induced'.

Labour No enema. Full shave. If you do not want shave ask doctor to write it in notes, otherwise done as matter of course. Partner 'very welcome indeed'. Amniotomy seems routine when admitted to labour ward. Epidurals available and seem to be given often. Can ask for half dose of pethidine. May be wise to do this as several women writing appear to have had large doses: 'I could not control my body or speak properly.' Midwives gentle, 'giving encouragement all the way through'. Woman wheeled to another room for delivery. Some midwives give careful explanation of episiotomy but several writers having normal deliveries described episiotomy done without consultation and without any opportunity to discuss it. 'Midwife announced she was going to cut me and before I could reply it was done.' If forceps delivery needed it is explained. Several women felt they were urged to push too soon and unwisely: 'If only a mother was more inclined and allowed to follow her instincts!' Baby given to mother to hold as soon as cord cut and then to father. Couple have time alone together.

Postnatal 'All day staff like one big happy family.' Night staff 'left a lot to be desired'. Poor communication between day and night staff and conflicting advice and information given. Mother allowed up after 5–6 hours. Some describe thanksgiving service: 'very moving'. Baby with mother from second night and is cared for by her from then on. She has free access to nursery: 'I wandered in and out and was never made to feel unwelcome.' Breast-feeding support given by auxiliaries who sit with mothers. Limited sucking time advised. One writer said information about her baby's jaundice was not volunteered: 'You have to *ask*.' Another writer minded very much that her baby was wakened by a 'surly nurse flicking fingers on his heels and making him scream. It was the last straw as I had had him awake with me all night and couldn't settle him.' Most writers said nurses 'took plenty of time to explain things' and there was 'jolly atmosphere'. Ample baths, showers, towels but no linen service on Sundays. One writer said she was made to 'feel like a criminal for stocking up with extra linen on Saturday'. Wards quiet at night. A mother who felt exhausted told sister, who cancelled all visitors and lunch, put baby in nursery, drew blinds, found screens to block out light. She was told she had postnatal depression and tranquillizers prescribed, but said she did not have depression, only needed sleep.

Flexible visiting. 'Not strict about number of visitors'; 'they are not hurried out'. Room where out-of-hours visitors can be taken. In single rooms partners can visit longer hours.

Suggestions More efficient antenatal clinic appointment system. Obstetrician should discuss with women possible side-effects on baby of any drugs given. More information given to women when in labour. Some women wished midwives had been able to spend more time with them in labour. Partners should not have to go out during examinations.

Burton District, Belvedere Road, Burton-on-Trent, Staffs HO

DNO writes: 'There have been many changes in the unit during past few years, partly due to changing patterns in maternity care and, of course, wishes and needs of patients.'

Antenatal New clinic opened 1979, gives more privacy. Less clinical appearance, i.e. warm colouring, carpeting, pictures on walls. Appointment system introduced. Patients no longer have to sit around in clinic partially undressed. Facilities for ultrasound scans. Evening parentcraft sessions. Expectant fathers encouraged to attend. Followed by informal discussion between expectant parents, consultant obstetricians, senior midwifery staff and health visitors. Monthly tours round maternity unit. There is closer integration of midwifery services in community and hospital. Community midwives do follow-up visits for patients attending consultant antenatal clinics.

Labour Fathers encouraged to stay with their wives throughout labour and delivery. Pubic shaves abolished in favour of perineal shaves, if necessary Prostin pessaries used for induction. Inductions 23%; forceps 10%; Caesareans 6%. Domino scheme introduced and community midwife accompanies patient into GP unit, where she conducts delivery, arranges for early discharge home and postnatal care.

Postnatal Mothers encouraged to handle their babies. Rooming-in practised. Patients given choice at night whether babies stay with them or in nursery and taken out for feeding. Demand-feeding encouraged both for breast- and artificially fed babies. For an experimental period of a year 1981–2, visiting hours extended to 2–8 p.m., own children allowed to visit. Some women find this 'tiring', but women who live at a distance appreciate it.

Fairfield General, Bury, Lancs HO

Antenatal For women booked in to GP beds antenatal care is given within GP unit, not in main clinic. DNO writes: 'We do not keep an induction rate list, but inductions are only performed here on medical grounds.'

Labour Forceps and Caesarean sections are approximately 25%.

SCBU DNO says there is 'free access to all parents and even Caesarean patients are taken to see their babies, 6 hours post delivery, in wheelchair.'

Mill Road Hospital, Cambridge

Teaching hospital. Consultant unit 'geared to complications, little support for normal mother and baby'. Also GP unit. Maternity block modern but old parts gloomy and 'a shambles'. Built 1838 as workhouse and poor-law infirmary with 250 places for 'prostitutes, spinning girls, vulgar youths, unruly vagabonds and rogues'. By 1900 infirmary for sick and destitute, mostly old.

During last war temporary theatre and X-ray departments set up in wooden huts – still there. In 1961 Ministry of Health agreed to re-site hospital by 1974. Tamara Ross, writing in *Nursing Mirror*, June 1980, comments on lack of space, with equipment and even offices in corridors. Lack of storage space, sisters having to share offices with doctors. No day room in antenatal ward; only a few chairs in recess at end of corridor. Walls damp. Roofs leaking. Buckets to catch rain. No labs, specimens have to be sent by taxi to Addenbrookes, 3 miles away. Shortage of single rooms, bathrooms and lavatories. Short-staffed, overcrowded.

GP unit Community midwives come in to deliver their own patients but writers note 'underlying friction between hospital staff and community midwives'.

Antenatal Writers said they saw different doctor each time. Sit elbow-to-elbow waiting and long waits for appointments after 10.30 a.m. Examinations in small cubicles separated only by curtains. Can overhear intimate details being discussed. Scans worried some women: 'nobody told me why'. One woman said scan was 'carried out in near silence'. Writers say however that they were 'always encouraged to ask questions', 'told anything I wanted to know', 'was examined sympathetically and thoroughly' and 'never felt rushed'. Nevertheless visits to clinic were very tiring. Shared care mothers see own GP between 3 and 6½ months. Chance to see round labour rooms in advance. Antenatal ward one bathroom for twelve women, no shower.

Labour Prostaglandins may be used to ripen cervix with amniotomy later. Staff efficient and friendly. Most writers described having enema. None after start of second stage. Epidurals available. 'I would have preferred to have my baby without all the technology used', but another woman said midwives understood that she wanted to give birth without drugs and tried to help her to do so. Midwife stays with woman in labour the whole time. Pethidine may be suggested but woman can refuse if she wishes. Most women describe having electronic monitoring but some only had this for a short time during labour and when all was well it was taken off. Fetal blood sampling may be done if signs of fetal distress. Midwife stays with woman the whole time. Students may be present at delivery but you can refuse. 'I felt like an animal during my internal examination with so many people present.' Strenuous, hard, long pushing is expected in second stage, though atmosphere is quiet. Genuine interest by midwives in avoiding episiotomy if possible but one writer said she was told by midwife on consultant unit that it was hospital policy for first babies. One mother discussed this with nursing officer and says she was told it was not so. She added, 'but I don't know of anyone who has not had one'. Community midwives deliver mothers semi-sitting with a wedge and several pillows and mother holds baby while placenta is delivered. Father may be asked to leave before suturing.

Postnatal Friendly, relaxed atmosphere. Staff enthusiastic but 'not very knowledgeable about breast-feeding'. Friendly auxiliaries. After delivery mother taken to ward to 'sleep' if it is night and baby to nursery: 'I lay awake re-living the birth. Could not sleep anyway as after second night babies are with their mothers 24 hours and inevitably there is one baby crying or someone walking around. Shattering!' Some women say they were given a great deal of help with breast-feeding by 'super' staff, but different theories on feeding. 'Demand-feeding on our ward meant 2–5 hours'. Also different views on whether babies should be given water and whether before or after feed. Conflicting views on what to do about engorgement. 'My painful breasts were manhandled by all and sundry as they attempted to get the baby to feed.' 'I felt the night staff thought they were running some kind of Borstal! One told me she "didn't fancy the idea" of breast-feeding.' Artificial milk brought up and left in ward for mothers to use if they liked. Paediatrician examines baby on bed in front of mother. 'What did annoy me was that whenever I asked a question about her I was told "Not to worry." I wasn't worried, I just wanted *answers*.' Very little chance to rest. On the other hand 'so few staff that you could do as you liked'. Temperature of nearly 80°. 'Salt available for sore perineum if you ask.' Two lavatories and one bath for whole ward. One woman said bidet on one ward was out of action for at least 6 months, thermostat faulty and new part not come.

Food 'dreadful', 'tinned pears and chocolate sauce' . . . 'staple diet of stew and icecream' . . . 'awful' . . . 'insufficient'. 'Cheese sandwich and jelly isn't adequate for a breast-feeding mother.'

Extended visiting hours first day. Visitors who arrive after hours may be admitted. Other family members can hold baby. Can arrange to go home following day if delivered by community midwife. Mothers and babies often transferred after 2 days to Primrose Lane, Huntington, if all is well.

SCBU Open visiting, mothers help care for their own babies. Single room where mother can take care of her own baby completely just before discharge, but only one of these.

Suggestions Friction between staff should not be communicated to patients. Redesign of labour suite so that women do not have to be moved for second stage. A few nurse specialists in breast-feeding and a breast-feeding counsellor. Better food of right type. Roughage including wholemeal bread and choice of bran breakfast cereal would reduce need for laxatives. Provision of more rooms in SCBU where mother can care for her baby.

★ **Kent and Canterbury, Ethelbert Road, Canterbury, Kent**   MO

Old building but well equipped and clean.

Antenatal Overbooked clinics; long waits. 'Sister incredibly helpful' and always finds time for discussing personal worries 'no matter how trivial'. All staff 'friendly', 'doing their best in difficult circumstances'. Writers describe routine scans at 16 weeks. Staff there 'casual' and not sensitive to women's feelings.

Labour Midwives 'gentle', 'sensitive', one writer said the doctor was 'arrogant'. Epidurals available and Caesarean section may be done under epidural, though father is not allowed to be present. One woman who had epidural Caesarean said woman doctor who gave the epidural 'reassuring', 'stroked my forehead'. Mother is shown baby immediately. After baby had been examined midwife put baby close to mother so 'our faces were in contact'.

Postnatal Feeding on demand. Baby can stay with mother day and night. All staff 'helpful', 'friendly', 'working well together', 'kind'. Mothers praise warmth and friendliness of both nursing and domestic staff. Baby can feed until falls asleep. People who had Caesarean sections said nurse arranged pillows so that she could breast-feed comfortably.

Suggestions More understanding of mothers' feelings by some doctors; 'they treated me as a sick patient and not a woman who had given birth. Nursing staff could teach them a lot.'

City Maternity Hospital, Carlisle, Cumbria

Antenatal Long waits, anything up to 2½ hours. Impersonal. Writers said they saw different doctor most times. 'This undermined my confidence as they all disagreed.' Staff 'pleasant, helpful, rather old-fashioned'. 'Seemed to prefer patients not to ask questions and accept what is said', but writers say that any wishes expressed by a woman are written in notes and respected by midwives in labour. Routine scans at 15–16 weeks and often later in pregnancy.

Labour 'Lovely, calm atmosphere.' Writers attribute this to midwives who are 'extremely helpful'. 'Couldn't do enough to make me comfortable.' 'Interested in natural childbirth.' 'Kind, encouraging, understanding, though very busy.' Routine enema, mini-shave, but both are explained beforehand. All women who wrote had had amniotomy. Epidurals available; if woman prefers not to have pethidine it is written in her notes. When pethidine *is* given it may be in large doses: 'I was so doped I was unable to push the baby out and had to have forceps.' Some writers criticize 'excessive zeal for latest technology' and 'too much interference from doctors in labour'. Some doctors were described as 'helpful'. Women sometimes found it difficult to get information from doctors. Monitoring seems to be used frequently and writers 'disliked being immobilized'. One woman said she was catheterized without being asked or told what was happening. Partners can be present throughout and are made very welcome. 'Sister made him tea and toast.' Writers advise having labour companion. One woman who had nobody with her says she was left alone 'for ages' without knowing where the bell was. Partner may not be allowed to be present for forceps delivery. Some midwives encourage women to sit up in second stage, though one said she was made to lie flat on her back and when she wanted to sit up the midwife told her 'babies come out of your bottom so you can't sit on it'. Another woman asked to be delivered in a semi-sitting position but was told that she must put her feet on the waists of midwives.

Writers appreciated cheer-leading in second stage and encouragement of 'natural rhythms'; 'no feeling of being bullied'. One woman said she was told by a midwife that the consultant had a rule that patients were not allowed to push for longer than 1 hour. 'The perineum wasn't given a chance to dilate. I was not allowed to pant through contractions.' Other writers said they had been allowed only 30 minutes pushing. Episiotomy is not done routinely and midwives are skilled at delivering with intact perineum. 'I was able to jump straight off that labour bed with him in my arms . . . thrilled!' Some writers were aware of conflict between midwives and medical staff. One woman objected when doctor told her to put her legs up in lithotomy stirrups so he could deliver baby. 'Sister argued with him.' He went away and she delivered baby without episiotomy.

Postnatal An amenity room with four beds. 'Very pleasant.' Other wards large and 'depressing'. Staff helpful, kind and patient and a lot of time given to help with breast-feeding. But on one ward nurses described as 'tense' and 'ridiculous rules'. 'Great emphasis put on some points of hygiene while other more obvious aspects ignored.' Elsewhere pleasant, relaxed atmosphere and friendly staff who are 'not too formal or fussy'. Baby can be with mother all the time. Night staff make cups of tea or coffee for mothers feeding their babies in small hours. But you may have to ask if you do not want baby taken to nursery at night. Feeding on demand. One writer felt 'helpless and weepy', was impressed by 'total support and encouragement from all staff' and was 'astonished by patience shown by midwives and students who spent long periods sitting on my bed helping me feed my baby'. 'Though I could not sleep they respected my wish not to take tablets.'

Suggestions Improve staff relations – get rid of hierarchy. Consultants should talk directly to mother and not just to student doctors. Improve food.

St Helier, Green Wrythe Lane, Carshalton, Surrey   MO

Old hospital, could do with massive face-lift inside and out.

Antenatal Busy. Allow at least 2 hours for visit and even then you may be pushed for time. 'No person-to-person feeling.' Not enough room for pushchairs or children's play. Writers seem to have seen the same doctor only about twice during antenatal care; 'only one doctor asked me if I had any problems or questions I wanted to ask'; 'Doctors treated me like a mindless zombie.' Writers said examinations were 'hurried' and 'impersonal'. Most writers said explanations were not readily given, one said 'everything was explained in detail. This could have been because I am a nurse.' Pessaries may be used to soften cervix before induction.

Labour Writers remark on staff shortages and how busy available staff are. Describe enema/shave. Midwives are 'efficient', 'kind', 'explain things'. But fathers are sometimes sent home; 'he was not even welcome to wait somewhere quietly'. This woman was in strong labour, but no one would send for her husband and he missed delivery. Oxytocin acceleration seemed to be frequent. Fetal monitors used. Epidurals available and 'top-ups given the minute I asked'. Caesarean section can be done under epidural and staff seem to like them that way. 'Theatre staff were enthusiastic, gave minute-by-minute account of what they were doing. Offered me baby to hold immediately and tucked her into bed with me. While we were waiting to go back my husband was holding her', but father is not allowed to be present at Caesarean birth. He can be there for forceps delivery, however, but not for amniotomy or when epidural is given. Doctors praised; 'kind and humorous doctor made me feel at ease'.

Postnatal Can demand-feed but discuss it with staff. Some writers said they were moved from one place to another without explanation; 'treated like cattle on one ward'; 'I felt the baby never really belonged to me'; 'I didn't feel free to have the baby at my bedside when I wanted to.' Writers said distilled water was provided for babies: 'given no explanation of why we had to do this'. One writer said 'in the booklet it states that the baby stays with you all the time from the fourth night on. We asked if we could keep our babies with us but were told no as it would keep other mums, bottle-feeding, awake.' Several writers described strict routines 'contrary to what they say in their booklet'. On one ward at least babies seem to be kept in nursery except at evening visiting. Mothers had to go to nursery to feed 'and there was not time for cuddling' but staff described as 'extremely kind', nursery nurses and student midwives helpful. One woman appreciated student midwife who attended her in labour coming to visit a few days later. Some writers said it was difficult to get information: 'I found you had to ask things all the time.' Staff divided over whether breast-feeding mothers should eat certain foods, e.g. strawberries. 'They kept pushing you as to if you had "been" – why didn't they give you things like bran and greens to help?' Day room for smokers; 'good idea because a lot of mums get nervous in hospital'. Babies must go to nursery on ward during afternoon visit so brothers and sisters cannot cuddle babies. Radio is played in nursery to 'help keep the babies content'.

SCBU One writer reports delay in allowing her to visit her baby even though SCBU staff were willing to come and escort her if ward was busy. SCBU is 'best thing about hospital'; relaxed atmosphere, individual help with breast-feeding and nurses spend a lot of time helping. Grandparents allowed to view but not touch. Fathers can spend time there too, including during feeds, and there are no rigid visiting hours for them; 'much better than on wards'.

Suggestions Better-planned antenatal clinics. Mirror in delivery room; 'every-body except the mother sees the birth'. Better communication and more information on postnatal wards and more staffing so there is time to help and give explanations. Improved food.

Chatham

All Saints, Magpie Hall Road, Chatham, Kent   M O

Old cottage-type hospital with long, large, overcrowded wards.

Antenatal Busy clinic. Care 'very good'; 1–2 hours wait to see obstetrician, but 'staff thorough' and 'caring' and this 'made up for the wait'; 'they are ready to answer queries'.

Labour Overcrowded labour wards 'noisy'. Woman who had Caesarean section said staff answered all questions about what was going to happen. After section baby was brought to her as soon as she came round from anaesthetic and was put to breast.

Postnatal Nurses give great help with establishing breast-feeding. Baby can be with mother at all times. Staff answer every question.

SCBU Both parents allowed in at all times; no restrictions. Father encouraged to help in looking after baby.

Suggestions More staff. More bathrooms. Longer visiting.

St John's, Wood Street, Chelmsford, Essex   M O

Very busy; large, 'uninviting'; 'bewildering'.

Antenatal Staff 'uncommunicative', questions are answered *if* you raise them; 'don't be reticent', one woman advises. Some writers were disappointed that their husbands could not be present during examinations or even sit in the waiting-room with them. Some said they felt as though 'processed through the birth machine'. Long waiting times. 'Disgusting habit of dumping empty specimen bottles in a bucket and one was expected to "fish out" your bottle from loads of others'. Some women who had shared care described only one visit to this clinic, others with GPs.

Labour Some 'super' midwives. Labour ward staff 'extremely kind'. Woman is never alone during labour. Several writers felt 'everything was done *to* me'; 'I wasn't consulted at all about anything'; 'it was all out of my control'; and were constricted and uncomfortable in bed because of monitoring equipment. Epidurals available and Caesareans can be done under epidural, but only when anaesthetist on duty. Woman who had Caesarean said, 'my husband woke me with baby in his arms'. He saw baby immediately after birth and was present while baby washed and weighed.

Postnatal Baby is with mother all the time. Day staff descriibed as 'helpful', 'considerate', but some unhelpful night staff. Theories on breast-feeding vary and writers say they got completely different answers to queries from different nurses and found this confused and confusing. Woman who had had Caesarean said her baby was 'dumped on my tummy' several times, then nurses apologized later. No day room to one ward and smoking is allowed on ward: 'I was annoyed that someone was allowed to smoke around my baby.'

Food 'absolutely diabolic', 'always badly cooked', 'not suitable for nursing mothers'.

Suggestions 'A little less bustle and a bit more consideration.' More thought should be given to breast-feeding advice. Stop allowing smoking on wards. Improve food.

St Paul's, Swindon Road, Cheltenham, Glos

Consultant unit and integrated GP unit. Shared care between consultants and' GPs and women go to antenatal clinic only for booking visit and in last four weeks. Fewer inductions than previously. SNO writes that 'induction performed only when strictly indicated'. Prostaglandins used as an alternative to amniotomy. 'Any diversion from the normal is always discussed with the patient.' Three full programmes of antenatal classes running at the same time, seven sessions per programme. Special classes for second-time mothers who can bring their other children. Breast-feeding class in early pregnancy.

Labour Shave/enema. More relaxed attitudes to electronic fetal monitoring recently. Acceleration with oxytocin was described by many writers; 'a drip to help me along after 8 hours'. Epidurals available and Caesareans done under epidural. Cassette players for music during labour. Bring your own tape or choose hospital ones. Father present throughout, including for forceps delivery and sometimes for Caesarean. Episiotomy rate 30%. SNO writes, 'if Leboyer-style deliveries are requested existing amenities would be adapted as far as practicable' . . . Alternative positions for delivery if midwife approves and mattress available to put on floor. 'Special arrangements can be made to cover all situations regarding support during labour.'

Postnatal 'Enlightened' attitudes to breast-feeding, though some nurses do not know how to help in practical ways. Babies in wards all day except for ½ hour when cleaners there, and with mothers through night if they wish. No 'interference'. Mother can pick up baby when she wants and feed whenever baby wants. 'Everyone I saw was breast-feeding' (actually 75%). Feeding can be done at visiting time but only with curtains drawn. Baby can be in bed with mother. If baby is not with her she can be woken to feed. Nurses described as 'brisk', 'helpful', 'kind', giving generous help and encouragement and there is minimum of routines. They are all very keen on breast-feeding. Some writers remark that there are too few lavatories and baths.

Visiting 3–4 p.m. and 7–8 p.m., but flexible; own children can visit.

Food 'not very nourishing for breast-feeding mothers'; 'a lot of stodge, biscuits, puddings, chips'.

SCBU 'Encourages mothers to spend as much time as they wish with their babies', according to SNO. Babies taken from SCBU to ward to visit mother if she is not well. Fathers welcome in SCBU and encouraged to handle baby. Babies' brothers and sisters can visit. Baby follow-up clinics with SCBU staff, so parents see familiar faces. Genetic counselling clinic.

231

Suggestions Partners should be able to be present for forceps delivery. Improved food.

St Peter's, Chertsey, Surrey   MO

Modern, clean, peaceful. Great strides forward recently.

Antenatal 'Impressed by friendliness and concern of doctors and nurses', but some writers say receptionists are not friendly. One said a receptionist made her leave her child in an unattended playroom with swing doors near a main road.

Labour All staff 'friendly'. Usually no enema or shave. Epidurals available on request. Pethidine appears to be used often and some women had dopey babies as a result. Delivery room, 'like large operating theatre'. Uncomfortable delivery table. Women tend to say they are 'rushed' through second stage delivery.

Postnatal Short-staffed; nurses busy and do not have enough time for everyone. Mothers left to own devices. Those nurses who want to help may be young and inexperienced, though some are very understanding. Greater flexibility now in feeding schedules. Writers said they would have liked more explanations. First-time mothers especially seemed to want more help. When advice is given it tends to be contradictory. Night staff vary; one writer said night nurse 'had most of ward in tears', 'left babies to scream' until auxiliaries came back from their break. One woman discharged herself after a similar incident.

Food 'inedible', 'appalling'. Several writers said their husbands brought in food for them.

Suggestions A special breast-feeding nurse to whom difficulties can be referred.

The West Cheshire, Liverpool Road, Chester, Cheshire   MO

Modern, purpose-built, with all up-to-date facilities. Nurses 'mainly young and unmarried' and 'tend to be unsympathetic to how a new mother feels'.

Antenatal Crowded clinic. Waits of up to 1 hour for 3-minute examination. Classes; for couples, informative, include tour of hospital. Birth plans accepted.

Labour Shave and enema no longer routine. Woman is in single room with partner. Fathers welcome and can stay for forceps delivery. Midwives 'encouraging'. Woman can choose any position which is comfortable in labour and for delivery. Writers advise making sure you empty bladder every hour or so, as some have catheter passed once bladder very full, causing possible delay in labour and unnecessary pains. Vacuum extraction often used in place of forceps. Women describe baby being put in cot by their side after delivery. Ask to hold baby if you wish.

Postnatal Baby can be with mother throughout 24 hours. Nurses do not always know who is/is not breast-feeding, who has had assisted delivery and therefore needs more care, know how to help with perineal pain or appreciate how uncomfortable it can be. Writers say most women have stitches. Many breast-feed and lots of encouragement and help given, especially by lactation sister. Apparently women are supposed to draw curtains round bed when breast-feeding; one says she was unaware of this until 'caught in the act by sister'. A depressed mother said she felt nurses did not understand and assumed that all mothers could cope. She went for bath and 'returned to third degree from nurse on my whereabouts "because your baby was crying"' and found this very upsetting.

SCBU Some writers described lack of coordination between postnatal wards and SCBU. Some on wards felt out of touch with their babies in SCBU. One who was told her baby was going there only overnight said she asked three times for her baby the following day, but was told nothing, so walked to SCBU at 3 p.m.: 'ghastly experience' after difficult delivery. When baby arrived back on ward he was crying. 'I had never done anything for my baby . . . a passing nurse asked if he was dirty. I replied I didn't know and she said, "well, change him" and passed on.'

Postnatal check-up Not always well managed: 'we sat with the baby stripped naked for an hour'. One woman was anxious on being told baby was fine except that his head was 'too big'.

Suggestions Stop 'pushing' epidurals. Do fewer episiotomies.

★ **St Richards Royal West Sussex, Chichester, W Sussex**   MO

Modern, clean, homely, relaxed atmosphere. 'Generates feeling of well-being.'

Antenatal Large numbers of patients. Children's playrooms; ultrasound scanning technician 'patient', spends time explaining what he is looking for and finding. Will take photo of baby as souvenir for mother if asked.

Labour Writers describe enema/shave. No drugs offered to mothers who have been to NCT classes unless they ask for them. Pethidine available and is sometimes given without previous examination. Several writers had had oxytocin acceleration of labour. Some felt they had been rushed through second stage; 'it seems expected of one to produce the baby as quickly as possible'. Episiotomy is not done routinely. Baby may not be delivered on to abdomen unless you *ask* first, but is left with parents after birth.

Postnatal 'I was able to do exactly as I wished with my baby for the whole of my 7-day stay.' Babies can be fed in bed. Plenty of help with breast-feeding; no water need be given but 'I found different advice given by staff on most subjects'. Babies are with mother all the time and can be fed if she wishes during visiting times. Staff, though rushed off their feet, 'most helpful' and 'kind'. Fair-skinned women may be advised to limit feeding time to 2 minutes each side to begin with and some queried whether this was sensible advice. Writers say that amenity beds are 'well worth the money' and a 'marked improvement on ward'. Extremely cheerful domestic staff. Exceptionally clean showers, lavatories, bidets and baths, rarely queues for baths, mother can have a bath at any time.

Visiting 3–4.30 p.m. amd 7.30–8.30 p.m. fathers only. Babies can stay in wards during visiting.

SCBU Two mother's beds available in it and mothers are encouraged to care for their own babies.

Suggestions Should be possible for couple to go out together for meal evening before discharge while staff babysit.

Querns Maternity, Cirencester, Glos MO

GP unit. Lovely old building with extensions of 'terrapin-type' rooms, set in lovely grounds on slight rise overlooking Cirencester. Complicated births go to Princess Margaret, Swindon, 15 miles away, but you can have a first baby here 'if you are determined'.

Antenatal No delays. Staff willing to answer questions. 'I always saw the same doctor at every visit, very pleasant, explained what he was doing and why.' Waiting-room with lots of toys for children. Staff happy to care for children while mother being examined or child can go in with mother. Good relaxation classes and fathers welcome; 'he did not wish to come to classes, but did and thoroughly enjoyed every one'. Evening visit to look over hospital. If husband cannot make this he can make another appointment.

Labour No inductions, although ARM sometimes done. Final decision as to whether to have amniotomy is left with woman. Mini-shave/small enema described by most writers. Woman is encouraged to walk about, use breathing learned in class. Meal is served in early labour if she wants it. She is told to ask if she wants any pain-relieving drugs. One woman who requested pethidine was asked by sister, 'Do you really want it? I don't think you've much longer to go.' Baby was born ½ hour after. 'Dull' delivery room 'though one hardly notices with the cheerful staff around'. Supported by cushions through second stage, partner's arm round shoulders, woman gripping under her knees. Midwives skilled at avoiding episiotomy. Writers say that nurses do not agree with full Leboyer-style delivery, but everything is quiet, calm and lights not bright. Baby wrapped and given to father to hold while placenta delivered, then handed to mother and midwife helps her to put baby to breast. 'When I asked the doctor if she was alright he replied that he hadn't seen her yet and then we all realized that everyone was so excited he had just stood in the background and let us get on with it.' Baby then taken away and mother wheeled to ward.

Postnatal Small wood-panelled wards. Under-occupied much of time. 'The nursery nurse is a dear. Nothing is too much trouble. She likes to introduce mother to baby by letting baby lie with just a nappy next to mother's breast and encourages mother to stroke and talk softly to baby . . . a beautiful experience.' Breast-feeding encouraged but bottle-feeding mothers not frowned on. Feeding usually 4-hourly but woman who intends to demand-feed should tell staff in advance and she can do so. One woman tried to get permission to be woken to feed during first 2 nights but was told she must have her rest. After the first night she insisted and was woken. Baby is given water if wakes between night and early morning feed. Very strict hour's rest after lunch, when baby is taken to nursery. Mother can visit nursery whenever she likes and take baby up to ward. Babies are not allowed on beds. Nursing chair next to each bed. 'A couple of times I fed her in bed. It raised an eyebrow or two, but nothing was said.' Nursery is at end of short corridor, large and bright with low nursing chairs for mothers feeding during the night. Small but warm bathrooms with plenty of salt available. Pleasant block of lavatories. Everyone eats around table overlooking garden at end of ward, including staff sometimes. Mother can be with baby when examined by paediatrician.

Food *delicious*, always hot, well-balanced and plenty of it, meal is kept hot if feeding baby. Choose from menu day before. Milky drink offered in evening. Tea-tray brought to mother while breast-feeding at night ('Wonderful!').

Own children can visit only two afternoons, Saturday and Sunday, ½ hour each day, but mother can go down to reception to see child at other times. Child may not see baby until mother returns home.

'Auxiliary always asks if there is anything you want washed when she brings round evening drinks'; 'I felt as if I had come home from a week's holiday in a hotel rather than a maternity unit. They were all my friends'; 'a cosy home-from-home and I was sad to leave it'.

Suggestions Visiting hours for children should be extended to more than a half hour on Saturdays and Sundays, and they should be able to cuddle their baby brother or sister.

Coventry Maternity Hospital, Walsgrave, Coventry

Consultant and GP units.

Antenatal Clinic 3½ miles from hospital; held in afternoons only. DNO writes: 'Positive action is being taken to improve the clinic facilities.' Women describe 'cattle-market' care and say it is 'horrific'. Two-hour waits. Husband/mother/ woman friend not allowed in to examination, different doctor every time. 'Tried to discuss episiotomy but was brushed aside with "That's a medical decision that only we can make. We know what's best for you and it's not your place to query our judgement . . . That's not your concern, it is up to the doctor to decide."' Though induction rate low – 12% in 1980 – women sometimes felt they had insufficient information to make up their own minds whether to agree to be induced. They said they were told that it was routine practice to give pethidine before amniotomy with induction, but this can be declined.

Labour 'Very relaxed, friendly atmosphere', 'everyone considerate', 'all the help and understanding I wanted', and a writer who had a baby there 4 years previously commented on improvements and said she no longer felt 'treated as an object in a baby factory' and that midwives were kind and helpful. But writers found it difficult to cope with sheer numbers of staff dealing with them. 'Nurses and doctors and midwives continually came and went.' When there were a lot of people around women did not always feel they had emotional support: 'no explanations, encouragement or advice during 17 hours'. Complete shave discontinued and now mini-shave only, but writer who asked not to have shave was told, 'You have to, I'm afraid', and it was promptly done. Women advise, 'Insist on the things that you feel are important to you.' Partner can be present throughout, including often for forceps delivery, and can hold baby afterwards. But treatment varies and some husbands were asked to leave before forceps delivery and some 'thrown out' every time woman examined. Electronic monitoring often used. 'I didn't like having my movements severely restricted.' 'I couldn't get comfortable . . . would have preferred sitting in a chair or more upright but I had the FHM on and that was why I was in bed.' 'Painful to have monitor button pushed into my side when contraction came.' Several women told to lie on their sides all through first stage found this uncomfortable and would have preferred to walk around. Pethidine offered but woman is not under pressure to have it. Writers apparently had large doses and said they were 'confused' or could not push. Epidurals available and Caesarean section done under epidural, highly recommended by some writers. 'To have my baby delivered under an epidural the next best thing to natural delivery.' Consultants seem often to recommend epidurals: 'I was not given much choice', 'Doctor wanted to use epidural; said I wasn't going to dilate quickly enough . . . midwives thought I had dilated more than doctor thought,' wrote woman who reached full dilatation 20 minutes afterwards. Staff shortages sometimes produce problems as with woman who had 22-hour labour and wrote that she wasn't offered washing facilities during this time beause of lack of staff and so 'felt awful'. Women describe pushing lying down on their backs, though some were allowed to choose their own position for second stage. Some said they were urged to push when they did not feel like it – 'staff were in too much of a hurry' – others that they could choose their own pace. Seems to depend on midwives. Some said they were told '1-hour time-limit on pushing', 'longer tires you and distresses the baby'. 'Difficult to push for as long and as hard as the midwife wanted me to.' Doctors and midwives praised for 'explaining all that was happening and calling my husband down to tell me what he could see as the head gradually appeared'.

Some women said that they had inadequate back support. They wanted to sit up to push. One asked for bed to be pushed up to wall and pillows brought, and said midwives were helpful. Writers who did not think of asking for this had less happy experiences. 'I wish some support had been at my back as I exhausted myself sitting up every time I wanted to push.'

Some insensitive care described in second stage. One writer said two midwives had a leg each: 'while I was pushing sometimes one of them would walk off leaving me off-balance'; 'First they told me to push and then said I mustn't, then changed their minds again. They would walk out of the door saying "Don't push" as I was struggling away trying hard not to'; 'The midwife was urging me to push when I did not have a contraction and I was unable to get into a proper breathing-pushing rhythm'; 'One doctor was saying to another that I wasn't pushing hard enough.' A senior member of staff 'persuaded me into pushing harder then brusquely ordered an episiotomy'.

Midwives gentle at deliveries. If you ask, lights are turned down and the baby delivered on to your abdomen. Can be breast-fed soon after. 'I was given the baby immediately and allowed to feed him. He was then cleaned up and handed back to me. They tucked him into bed with me and took us up to the ward with him feeding merrily.' Good midwifery care described in **GP unit**, though here again, 'I wanted to push with urge but midwife wanted me to push for whole of contraction.'

Some long waits to be stitched and women describe waiting 2 hours and stitching taking over an hour 'with my husband outside separated from me and the baby'. Forceps rate 13%, vacuum extraction 2%, Caesarean section 9%. 'Some doctors did not appreciate how painful episiotomy could be. The doctor laughed it off. Eventually the SNO saw me. Stitches were then removed. I felt much better.'

Postnatal Overcrowded wards and staff shortages mean that nurses have insufficient time to help with breast-feeding. 'Mothers need to be strong-headed and determined.' Some said staff were 'caring, friendly and gave me a lot of support' and that they had 'nothing but sympathy and kindness from the staff'. Others talked about 'bossy' nurses. 'There were lots of rules which I ignored, but they intimidated younger and less confident women.' Demand-feeding practised, but baby may not be allowed in bed with mother though some took no notice of this rule. DNO says 'Babies are roomed in during the day and also at night if the mother wishes this.' Iodine bubble-baths used for perineal pain.

Forty-eight-hour discharge can be arranged but some women met with resistance in trying to organize this.

SCBU A writer who had 48-hour separation from her baby says she was allowed to see him only twice in that time. 'Nurse didn't have time to let me breast-feed or help me express. He was bottle-fed against my wishes.' Result was engorged breasts, trouble in starting to feed and that she felt 'baby was not mine'.

Suggestions Some (male) obstetricians could be more 'approachable'. Women should not be put under pressure by being offered pethidine repeatedly.

Partners should not be sent out every time doctor examines. Look at ways of reducing stress put on women in second stage. Some women who were handed baby only *after* cord cut would have liked to hold baby before this.

St Mary's Maternity Hospital,
Lodge Road, Croydon, Greater London

'Dingy, dark, cramped hospital. Gloomy corridors, most wards badly lit.' *Antenatal* DNO writes 'The inadequacies of this clinic are recognized but a new purpose-built clinic is to be started on the Mayday site'. (See Mayday Hospital, Thornton Heath.) Toys available for children in the waiting area. Electronic fetal monitoring may be done.

Labour Three beds in first-stage room; also day room which women can use while in labour. No pain-relieving drug is given to a woman against her wishes. Epidurals not available. DNO says that 'Modified Leboyer-style deliveries are undertaken if requested.' Episiotomies not routinely done.

Postnatal Demand-feeding encouraged. Baby can now be with mother all the time. Women can care for babies as they like. Ward staff mostly 'helpful', 'cheerful', 'sympathetic', 'morale high in spite of run-down appearance of hospital'. Babies demand-fed whether by breast or bottle. Some writers hated being woken at 5.30 a.m. 'shaken awake roughly'; 'my feeble attempts to avoid this by writing notes to say when I'd finished feeding baby and sticking them on my thermometer were totally ignored'. Not enough baths or wash-basins and no bidets. Writers felt hospital was under-staffed at night: 'nobody could be found between 2 a.m. and 4.30 a.m. most nights'.

Opinions on food vary. There is no choice, but some writers thought meals were imaginative, wholesome and sensibly planned. Vegetarians, however, complained of minute portions and described breakfast as being boiled egg, lunch omelette, and supper two fried eggs: 'staff wondered why I was constipated'.

Women delivered at Mayday may be moved here 1–2 days after birth. 'I found this upheaval 2 days after giving birth very disrupting and exhausting. It is bad enough to have to get used to the routine in one hospital without having to go through the process twice in one week.' 'My husband was able to "spring" the baby and me from St Mary's only 6 days after the birth. I cannot see why the full stay of 8 days has to be so rigorously adhered to. If I'd stayed in hospital any longer I would have needed to be hospitalized again for sheer exhaustion and lack of sleep.'

Suggestions Do not get mothers up so early. Improve decoration, bathing and washing facilities. Extend visiting to every afternoon. Restriction on *numbers* visiting would make visiting time 'less exhausting in cramped, stuffy, little wards'. Better training of catering staff to cope with vegetarian meals.

Cuckfield, Sussex MO

'Excellent' care from 'helpful', 'encouraging' staff.

Antenatal Most women who wrote had been induced when one week past due date and felt they had no choice. Prostaglandin pessaries were used for induction and waters broken about 3 hours after but they said they were asked first whether they would have amniotomy.

Labour Warm reception from all staff. Several writers said they were not shaved and did not have enemas. Midwives praised; help with breathing, are 'calming', 'not patronizing', 'seemed able to read my thoughts'. 'There was real communication.' Woman is able to walk around in first stage. Father encouraged to help, to massage back and support emotionally, though may be told to wait outside during admission procedures. Pethidine/gas and oxygen offered and may be advised, but mother can decline. Electronic fetal monitoring used frequently. Partograms used. Some mothers wished they could have more pillows in second stage. Midwives may ask woman to put one foot on her hip and other on her husband's. May lift woman so she can see baby's head after it is born. Episiotomy is not done routinely. Delivery quiet and lights dimmed; 'a great help'. Baby put straight on mother's body, then wrapped and handed back to be put to breast. Some writers said couple had time alone together, others that midwife suggested that husband leave shortly after so that mother could rest – 'the last thing I felt like'. Mother and baby may be wheeled to ward together, though some babies were taken to be bathed and mother was taken to ward. Some fathers here have cut cord. Writers suggested that Caesarean section rates here were on high side.

Postnatal Large wards, mostly full. All staff described as 'kind'.

Suggestions Better back-support available in second stage so that woman can be upright if she wishes.

West Hill, Dartford, Kent MO

Antenatal 'Cattle market'; 'overcrowded'; 'cramped'; 'poor organization'. Writers say appointments system does not work well. Partners are discouraged from prison'. Women who were happy to feed their babies at set times and common and some writers said that this waiting time could be better used. When one writer complained she says she was told, 'it's you who wants the baby, so put up with it'. Some doctors 'aloof', 'try to suppress questions'; 'one continually discussed my case with a student and I didn't get a chance to ask anything'. Woman who had scan would have liked to know what it revealed. Staff sometimes 'unhelpful', 'ill-mannered' (e.g. don't say please and thank you) and some nurses 'condescending', e.g. 'where's your wee?' Writer's felt 'processed'. Woman who looked at her file was 'found out' and reprimanded in front of other patients. Some writers said there was poor coordination with GP. One who wanted to know if she had rubella anti-bodies could not get

Doncaster

information. Writers said they were advised to book for 10 days for first babies otherwise 'you won't be able to cope'. Forty-eight-hour discharge possible, but you have to be firm if this is what you want. When one woman started labour 2 weeks early her husband simply said, 'Relief! No more visits to the clinic.'

Labour Writers say they had mini-shaves/enema. Partners excluded for this. Midwives 'kind', 'charming', 'enlightened', 'relaxed and friendly'. Pethidine offered. In second stage told to get three pushes into each contraction, which some women found was not helpful. Also were told to start pushing as soon as contraction began. Doctor also urged this. One woman said she would have liked to get into her own rhythm. Plenty of pillows, but with plastic covers, which slip; partner then has to replace them. Father can usually be present for forceps delivery.

Postnatal Mothers supposed to be in bed for 6 hours after childbirth. Ward busy and understaffed. Ask if you want attention. Twenty-four-hour rooming-in after first 4 nights but 'deviousness and insistence helped me keep my baby the second night'. Others say babies in nursery are given dextrose. Conflicting advice about babies crying; 'I was told off for carrying my child around.' Other nurses suggest cuddling baby in bed. Others again say babies must not be on mother's bed. Though feeding is on demand, it is strictly timed. Mother who said she fed every hour if necessary, though told this was 'too often' and that she must not feed longer than 3 minutes, did so nevertheless; 'the best policy is to get on with what you have decided and ignore raised eyebrows'.

Suggestions Antenatal clinic 'staff should be educated to realize that patients are adult human beings, interested in doing the right thing for themselves and their babies'. Questions should be encouraged. More cushions in delivery-room. Some mothers would prefer not to have baby in nursery first night and would have slept better with baby within reach. Repair clanking noise in heating system in delivery room. Ten-day postnatal stay should be reduced to 5.

Doncaster Royal Infirmary, Doncaster, S Yorks   MO

Antenatal No appointments times; sometimes wait of 1½ hours plus. Toys for children have been removed. Encouraged to ask questions but no guidance with breast-feeding in antenatal clinic. 'The talk during parentcraft classes was unrealistic, emphasized how easy breast-feeding was, without any advice on how to overcome possible setbacks and problems.' Film show every month to which partners invited. One writer suggested, 'Some talks should be done at the beginning of pregnancy about caring for yourself, eating the right type of food and there should also be more discussion on breast-feeding.' Clinic 'overbooked and under-staffed'. Staff 'gentle and pleasant' but 'you cannot make any relationship with them'. No time to discuss problems. 'The hospital mass booking system makes you feel like a cow.' One woman said she would have liked some privacy so she could feel free to discuss problems without fear of being overheard. Several women admitted for induction said that there was no possibility of discussion: 'the doctor I mostly saw was foreign and his English was difficult to follow. The impression given was that of a troublesome production line, made up of imbeciles.' Some writers said their husbands were informed about their reasons for induction but they themselves could not share in making decisions about care.

Antenatal ward: 'Care could not be faulted' but some writers felt they needed some psychological support; 'I found separation from my 2-year-old very difficult and the worry about him was sometimes intolerable, but no member of staff showed much concern over this' and she had no opportunity to talk it over.

Labour One woman who had her first baby in this hospital a few years ago said that it had 'greatly improved'. Epidurals available. For some reason most women wrote about ante- and postnatal care and seemed to feel they were processed smoothly through labour, without having any choices.

Postnatal Some writers said they felt they were expected to be very passive; 'when I left the consultant thanked me for being a good patient. I suppose because I did everything asked and made no trouble, but I was desperately unhappy.' Several women indicated that they wished relationships with staff could have been more personal. Advise Domino scheme, which is in operation here, in preference to consultant care.

Suggestions Appointment system in antenatal clinic to reduce waiting time. Somewhere for children to play in clinic. More understanding of psychology of birth.

Russet County, Somerleigh Court, Dorchester, Dorset MO

'Efficient place'; 'care for well-being of both mother and baby'.

Antenatal 'Any questions I had were answered fully' but different doctor seen most times. 'Good antenatal classes run by midwife and a Health Visitor but initial biology lesson repeated so often that I could have taught it to a class of 14-year-olds quite adequately.' Breathing taught. Realistic description of hospital procedures. Visit to labour ward useful. Labour rehearsal with partners helpful, giving them an idea of what to expect. Monitoring and acceleration explained.

Labour Partners may be sent away for prepping, otherwise present througout. Writers said they had mini-shave/suppositories/bath. It sounds as if labour is frequently accelerated with oxytocin. One writer who was admitted at 10 a.m. with slight contractions and waters dribbling was immediately put on drip. Electronic monitoring also used. 'It was on the blink and emitting piercing whine . . .' 'Midwives were reassuring about the state of the baby.' Pethidine sometimes given late in first stage. One woman described being given second 'small' dose and having to be woken up to push. In second stage woman is propped up with pillows and helped to sit up. Episiotomy not done routinely. Baby is checked and then handed to mother immediately, and then taken away to be weighed, returned to mother and she is encouraged to put baby to breast. Couple have some time together with baby, but if night baby then goes to nursery. Woman who was delivered at midnight said she was not cleaned up and taken to ward until 3 a.m. Auxiliaries told her they had to clean and change babies in nursery first. Her husband had left at 1.30 a.m. and baby was in nursery.

Postnatal Baby is by mother's bed in day and in nursery at night. Reports from 1979 indicate that for first 2 nights baby is given bottle, but baby is brought to mother for feeding after that. Demand-feeding can be practised if you decide in advance and tell nurses; otherwise several mothers describe 4-hourly routine. (Has this changed?) One writer said that not many women chose to have babies with them at night. Nurses 'helpful', 'cheerful'. Always prepared to answer questions. Excellent night sisters do round of each ward chatting to every mother. One woman was annoyed that her baby was examined in her absence and without asking her permission, 'I went for a bath and returned to find my baby crying in a damp cot with his nappy removed and a paediatrician cheerfully said, "I'll leave you to sort him out."' Queues form for lavatories in morning even when wards not full.

Suggestions Baby should be given paediatric examination in front of mother and she should be able to have discussion with paediatrician. More lavatories.

Eastbourne District and General, Eastbourne, E Sussex   MO

Large, brand-new buildings, well-designed, spacious, clean but impersonal. 'Lovely, purpose-built maternity wards with large windows overlooking fields.' 'Latest equipment, but I felt lost in the efficiency.' Several writers found atmosphere unfriendly.

Antenatal 'Brisk', 'efficient', 'a succession of doctors and I don't know who else busy asking questions and filling in the sacred forms'. One writer said she felt awkward asking questions and when staff tried to answer them 'they always seemed to suggest that the pregnancy was their problem, not mine' . . . 'When I mentioned Leboyer I was taken aside by sister and told birth would be painful and I would need pethidine and gas and oxygen. Not very encouraging!' Opportunity to visit wards.

Labour 'Succession of nurses and midwives, none of whom I had seen before or saw again after the birth.' Partner can be there throughout. No help with breathing from staff, but 'repeated offers' of pethidine. 'Midwife suggested if I didn't take pethidine I wouldn't be able to manage later on . . . I wish I'd had the wits to ask for only a very small dose.' Strict rules about not doing frequent vaginal examinations, so some writers said the baby's head was on perineum before midwife realized mother was fully dilated.

Postnatal 'I was bewildered when my baby was taken away for 3 hours just after birth. When the nurse eventually handed her to me she would not allow me to just cuddle her, but insisted on putting her to the breast. She tried to ram my nipple into the baby's mouth. The baby started screaming. I felt like a machine. After about 5 minutes I started crying.' Nurse left, another nurse came and took baby away. Brought next feeding time. 'Another nurse said, "ah, you are the mother who doesn't want to feed her baby." I burst into tears again. She came back, apologized and helped me feed the baby.' Demand-feeding allowed but 'a big inconvenience to their routine'; 'I never had any problem feeding, only with the hospital staff.' One writer who fed her baby again when the baby cried immediately after a feed was told by nurse she would make the baby ill: 'Sister said baby would get stomach-ache and told me I was a bad mother.' 'I was torn between my instincts and the conflicting, rigid demands of staff.' Valium was prescribed, which she refused: 'they had so much power and were so superficially polite'. Leaving was 'like being released from prison'. Women who were happy to feed their babies at set times and leave them in the nursery at night liked the hospital. These reports came from 1979, so it is worth asking if things have changed. Writers said there were 'many staff coming and going', that it was 'difficult to get explanations', and that mothers were not informed when paediatrician examined their babies. 'I only saw the doctor once by accident when he examined the baby and he didn't say anything to me, only to the nurse.' Physiotherapist 'friendly', 'constructive'. Mod. cons. greatly appreciated.

Suggestions Doctors interested in caring for emotional as well as physical health. More flexibility. Much more information available to mothers, especially about feeding.

Chase Farm Hospital, The Ridgeway, Enfield, Greater London

Consultant and GP units. Insufficient reports from mothers were received about consultant unit to include it here, but SNO kindly provided statistics for 1980; induction rate 29%, forceps 14%, vacuum extraction 0.7%, episiotomy 48%, Caesarean section 13%. She writes, 'there have not been any changes of policy since last insertion in your book'.

★ *GP unit* Antenatal care shared between GP and midwife.

Labour Writers say they got to know midwife well during pregnancy and she was called when they were admitted in labour. 'It was like being greeted by an old friend.' Relaxed and happy atmosphere. Writers most appreciated continuity of care.

Postnatal Own midwife comes in to check mother and baby, own GP if there are problems. No rules. Can demand-feed. 'The assumption is that you know what you are doing' and that 'you are just there for a few days' rest and staff are there to relieve you of physical work, give advice if needed and check that all is well with mother and baby'. Atmosphere of complete freedom. 'The staff were our friends.' 'I felt as if I was staying in a very superior hotel.' 'I can't remember hearing a single "don't" during my stay.' 'We were left to sleep until the babies woke in the morning.' 'Night sister sat down with us at breakfast and chatted about her work. Midwife told me about her coming holiday. They get their work done in spite of being short-staffed.' Whole family encouraged to get to know baby. Unrestricted visiting, children welcome. Some writers contrast their stay here with other hospital experiences. One was very surprised that 'none of us got the "weeps"'.

Epsom District, Woodcote Road, Epsom, Surrey   MO

'Fairly modern', 'not cramped', 'bright wards', 'clean', 'cosy'. Understaffed.

Antenatal Booking-in clinic involves longest wait, about 1½ hours. Usual wait about 1 hour. A few toys for toddlers. Rare to have same nurse doing several things to you, yet all reassuring, 'cheerful'. 'I was welcomed by the reception-ist, then the nurse and finally the registrar or houseman, and this friendliness outweighed any long waits.' 'I felt I was more than just a name on a list because they remembered my name.' Women disliked waiting around 'sometimes in cold with scanty gown on'. Though some registrars described as 'brisk', 'they allowed me to hear my baby's heartbeats'; 'the pelvic X-ray was shown to me and explained, but in medical terms I could not understand'. Several writers described induction with prostaglandin gel overnight, prostaglandin tablets in morning following ARM.

Labour Partner can be there all the time, is encouraged to mop face, etc. Woman is able to walk about in first stage. Pethidine sometimes encouraged, though other woman said drugs were not 'pushed'. Two writers said they were told by midwives they were receiving standard dose 200 mg Phenergan, and warned if you want lower dose, be very firm about it. Some writers said they were given pethidine they did not want, others that it was given much too late at onset of second stage. 'Midwife was most cooperative in letting me do what I felt happiest doing.' 'All my questions were fully answered.' 'I felt among friends,' said one writer, commenting on 'sincerity' and 'warmth' of staff. Baby given to mother wrapped; couple have extended time together with baby after delivery, but partner must leave room during stitching.

Postnatal Breast-feeding strongly encouraged and nurses helpful. Baby is with mother all the time, except that baby expected to go to nursery first 2 nights. Mother who said she wanted baby with her encountered no objections. Several writers advise amenity bed, private room on ground floor with french doors opening on to terrace and lovely gardens . . . One said she enjoyed 'happy, easy atmosphere', but didn't think she would have had such a restful time on ward. Woman can get up 6 hours after delivery. Nurses 'caring' and 'kind'; no agency staff employed. Mother can care for baby as she likes, without interference but nurses willing to help if required. 'They did not try to take over our babies. We were allowed to do whatever we felt right.' *But* different shifts have different methods and ideas, and there is no continuity. First-time mothers were confused by conflicting advice. The leaflet states that all babies are demand-fed but not more than 3-hourly. 'Wake baby after 6 hours sleep during day'. Feeding time limited to 3 minutes each breast first day, 5 minutes second, 7 minutes third, 10 minutes fourth. 'Please try not to feed at meal times.' After Caesarean section baby is in nursery until seventh day. Mothers may have one cigarette after each meal, but may not smoke in lavatories, bathrooms or shower rooms. A woman who decided to bottle-feed said nobody queried her decision. One suffering from 'baby blues' said everyone was most sympathetic. Pain-killers and sleeping tablets offered but 'not pushed'. Some writers found it difficult to get baths because 'half the time there was no hot water'.

Food 'average', 'little choice', 'inadequate for breast-feeding mothers'.

Restricted visiting, only ½ hour in afternoon and 1 hour evening, but writers say staff are 'easy-going' and 'stretch it out a bit'. Own children may visit in afternoon. Forty-eight-hour discharge possible.

SCBU Parents encouraged to visit whenever they can; 'this gave us more time together'. Are encouraged to cuddle, feed and change baby and can stay as long as they wish.

Suggestions More continuity of care. One writer, who said she 'missed my husband, son and my link with the outside world', was among those who wanted extended visiting.

Royal Devon and Exeter (Heavitree), Gladstone Road, Exeter, Devon   HO

Consultant unit. DNO writes: in delivery suite 'the decor is pleasant, incorporating double-glazing, curtains, wallpaper; taped music and a radio is incorporated with the nurse-call system. Telephone points and a trolley phone' . . . Mothers are encouraged to have husband, relative or friend with them during labour and at deliveries. Epidural anaesthesia available . . . Induction rate 23%; forceps 16%; Caesarean section 13%. Women can be transferred to GP unit near their homes if they wish after delivery.

SCBU DNO writes: 'Every effort is made to keep mother and baby as near to each other as possible so that parents can share in their baby's care.'

Blackbrook Maternity Home, 32 The Avenue, Fareham, Hants   HO

GP unit. Eleven miles from St Mary's in Portsmouth and linked by motorway; old Georgian house lying in its own grounds; friendly, relaxed and peaceful atmosphere. Has Resuscitair and incubator for transferring sick babies.

Antenatal Clinic once a week; visited by consultant. Some home births done by midwives working here. No induction, but occasional oil/bath/enema by community midwife. Nursing officer writes: 'Mothers receive almost continuous individual attention when in labour. Husbands are allowed to be present and encouraged for the delivery, although in the early stages of labour before the mother is in the labour ward they tend to go home and come back when they wish. Sonicaid [ultrasound] available. Episiotomy rate 23%.'

Postnatal Nursing officer writes that breast-feeding on demand is 'permitted, although most patients seem happy at having the baby fed at routine times. It is optional whether babies are roomed in . . . they are usually in the nursery all the morning as the mothers sleep to make up for early rising and staying up to feed the babies in the evenings; 85% of mothers breast-feed. We find this sleep is helpful as otherwise when husbands come in the evening the mothers are exhausted and sometimes tearful.'

Visiting 3–4 p.m. and own children can come. Nursing officer says that: 'Relatives who have difficulty visiting during the set hours are usually let in at any time.'

Community midwives can book their patients in and take them home after 48 hours. Women delivered in St Mary's at Portsmouth are transferred here for postnatal care.

Gloucester Maternity, Gloucester

Consultant and GP unit. Husband, relative or friend can be present during labour and delivery. Several women said they had 'a very good response from midwife when I told her I had been to NCT classes'. Mini-shave/no routine enema. All staff introduce themselves. Woman may be asked if she agrees to electronic monitoring and specific reason given for its use. Writers liked the way their partners were kept informed of everything and told what to do to be most helpful. And said that at no time were they asked to leave. Midwives will delay clamping cord until it stops pulsating.

Postnatal DNO says babies roomed in 24-hours a day and are fed on demand. Baby may be tucked in bed with mother. 'Nobody touched the baby without asking me first.' If mother is feeding at mealtime her food is kept hot or brought to her in bed. Most mothers breast-feed.

SCBU Open visiting for parents; own children and grandparents can visit; mothers encouraged to help with their baby's care; two overnight rooms for mothers.

Suggestions Food needs improving/more of it.

Blake Maternity Home, Ham Lane, Elson, Gosport, Hants HO

GP unit. Unit was redecorated in 1980.

Antenatal Two consultant clinics a week and two midwives' clinics. Shared care with GP. No inductions. Nursing officer writes, 'Episiotomy is only performed when an obstetric indication warrants this procedure.'

Postnatal She writes, 'We have implemented changes, we encourage each mother to treat her babe as an individual, by demand-feeding and handling their babes themselves, with support from the midwifery staff.'

Northgate Hospital, Northgate Street, Great Yarmouth, Norfolk HO

Old, single-storeyed building.

Antenatal Community midwives visit all mothers in their homes twice, or more if required. Mothers have their midwife's telephone number and, says DNO, 'are encouraged to ask for support and advice whenever they feel the need'. Ultrasound scanning available and all screening tests for high-risk pregnancies. Mothers seen at least three times by one of three consultants. Parentcraft and relaxation classes and tour of maternity unit. Films and discussions for both parents and group discussions on breast-feeding. Midwifery sister who coordinates midwifery programme also does counselling on postnatal ward.

Labour DNO writes: 'The rate for induction and augmentation remains stable. There has been no increase in the rate of forceps delivery and very little increase in the rate of Caesarean section.' Forceps/Caesarean sections 28%, for medical reasons. Electronic monitoring is used selectively. Partner can be present throughout labour. Mother can hold and feed her baby after delivery.

Postnatal DNO writes that 'the atmosphere everywhere is as relaxed as it is possible to achieve in a hospital situation. Babies stay by their mother's bedside, although the mother may request that the baby goes to the nursery at night and is returned for feeding. Babies are fed at their request and complements given only when absolutely necessary.' Twelve-hour to 10-day discharge can be arranged in advance. DNO writes: 'The midwives are fighting hard to maintain their status and to regain some of the ground they have lost due to medical advancement in the past few years.'

Grimsby Maternity Hospital, Second Avenue, Grimsby, S Humberside

Consultant unit Old building.

Antenatal Care shared with GPs. 'Apparently all the women waiting had been given the same appointment.' Women describe long waits and may be left alone in examination rooms for about 10 minutes before doctor comes in. Writers found doctors unsympathetic: 'It seemed the doctor resented me

247

Grimsby

taking any of his time.' Husband is allowed to attend when woman has scan 'though not while I was getting dressed'. 'Working of scan was explained fully to us both and we were invited to look at the screen.' Some women found it difficult to raise subjects for discussion with obstetrician: 'It was slightly frowned on to inquire about anything like episiotomy. After all, I wasn't the first person to have a baby!' Couples invited to visit hospital to be shown round. DNO describes all staff as friendly 'and try to give mothers individual attention throughout their pregnancy'. She says that labour is induced for medical reasons only; 18% induction rate.

Labour Women describe full shave/enema. Fathers encouraged to be present during labour and delivery but may be told to wait outside during admission procedures. May also be told to go home and rest if nothing much is happening. If night woman may then be given sleeping tablet. Some writers thought midwives hostile to NCT. One woman who said she had been to NCT classes says she was told, 'Oh, one of *those*!' Walking about in first stage encouraged but amniotomy seems to be done routinely. Pethidine is offered, apparently in large doses: 'It completely knocked me out.' Some women said that it was given without them asking for it. Electronic fetal monitoring may be used. One woman says she thinks someone should have shown her husband how to rub her back. Dilatation chart on wall was explained to couple by 'very sweet, efficient midwife'.

Second stage. Women are encouraged to push with feet on midwives' hips. Some were disappointed at not being allowed to sit up to push and not being able to see their babies born. Partner is sent out before forceps delivery. Episiotomies not routinely done. Modified Leboyer delivery arranged when requested. Husband may be asked to leave before stitching. 'I do think the doctor could at least have spoken.' 'With the main lights off and just a light on my tail end, he reminded me of a watch-mender.'

Postnatal 'Most of the staff were smashing! They put their arms round you on weepy days.' Babies are by the mothers' bed during the day, but DNO says that 'Most mothers ask for them to be taken to the nursery at night. They are wakened to feed their babies at night if they wish.' Grimsby is School of Midwifery and DNO emphasizes that students are taught 'to treat each mother as an individual within a family unit'. Writers say that when shifts change information is not passed on well enough to next nurse, both in labour and on postnatal wards. Simplest to keep baby with you if you have single room as there is shortage of space in main wards. Pain-killers 'given out freely'. Ice-packs or heat lamps available on request for perineal pain. Cups of tea often brought round. Women can smoke on wards, but 'not over baby'. Writers describe shortage of baths: 'a day-long race to get a bath'. Bidets available. Depression treated with much sympathy.

Fathers can visit at any time and own children in the afternoons. Visiting for others 3–4 p.m. and 7.30–8.30 p.m.

Food 'edible but that's all'. When baby is in nursery mothers can go in whenever they wish.

Mothers and babies may be transferred to Croft Baker Maternity Home, Cleethorpes, for postnatal stay.

SCBU Visiting is encouraged and DNO says that 'Mothers handle their babies as much as possible'. 'Whole family can go in wearing gowns, masks, slippers, they all cuddled the baby.' Baby is brought to mother for feeds if she does not want to go down and if baby is well enough.

Suggestions Better coordination between shifts. Partner should be able to be present for admission procedures and forceps delivery: 'I mean he is going to see it all anyway, isn't he?' He should be offered drinks during labour. Cleaners need guidance about what they say to new mothers – 'Set off bouts of weeping' when they criticize. More bathrooms, evening visiting fathers only.

Mount Alvernia, Guildford, Surrey   MO

Private hospital, owned and managed by nuns. GP patients and private patients with consultants. Facilities for Caesarean sections. Comfortable.

Labour Midwives, especially nuns, 'sympathetic', 'kind', 'understanding', 'eager to discuss things with mothers', but not used to women with NCT-type preparation and attitudes. 'Assumption that woman is most concerned with adequate pain relief.' Husbands welcome and encouraged to stay throughout unless labour is prolonged. One writer mentioned limit on pushing of 10 minutes for no clear reason. Episiotomy appears to be done rather frequently. 'Everyone seems to have stitches.' Baby delivered on to mother's abdomen and given to parents straight away. Suturing is done immediately.

Postnatal Demand-feeding approved of in principle but not in practice, e.g. not at meal times. Babies supposed to be in nursery at night and during afternoon rest hour. Mother who has single room can keep baby with her 24 hours, however, if persistent. Some writers said babies in nursery at night may be left to cry if feed not 'due'. Overworked night staff 'inflexible but well-meaning'; 'looking after your own baby at night is discouraged'. Conflicting, inaccurate, often discouraging breast-feeding advice, e.g. 'He's a large baby so you'll not have enough for him; you'd better give a top-up' and 'He's a small baby so he needs plenty of food; you'd better give a top-up.' ('Test-weighing was a torture.') Writers say nearly all babies have complementary feeds from first day 'while we're waiting for the milk to come in'. Routines rigid. Nursing care good. 'Staff give impression their job is to look after your baby *for* you', and all seem to agree they got opportunity to rest. Some felt they could not recommend Mount Alvernia to first-time mothers wishing to breast-feed and if they do decide on Mount Alvernia they should get all the information they can about breast-feeding before going in. Food very good. Long visiting hours. No special care facilities for babies.

Suggestions Women should be treated as new mothers, not as patients needing rest'.

Guildford

★ **St Luke's Hospital, Guildford, Surrey**

Old buildings but very clean. Overcrowded. Many improvements in this hospital in last few years. Inconvenient layout in maternity wing. Labour ward reached only by going through antenatal ward and postnatal ward one floor above SCBU. Community midwives work here too.

Antenatal Staff friendly. Women can visit labour and postnatal wards in advance and equipment is explained. Saturday morning, the husbands too can ask questions. Nurses considerate, kind, though working at high pressure. GP patients visit once only at 36 weeks. Wait of about 15–20 minutes. Waiting area is line of chairs at back of changing rooms. Examination rooms down either side and opening into waiting area. 'Too many people get passed from one person to another and can't get questions answered.'

Labour Partner welcomed throughout, though some writers said that physical contact was discouraged. Most writers said they had freedom of choice about whether to have drugs and which, though a few said they had no choice 'they were given'. Epidurals available. Everybody praises midwives: 'pleasant, friendly, understanding, courteous, sympathetic, patient, though over-worked'. They are well informed about breathing techniques and 'understand mothers' feelings'. Much freer attitude now about positions for labour though most women were delivered lying on their backs. Electronic monitoring may be used but writers said they were under no pressure to have it. Midwives tried to avoid unnecessary episiotomies.

Postnatal 'Free and easy atmosphere'; 'staff do all they can to make everyone happy'. Nurses very busy but supportive, encouraging, helpful, especially with breast-feeding. Baby is with mother all day, in nursery at night. Night feeding discouraged first 3 nights. Thereafter mothers woken. After 3–4 days mother may move to side ward and have baby with her all the time. Staffing levels at night 'ridiculously low', 'totally inadequate'. Demand-feeding. Writers say some auxiliary staff bottle-feed at night in spite of hospital policy that mothers should be able to breast-feed at night if they wish to. So discuss your wishes with *all* people caring for you and the baby. Women who bottle-fed said they were under no pressure to breast-feed and were grateful for this. Beds uncomfortably high for women who had stitches. Mothers can hold their babies at evening visiting time. Allowed to keep own Guinness, milk, orange juice, yogurt in kitchen fridge. Can wander into kitchen whenever they want. In day room smoking is allowed: 'pretty awful'. Shortage of bathrooms and washing facilities and queues form. No bidets.

Short visiting times – 1 hour in the afternoon, 1 hour in evening, husbands only 'at time when many are putting other children to bed'.

SCBU Mother is taken to see baby in unit before going to ward. Encouraged to express milk and use pump. Expressed milk bank and expressed milk only used in SCBU. Unit is highly praised.

Suggestions Midwives should not be so overworked. Midwives' encouragement of fathers should extend to massage, holding the woman in labour and supporting her in his arms. Fathers should not be 'ushered off home' soon after birth. Cleaning materials should always be set out in the bathrooms. More bathrooms are needed. Improved soundproofing between Hillier Ward and labour and delivery rooms.

Halifax General Hospital, Salter Hebble, Halifax, W Yorks

Consultant unit and GP unit. Friendly atmosphere.

Antenatal Scan at first visit. Some women were not allowed to see screen, technician 'too busy'. Writers say that amniocentesis is offered to everybody but can be declined. Clinic 'very impersonal'. See on average six different members of staff on each visit and different doctor every time. 'I felt dehumanized.' At least one consultant 'charming' and 'always tells his patients everything'. Waiting time 2½–3 hours, '1 hour undressed'. Insufficient privacy. Treatment discussed 'only if I butted in'; 'too many bits of blood given to too many people. Why couldn't one sample be taken and divided for test purposes?' Inconsistent advice, especially about breast-feeding. Emotional needs not considered. Mother who is herself nurse said, 'Everyone told you something different. I heard one midwife saying "Well, dear, if you have a girl this time you will find it easier to feed. Girls are always better suckers."' One woman actually enjoyed going to clinic: 'I asked lots of questions which were always answered cheerfully.' (Did she have the charming consultant?) Some writers describe long journeys to get there and back again after and found it exhausting at the end of pregnancy.

Antenatal ward. Writers said that sometimes they did not see doctor for a week. One writer felt she deteriorated from 'total lack of physical activity'. Only doctors have authority to discharge, so 'once in it is hard to get out'. One writer admitted for leaking waters said she discharged herself when they stopped leaking against strong disapproval. Women allowed home at weekends if not ill.

Labour: consultant unit Enema, shave. Partner must wait outside. Midwives 'kind', 'pleasant', 'chatty'. Electronic fetal monitoring used frequently. Partner allowed in only after this is set up. One woman says she was told that her partner could not come in unless she was married to him. Women say they were urged to have pethidine, which is sometimes given just before onset of second stage. One who declined says she was told, 'You're one of those heroes, are you?' Labour rooms contained stools. One can walk around before being electronically monitored. One writer says she spent her whole labour on the stool and recommends this. Moved to another room for delivery. Pushing against midwives' hips seems to be common. Ask if you want help with putting baby to breast after delivery. Father can cuddle baby and couple are left with their baby for short while. Then baby to nursery and partner sent out during stitching. Women describe suturing sometimes done before local anaesthetic had time to be effective. Some said baby was separated from them for several hours.

Labour: GP unit Full shave/enema. May be offered Mogadon if in early labour and night time and partner told to go home to rest: 'I felt abandoned. The lights were out and I was alone.' Pethidine offered but drugs not 'pushed'. One woman felt she accepted pethidine only because she had inadequate company and support. She started to hallucinate and said, 'I felt angry at being so drugged.' When midwives saw she was distressed stayed and talked with her and she relaxed. Usually midwife seems to pop in and out. If you want someone with you, do not let your partner go home. Plenty of drinks provided, including Ribena. Moved to another room for delivery. Father does not have to wear mask or gown and can hold baby straight away. Delivery quiet and informal. Midwives vary with regard to episiotomy. Some do them frequently, others are expert at avoiding them. Say if you do not want episiotomy. There may be a long wait for GP to come to suture. Some writers asked why midwives can't do their own stitching. Given baby to hold and suckle after delivery.

Postnatal 'All staff, tea-ladies included, very helpful'. An old auxiliary nurse particularly mentioned for help she gives mothers for getting baby fixed on breast. Women who delivered early morning could not get to sleep and would have appreciated being in single room for a few hours. 'I got no sleep for 24 hours.' Writers say it is better to be in side wards than in main wards and suggest that if you get overtired you ask to go to side ward to sleep. Staff nurses extremely helpful with breast-feeding, especially those who have breast-fed their own babies. Can be woken in night to feed baby. Writers describe breast-fed babies being given glucose water at each feed.

Food tends to be starch, sugar, fat. Two vegetarians had bad time. Writers advise having someone bring in dried or fresh fruit, honey and perhaps muesli.

Forty-eight-hour discharge possible.

Suggestions Women on antenatal ward should be encouraged to go for walk. Partner should not be sent out at any time. Midwives should tell woman in labour how she is progressing. Greater care about suturing. More fresh vegetables, salads, fruit, whole foods.

Harpenden Memorial, Carlton Road, Harpenden, Herts   MO

GP unit. No facilities for complicated deliveries. GP/own midwife do delivery together. Small unit. 'Very friendly atmosphere', 'homely'. If complications develop woman is moved to Luton and Dunstable or St Albans City. Writers felt they had excellent care and attention.

Antenatal No antenatal clinic at hospital; attend GP's clinic; mothers see the same people throughout antenatal care and delivery. One visit before birth to maternity ward for 'sister's clinic'. Shown around delivery rooms and ward and hospital procedure explained; 'all questions answered'.

Labour Woman induced with ARM and 'tablets to suck' when two weeks overdue said it was all 'great fun'. No oxytocin drip used. Mothers can stroll around in first stage; light meal provided if hungry. Midwife listens to baby's heart, not machines. Midwives encourage natural birth. Pethidine offered but not 'pushed'. Partner may be asked to leave room when woman empties bladder (on commode), may be asked to hold behind woman's head for second stage and hold up one leg. Baby handed to mother after being wrapped. 'I demanded food, given a huge bowl of Rice Crispies, lovely!'

Postnatal Breast-feeding encouraged and all help one could possibly need. Mothers care for their own baby. Writers speak enthusiastically of atmosphere on postnatal wards, say they are not aware of any routines, that 'nothing is too much for the people who work here, from the domestics to the doctor'; 'everyone friendly' and 'interested'; 'I felt very special'; 'care is second to none'. Community midwives call in for chats and GP visits every day. After milk comes in mother can be woken in night to feed and is given glass of milk herself. It seems that babies were in nursery for much of the time except at feeds and visiting. Food 'fantastic'.

Suggestions Partner should not be sent out at any time during labour. One woman, who said she 'didn't sleep a wink' through night after birth because her baby could not be with her though she asked, suggests that it should be a mother's right to have her baby with her then. Women should be able to have babies with them all the time, if they wish. Some writers thought that 6 a.m. was too early to be woken and suggested that mothers should be allowed to sleep on if they could.

Carlton Lodge Maternity Home, Leeds Road, Harrogate, N Yorks
MO

GP unit. 'Homely', 'like a private house', 'non-institutional furniture, pictures and pot plants', 'spotlessly clean'; 'I felt like a guest in a private home'. Writers comment on courtesy of staff. Arrangements can be made for shared care between usual GP and one who uses home.

Antenatal Appointments system works! Woman sees one or two members of staff only. Consistent advice given. Encouraged to ask questions and breast-feed. Plenty of help. No inductions done. (Must go to Harrogate General if induced.)

Labour Care is from one midwife assisted by auxiliary throughout. No enema, mini-shave. Partner made 'most welcome', but may be asked to leave room during prepping and stitching, though given tea outside. Need not wear gown or mask. Midwives 'gentle', 'kind'. All staff 'very supportive'. Drugs not pressed, but offered 100 mg pethidine. Mother can listen to fetal heart herself.

Water provided with bendy straw, mother's face wiped during second stage. Can use acupuncture in labour if wished and much interest is shown. One woman who went in with ruptured membranes, but no contractions, says nothing was done for 24 hours and her husband could stay the night, which was much appreciated. Several writers said they wore their own night-gowns for delivery. Baby can be suckled immediately after birth.

Postnatal Excellent help with breast-feeding. Mother not allowed to have baby with her rest of day on which born ('I was told this was because my room was not as warm as the nursery'), but is made welcome in nursery. Baby is brought to her for feeds and when other children come to visit in afternoon. 'Postnatal care is totally directed at establishing mother–infant relationship, and father is very excluded.' Staff 'interested' and 'concerned', 'never intrusive', but 'very much like being back at school' which one woman found 'oppressive'. Emphasis is on mother having rest: 'I had one very bad night with the baby and it was arranged for me to sleep late the following morning.' No artificial feeds given to breast-fed babies. Feeding on demand. Mother is woken at night to feed, but baby must be in nursery. Even so most writers do not seem to have felt 'taken over' and said things like 'the baby belonged to me from the very beginning'. One writer who had no visitors at evening visiting time said baby was brought to her then, 'a nice touch'. Domestic staff 'pleasant' and contribute to happy atmosphere. Separation from partners caused emotional strain for some women and they felt there should be more provision for fathers.

Suggestions Some writers who 'smuggled in own food' more fibre, fresh fruits and raw vegetables. More bathrooms.

★★ Northwick Park,
Watford Road, Harrow, Middlesex   MO

High-tech plus very good emotional support. Large, modern hospital, clean and bright; 'happy atmosphere'; 'staff very helpful'. 'Improving by leaps and bounds.'

Antenatal Midwives' clinic exists where woman sees same woman throughout unless she is on holiday. 'I looked forward to my visits'; 'was never kept waiting more than 30 minutes'. Depends on consultant whether mother is likely to have scans or not. Some writers described 'watchful expectancy' when went over dates, less induction. One was told by midwife that consultant did not like to interfere with course of nature. When labour is induced prostaglandins often used. Antenatal classes 'excellent' but apparently different women turn up each time so they cannot get to know each other. Tour of labour and delivery suite and shown equipment. Watch baby being bathed.

Labour 'Smiling midwife' greets mother. No enema, no shave. Several writers said their partners had to wait outside when a doctor came in. One woman, alone after staff had gone out, fainted and came round surrounded by midwives asking how it happened. She feels that if they had not forgotten to get her husband in again this need not have happened. Doctor said husband was sent out in case he should think doctor was 'mauling his wife'. Electronic monitoring used including telemetry. Labour is now less frequently accelerated with oxytocin, and it is expertly given. Writers say 'wonderful attention throughout' and 'the atmosphere made me feel very relaxed'. Wheeled to different room for delivery. American plastic delivery chair available, though some women find it too rigid, and immobilizing and narrow when they are trying to hold the baby afterwards. Told to 'push whenever you like.' Far fewer episiotomies are being done. Baby is handed to mother after delivery and can be put to breast immediately. Partner may be asked to wait outside during stitching: 'Why, I don't know, since he'd seen the birth and the cut.' Couple have time alone with baby – 'as long as we wanted'. Mother wheeled to ward with baby. Baby is weighed on ward and brought back.

Postnatal Totally demand-feeding. Baby is with mother all the time from beginning, but in nursery first night if she wishes. 'They let you get on with it.' Mother can bath her baby whenever she likes, feed and change whenever she likes and baby is not taken out at visiting times. Help with breast-feeding if needed though 'some nurses are not happy with demand-feeding and warn: "Not too long, dear, or you'll get sore nipples."' Writers advise, 'Smile and ignore them.' Sister of Frances Ward very highly praised, especially her attitudes to breast-feeding and her help and influence on whole nursing staff. Electric breast pumps available and kind where mother can control suction herself. Afternoon rest encouraged. Plenty of bathrooms, 'mostly good'. Fathers can visit any time between 9 a.m. and 9 p.m., except meal times.

Suggestions Partner should never be made to leave woman during labour. While mother is being stitched baby should be in her arms, not across room.

Buchanan, St Leonard's-on-Sea, Hastings, E Sussex   MO

'Not very homely'; 'fairly friendly'; 'plenty of rules'; 'well run and staffed'.

Antenatal Women having shared care have two check-ups at hospital only – 'very impersonal'; 'they take ages'. Describe standing in queues. Say they never see the same midwife twice. Woman who had not realized she had to take specimen said, 'The nurse lost her temper.' One woman, who said she felt 'just another mum, not special' when she visited the clinic, said nurses were not prepared to answer questions, but said 'ask the doctor', who was far too busy. One doctor 'appeared quite hostile when I said I was very healthy and felt on top of the world'. This impaired her confidence. Other writers say that doctors are 'brusque'. Same women said they were *told* they were to be induced and *told* they were to have epidurals: 'When I saw the consultant I said I wanted everything as natural as possible. He said, "What do you know about it? We know best."' This poor communication led to some writers losing confidence. 'I could not trust that my wishes would be respected.'

Antenatal ward: woman for whom tranquillizer prescribed for hypertension wrote, 'Two hours after receiving this drug I ran screaming across the ward, "Everything is going inside my head!" No one took a blind bit of notice.' She was given more, with similar side-effects, and hallucinations.

Labour Enema. Some said that midwives were keen for them to have as natural a birth as possible and helped with breathing, but this seemed to depend on who was on duty. Some got on very well with one midwife, but then shift changed. 'My husband felt lost and didn't feel his help was needed.' Two writers said they were told to push in second stage when they were having no contractions. Episiotomies not done routinely and midwives skilled at delivering without them. But 'I sat up to see the head but was told off for disturbing the drip.' Mother and father given the baby to hold after it has been cleaned 'for about 5 minutes'. Father is then sent away, mother and baby to postnatal ward and baby may be taken 'to be cleaned up'. (Again?) If night time, mother given drink and sleeping pill.

Postnatal Some writers did not have chance to breast-feed after delivery: 'I thought I would be able to put her to the breast, but she was never brought back that night.' Demand-feeding not advocated. Mother can be woken for night feeds 'but I should have liked her with me at night as well as day time'. 'Staff have little sympathy for girls who have difficulty breast-feeding. They are told to give complementary bottles or change to the bottle.' Several writers say they found routines tiring. One woman with stitches said she got 'little understanding'.

Food 'not bad'; 'not enough'.

Visiting 11–12 a.m.; fathers only, 3–4 p.m. and 6–7 p.m.

Suggestions More explanation about progress of labour. More explanation about drips. Partner should not be sent out during vaginal examinations. Baby should be given to mother before cord cut and be put to breast if mother wishes. Demand-feeding should be encouraged and rooming-in at night for all mothers wishing it. Fewer tranquillizers.

Maternity Unit, Hereford County, Hereford

Consultant unit and GP unit.

Antenatal Waits of up to 3 hours 'an ordeal': 'you have to queue in a corridor to see a doctor'; 'Everyone is treated like a child'; 'I felt I should be running round saying "I'm so sorry I am having a baby – it won't happen again."' 'One woman was told off in front of us for not bringing a specimen.' In contrast one writer says her consultant was 'always ready to answer questions and have a chat'. On the whole, care sounds efficient, but women seem bewildered by tests and a few frightened of the doctors. Writers say they see different doctor each visit. Conveyor-belt routine. No facilities for children. Woman who asked about Leboyer delivery says she was told 'she lived in the clouds': 'It only happens in films'. Women describe frequent scans. This may be because hospital receives high-risk cases over wide area. Nurses, however, are 'cheery' and 'helpful'.

Labour Shave. Some women were asked if they wanted enema, which is not routinely done: 'I had bath with constant flow of people coming in and out.' If it is night woman in labour is required to fill in menu card for next day. Single first-stage rooms. Husband, mother or close relative can be with woman throughout labour and is offered tea/coffee, but may be asked to leave if delivery not straightforward. Some writers said staff were 'marvellous' and 'worked together as an obviously very happy team'; 'gave great confidence in their expertise'. Midwives are described as 'kind', 'sympathetic', 'will give all the time in the world to talk things over'. And one writer said doctor 'jollied me along'. Sonicaid (ultrasound) may be used to monitor fetal heart rather than clip on baby's head. Several writers seem to have had rather large doses of pethidine and felt 'totally out of control' and sometimes to have been given it rather late in first stage. Advise asking for mini-dose. Women feel that episiotomies are done more or less routinely. Can sit propped up for delivery. The baby can be delivered up on to mother's abdomen. Midwife will wait till cord stops pulsating *if you ask*. Women describe how held baby naked till end of third stage and then midwife wrapped baby. Couple left with baby for about an hour to get to know each other. Partners then go home and baby is bathed.

Postnatal Large noisy ward (especially at night). New bidets, lavatories, showers, baths. But toilet facilities used by smoking mothers *and* staff: 'ashtrays piled high with cigarette stubs'; 'stank of stale smoke'. Nurses 'friendly', 'very supportive and one couldn't have had more care', though they are sometimes 'overwrought' with work. Rooming-in and apparently policy of feeding on demand, but nevertheless some women found routines very tiring: 'I was glad to come out after 6 days, exhausted . . . babies had to fit in with the hospital routine, which was almost impossible.' Atmosphere generally informal, depending on sister in charge. Woman who had Caesarean section thought care was 'appalling'. She was in bed at opposite end of ward from nursery and lavatories and was told to look after her baby the second day after her operation; says staff were too overworked to give assistance and bring her baby to her and that she had to carry her herself while feeling faint and ill. Several writers in GP beds said they enjoyed stay – 'I felt special' – and remarked on pleasantness of staff.

Food excellent though some women said it was not well adapted to needs of lactating women. Printed menus. Pleasant dinner ladies. The woman who had Caesarean section was unable to face beef curry followed by plums and custard immediately after her operation. Thought she ought to have been offered something more suitable.

Rule is that when woman is moved to another hospital nearer home for postnatal care she must be in hospital vehicle with radio contact with hospital. Yet hired cars are used, some of which have no radio contact and may be less comfortable than own car. The woman who had Caesarean section said no pillows were provided and it was painful to hold baby on her lap for 42-mile journey.

Forty-eight-hour discharge possible if all well with mother and baby.

Visiting daily 3.30–4.30 p.m., two visitors only, and 7–8 p.m., husband only or close relative. Own children in afternoon at discretion of ward sister.

Suggestions Women should not have to wait in corridor in antenatal clinic. More staff who have time to talk over problems. All midwives should learn skills of encouraging women in labour. Doctors 'should keep themselves abreast of the times and learn about new ways of doing things', e.g. Leboyer, Odent, moving around in labour, upright positions and mother lifting her own baby out. Improved general standards of cleanliness in lavatories and nursery.

Hexham General, Hexham, Northumberland

Modern unit, 'very friendly atmosphere'. Community midwifery service run from hospital, so good relations with Community midwives and with local GPs. Most staff have been there for years. Nursing officer writes that 'The Consultant in charge is always concerned with the patient's point of view and the service is therefore quite flexible.'

Antenatal Visit only at 34 weeks for GP patients.

Labour Half-shave, enema, bath. Midwives may listen to babies' hearts themselves. Fetal heart monitors also used. When using the monitor women say they have to lie flat on their backs, which is painful. One whose baby had been passing meconium said, 'The midwife and doctor left my husband and I alone with a fetal heart monitor for about 1 hour, the point of which I have no idea as there was no one to monitor it but us.' Excellent anaesthetist cover. Staff 'helpful'. Drugs not 'pushed' and usually little intervention. Mother is encouraged to watch delivery.

Postnatal Woman who was left alone 'a long time' in labour ward after delivery said bell was not plugged in and she was cold. Paediatric specialist visits regularly. NCT has, says nursing officer, 'very pleasant and open contact with the unit'.

★ Wycombe General, High Wycombe, Bucks   MO

'Welcoming', 'friendly atmosphere', 'informal', 'relaxed', 'modern, well run, very busy', 'light and airy' hospital. Staff 'can't be more helpful', are 'considerate', 'enlightened' and 'deserve nothing but praise'. Two ante/postnatal wards are each broken up into four-to-six-bed bays, some ante- and some postnatal.

Antenatal Long waits, 2½ hours common. If possible arrange appointment before 9.30 a.m. Tea bar in main part of hospital and no way of getting refreshment in clinic. May have scans.

Antenatal ward. Staff 'cheerful', 'nothing seems too much trouble'. Women say they are treated as individuals and intelligent, responsible persons, and that staff always use their names: 'If you ask questions everything is explained.' Auxiliaries stop for chat. Impromptu talks on baby care provide opportunity for discussion. Own children visit, can have cuddle on bed. Visiting 2.30–4.30 p.m., 'could be tiring', and 7–8.30 p.m. Children can come in evening if more convenient; 8–8.30 p.m. for husbands only. Several women described induction routinely at 14 days past due date, but some have asked for labour to begin naturally when monitored then and, if all was well, allowed to start labour spontaneously.

Labour Shave often omitted; electronic fetal monitoring may be used. Epidurals available on request any time and Caesarean section done under epidural: 'They were careful to ask if I really wanted an epidural and didn't pressure me at all.' When labour induced 'prostaglandin gel first'. Some writers said they wanted their partners with them from the start. One was told that her husband could stay throughout, but said that on arriving at unit at 8.30 a.m. he was sent home till 1.30 p.m. when labour was established. She was therefore lying with drip for 5 hours on her own while he tried to work at home: 'we were both upset when he could have been sitting beside me and talking to me'. Midwives praised: 'She kept me informed at all times of what she was doing.' Woman keeps her own bed in labour room and on to postnatal ward and her locker is wheeled with her. 'You are surrounded by your own bits and bobs.' Partner treated as natural companion, not sent out during examination. Woman is encouraged to walk about in room and down corridors. Some writers felt under pressure to have labour speeded up by drip when contractions slowed down. During the second stage several writers said the midwife let them pace themselves. Lights dimmed for delivery. Some women were told episiotomy was to be done: 'I expected to be told and it shocked and upset my husband to suddenly see a pair of cutters go into me. Some felt they had unnecessary episiotomies: 'The labour was proceeding well'; 'There was no strain.' Mother can suckle baby on delivery table and couple have good time to get to know their baby: 'They were quite happy for my husband to walk up and down cuddling his son and talking to him.' Baby wheeled to ward with mother and stays with her until 11 p.m.

Postnatal Several women said it was difficult to get sleep on ward after delivery if it was daytime. Lots of encouragement with breast-feeding. 'You do whatever you want'; 'It's your baby and they really mean it'; 'No question of being afraid of doing the wrong thing'; 'Mothers care for their own babies though nursery nurse is available to discuss things with if needed.' Babies can be fed in or out of bed; no restrictions. The nursery is noisy, with blaring pop music on radio, glaring strip lights, circle of chairs; 'Not an environment in which to relax and feed a baby.' Top-up bottles may be suggested for restless baby at night. Mother can refuse, but may meet disapproval.

Meals good. Choice of menu and size of portion. 'If you like a good breakfast order *large* portion.'

Day room used only by smokers. Private rooms available for mothers: 'I felt quite at home'; 'exceptional unit'; 'very friendly'; 'they go to great lengths to help mums feel part of a team'; 'you feel you can ask about anything'. Staff sympathetic about pain and concerned to help others be physically comfortable.

SCBU Five star. Care for whole family. Camp beds for fathers.

Suggestions Antenatal clinic more efficient. Rush and bustle of postnatal wards should be reduced so that mothers get more rest after delivery.

★ North Herts Hospital, Bedford Road, Hitchin, Herts

Old but extremely clean. Staff at all levels 'super'. Very pleasant ward/rooms, air of friendliness and helpfulness.

Antenatal Women describe discussions with doctors about drugs used in labour and methods of delivery: 'I feel sure that before long they will enter into discussions about episiotomies.' Consultants/midwives always willing to answer questions but 'you have to be quick and brave enough to ask'. Even so, it 'feels a bit like being on a conveyor belt, quick-in, quick-prod, quick-out'; at least the 'quick-in' is a good thing! Staggered appointments reduce waiting to minimum. Toy box and books, NCT playgroup leader so mothers can relax. Induction rate 8–10%.

Labour Suppositories can be declined. Woman can wear own nightdress if she wishes. Partner can stay, including through admission procedures. Head of midwifery writes: 'labouring women are encouraged to be up and about and in whatever position they feel comfortable for the first stage'. Not more than 10% have labour accelerated. 'Absolute understanding between midwife, student and me. No drugs offered at any stage. They knew I was an NCT addict.' 'Whole thing very intimate'; 'constant reassurance and praise'; 'they inspired confidence'; 'I look back on labour as a team effort, me as Captain!' One woman objected that she was given no warning that episiotomy was going to be done. Another wrote 'midwife said episiotomy was essential. I was happy to believe this because of her friendliness and honesty.' Baby is delivered on to mother's abdomen and remains there,' writes head of midwifery, 'for as long as she wishes and put to the breast as soon as she wants.' Forceps delivery rate 10–15%, Caesarean sections less than 10%, vacuum extraction 1–2%. Baby is weighed, examined and cleaned in the delivery room, remaining with mother, and both go to ward together.

Postnatal Rooming-in and demand-feeding. Mother cares for her baby in her own way, but help and advice always available. One writer said that some nurses and midwives could do with experience of childbirth, being more understanding of mothers' emotions. Conflicting advice about sore nipples given. Some women refused to allow their babies to have dextrose and the doctor was 'perfectly happy' about this. 'No stupid rules.' Fathers always welcome to handle babies at visiting times. Head of midwifery says that 'Flexibility of lengths of stay is proving very satisfactory' . . . 'If parents have a malformed or stillborn baby the husband is welcome to stay overnight with his wife.' Food 'not brilliant'.

Suggestions Consultants could make themselves 'far more approachable'.

Princess Royal, Huddersfield, Yorks   MO

Antenatal Writers advise asking for early morning appointment as there is less chance of long wait at this time. Clinic like 'assembly line': 'care impersonal'. Questions about pregnancy not encouraged. 'Some of the staff passed me off as neurotic because I had the courage to ask questions and query decisions.' No facilities for children – writers said they were expected not to bring them. 'I would like to have seen the same midwife at each visit'; 'I saw so many midwives (six at first visit) that most of the consultation was spent with them reading from my notes. Each one gave me a different date for the baby's arrival and my overall feeling was one of confusion and lack of continuity.' 'Since I went to the antenatal clinic on the same day each time I think it should have been possible to limit the number of doctors I saw to two or three.'

Labour Lack of continuity extends to labour; 'only continuity is that of written notes'. See entirely fresh staff on labour ward. 'Nurses too overworked and understaffed to have time to discuss things with patients'; 'Asian women very badly looked after if they cannot speak English.'

Postnatal Good emotional support. Domino delivery with 6–8 hour stay after delivery possible.

Suggestions System should be changed so that staff who care for women antenatally can be present during labour and delivery.

Hull Maternity, Hull, Yorks   MO

Antenatal Clinic described as 'chaos'. Mothers sometimes have to stand because all seats in waiting-room taken. Crowds outside consulting rooms. When seats are full women sit in changing cubicle nearby, so that women needing to strip have difficulty in finding empty ones. 'Mass of fuming ladies who may have to wait 3 hours.' But doctors and nurses 'very friendly', answer questions readily and are trying to do something about appointment times. There are 'ultrasound scans galore'. Rarely see same doctor two visits running; 'hackles rise when asked what blood pressure is or use technical term'; doctors discuss patients in their presence, but exclude them from conversation. And women are not asked if they mind being examined by medical students. Good preparation classes include relaxation, tour of labour wards and open forum with consultant paediatrician.

Huntingdon

Labour Partners welcome. Everyone who wrote had had electronic fetal monitoring. Some writers felt that birth here was too technological and one said that doctors 'managed to ruin the marvel and thrill of the birth experience'. Epidurals often suggested. Baby is handed to mother immediately at delivery.

Postnatal Staff 'always kind', but some quickly give up on breast-feeding. SCBU 'superb'.

★★ Primrose Lane Maternity, Huntingdon, Cambridgeshire

Reprieved from threat of closure. Small, modern, single-storey GP unit. Women often moved here with their babies from Mill Road, Cambridge, after 2 days.

Antenatal Long waits, at least 1 hour, nowhere for children to play. Not enough seats; 'Once past these hurdles examination is friendly.' Women say they are helped to feel involved with the unborn baby. 'When the doctor and midwives had felt the baby's position they always asked how I thought it was lying. One doctor drew a circle on my bump and said that if my husband put his ear there he should be able to hear the baby's heart-beats.' 'Drew on me the outline of baby's position complete with features.' Very friendly staff always available to give help and chance to talk to midwife before and after seeing doctor.

Labour Epidurals available. Care given is personal and intimate. Women said that staff were keen to help them have the kind of birth they wanted.

Postnatal Own community midwife and GP visit. Breast-feeding encouraged; midwives and nurses sit with mothers and help. Baby with mother from 9.30 a.m. till 9.30 p.m. Mothers go to nursery to feed at night. Breast-fed babies get bottle if mother wants to sleep. Encouraged to cuddle and get to know baby. Writers thought it was a friendly place. Many staff have children of their own. Community midwives are said to be marvellous and to give 'good psychological care'. 'Help when you need it yet you can do your own thing.' Food 'not good' . . . 'tendency to starch'. Each woman has lockable wardrobe.

Suggestions Improve food.

Maternity Unit, Heath Road Wing, Ipswich Hospital, Ipswich, Suffolk

Consultant and GP unit. Hospital built in seventies.

Antenatal Writers describe 2–3-hour waits. 'Husbands actively discouraged from waiting with their partners'; 'undressed in cold room'; 'examined by houseman who seemed to believe that my IQ was way below average'; 'lectured by severe sister'. As one woman said: 'It dampened my feeling of delight to be pregnant.'

Labour Most writers mentioned they had shave. Midwives 'considerate', do not 'pressurize' women to have drugs. Most staff understand NCT-type preparation for birth and respect it. 'Midwife asked if I was NCT-trained and said, "Oh, good! They know exactly what to do. It's marvellous!"' Some midwives think NCT 'over-dogmatic' and are less supportive to NCT mothers. Partner can be there all the time. Descriptions of happy atmosphere at delivery and time for both parents to get to know baby after. Minimum lighting in delivery room. Father given baby to hold and can hold baby while mother stitched. But a few writers did not have a happy experience; 'My husband and I would have greatly appreciated the opportunity to have a cuddle with our baby . . . everything was so rushed after delivery. The baby was whisked away, my husband invited to leave and I was left on my own. What an anti-climax!' 'No one to share my feelings of elation and personal triumph.' Some women were hungry after delivery but no food available: 'I was given a cup of tea but wanted something to eat. I could have swallowed a horse!'

Postnatal 'Care cannot be faulted. Help is always there when asked for but not pressed.' But some writers said that staff were 'authoritarian', one felt treated 'like an idiot, given no credit for knowing anything about baby care'. Father soundly reprimanded for sitting on wife's bed. Food ordered in advance. One woman, admitted on Sunday, had to take whatever food was left over on Sunday and Monday, as this food was ordered Saturday and she was not there then. 'Sheets and nappies ran out every afternoon.' Some women described long wait for clean supplies. Forty-eight-hour discharge can be arranged.

Suggestions Create more continuity of care.

Keighley – see Steeton

★ Helme Chase, Burton Road, Kendal, Cumbria   MO

Women having second babies here say there have been enormous improvements over the last 4–5 years. SNO is much praised: 'very human', 'easy to talk to', 'friendly'. Midwives 'inspire confidence' and are 'kind' and 'friendly'. Many have been there for years.

Antenatal Questions answered honestly by most staff. Writers advise say what you want and you are likely to have your wishes respected. Cheerful waiting area; care personal; staff look after children if necessary. Most writers describe waits of less than ½ hour, but there were some longer ones. 'Wonderful nurses.' Scans done at Lancaster Infirmary.

Antenatal wards – when weather suitable women can go out in grounds and attend antenatal classes. If not ill allowed home at weekends. Own children can visit every day.

Labour When inductions done, oral prostaglandin tablets may be used. Own midwife meets woman at door and accompanies her to labour room. Writers usually had enema/shave. Partner can be present throughout. Midwives 'give plenty of encouragement' and are 'kind', 'calm', 'helpful'. Progress of dilatation explained. A couple who went in with two other children were encouraged to stay together and staff said they were happy to look after children. Episiotomy not done routinely and midwives skilled at delivering without need for stitching. After delivery baby given to parents to hold and mother encouraged to put baby to breast. They have about an hour to get to know each other: 'We were made to feel very special.'

Postnatal Great deal of help to establish breast-feeding. Night sister specially praised for her 'very commonsense approach'. 'Friendly', 'homely' atmosphere. Baby with mother all day after second day. Breast-feeding mothers asked if they would like to get up to feed in night and nurse, 'joy of joys!', brings big mug of tea. Food plentiful, well-cooked: 'It is like a five-star hotel.' Efficient, friendly auxiliary staff. Husband and other children can visit any time and cuddle and get to know baby.

Suggestions More lavatories, especially on antenatal ward. More staff.

Maternity Department, Queen Elizabeth Hospital, Gayton Road, King's Lynn, Norfolk

Department in new District General Hospital, opened 1980. Pleasant, light and airy.

Antenatal Small clinics with effective appointments system. Waiting times usually short. DNO says 'children are welcome and creche facilities available if required'. Craft and relaxation classes each weekday, with some afternoon and evening classes. Individual help for prospective adoptive parents. DNO says induction for medical reasons only.

Labour Single room for labour and delivery. Partner encouraged to stay throughout labour, including during examinations and complicated deliveries, at discretion of midwives or obstetricians. Women may choose whether or not they wish to have drugs for pain relief. Epidurals done, including for Caesarean sections. Father may be present. Baby given to mother to hold after delivery and father can cuddle baby too. If mother is going to breast-feed midwife helps put baby to breast. Baby stays with mother and goes with her to postnatal ward.

Postnatal Rooming-in. All babies fed on demand. Nurses generally sit down and talk over problems, are 'patient' and 'encouraging' with helping to breast-feed. Mother can care for her baby herself. Baby can be dressed in own clothes.

Visiting 1 hour in afternoon, when own children can come. Evening visiting of 1 hour for husbands only. If baby in special care mothers can visit any time. Children can visit their brother or sister.

SCBU Two overnight rooms available in SCBU for mothers.

Kingston Hospital, Kingston-upon-Thames, Surrey MO

Busy, well-equipped hospital, 'rather depressing old buildings' and some modern ones. Understaffed. Domino system operates here, including for first baby if you wish.

Antenatal A lot of criticism of antenatal care here. Two-hour waits in crowded clinic 'an endurance test', 'unbearable heat'; 'all very public', but 'everyone very kind'. Severe staff shortages lead to long waits in claustrophobic cubicles. One writer who tried to find out hospital policies about management of labour says she was 'fobbed off' and no one told her anything. Nursing staff are harassed by overwork. Most writers had had scans. Women can tour labour wards beforehand, but not their partners. Midwife clinics are held in local 'cottage' hospitals.

Antenatal ward. If not ill allowed home at weekends; 'told to treat the place as an hotel by doctor'. All questions answered at length. Induction rate appears to be high. Prostaglandin gel used. Advised beforehand to have epidural.

Labour Personal preferences can be discussed with staff beforehand. Birthing room. No shave or enema. Epidurals readily available. Partner can usually stay for all procedures. He is 'one of the team'. Electronic fetal monitoring used, but not routinely. 'The machine broke down and though a technician came and tried to mend it, it was still not working properly. No one seemed to understand and then *we* explained how.' 'I was strapped up to every imaginable piece of machinery . . . very boring.' Woman is encouraged to walk around in labour. One writer said 'labour room had lovely view'. One had a visit from a woman checking venetian blinds during labour and found this distracting. In second stage a writer said 'I felt the midwife was doing things *her* way rather than my way.' But 'the doctor waited till I was in a good position to watch my baby being born'. Modified Leboyer-style delivery can be arranged, blinds pulled down and everyone is quiet; alternative birth positions are allowed. Some writers said they were not handed their babies immediately after delivery but had to wait while baby was given 'a test', others that they could feed a few minutes after delivery. Parents have time with their baby and are not turned out of delivery room.

Postnatal Baby is by mother's bed 10 a.m. to 10 p.m. Writers advise asking for lactation sister if you need help with breast-feeding: 'wonderful lady who manages to find time for everything. Gives lots of encouragement.' Nurses 'friendly' but some agency night nurses less so. If a woman has been on antenatal ward staff come to visit her postnatally; much appreciated. If you ask, questions are answered. Ice packs provided for perineal pain. One writer who said there was no 'tender, loving care' said 'one sister wouldn't let me cuddle my baby between feeds and wouldn't give a reason, but none of the rest of the staff agreed with her'. At night mother can be woken when her baby wakes and some night staff are particularly good: 'I asked for a glass of water when I was feeding and the next night found a glass of milk waiting for me.' Nurses sit and chat with mothers during night feeds. Wards 'grey' and 'dismal'; lavatories 'filthy'. Not enough baths and those that are there are 'old and rusty'. Smell of food 'offensive'. Evening visiting for fathers only.

Suggestions Some continuity of care. 'Treat women as human beings capable of thinking.' More staff. Improve interior decoration and provide shower rooms.

Kirby Muxloe – see Leicester

★★ Royal Infirmary, Ashton Road, Lancaster

Modern unit (opened 1976). First-class facilities, 'well organized', pleasant wards. Staff 'friendly', 'considerate', 'understanding' and 'sympathetic', including auxiliaries. SNO writes: 'We endeavour to be flexible in our policies. All ladies are treated as individuals. Community midwives deliver their own patients here.'

Antenatal Women attend midwives' booking clinic before seeing consultant. Can spend at least 30 minutes with midwife in relaxed atmosphere to discuss any aspect of care. 'Everyone made me feel so welcome.' Reasons for tests, and also for induction when it is proposed, carefully explained and all questions fully answered. Consultants 'not at all aloof', 'friendly' and 'understanding'.

Antenatal ward. Some preparation given to women unable to attend classes. Some writers said that partner was allowed to visit outside visiting hours every day. 'I was brought little presents by some of the staff occasionally'; 'staff offered to shop for baby layette for me'.

Labour Partner can stay throughout. 'Staff always eager to explain things' and 'extremely helpful'. Choice of pethidine or epidural; 77% normal deliveries; 8% forceps; 14% Caesarean sections. Writers who had Caesareans commented on 'cheerful atmosphere' in theatre and said that procedures were explained. Baby goes to mother for cuddle immediately after delivery.

Postnatal Good help with breast-feeding by supportive midwives: 'amount of time staff prepared to spend with individuals remarkable'; 'when I thought I'd never do anything right the staff always found something positive to focus on'; 'nurses usually instill confidence' – but there is problem with conflicting advice: 'I was bombarded to utter confusion by each nurse giving me their view on feeding.' Women who chose to bottle-feed did not have such a happy time; one said staff were 'rude' and made her feel 'miserable'. Nurses 'frequently come to chat' with mothers. After Caesarean section baby is in nursery at night, but brought for breast-feeding. One woman whose baby was brain damaged said 'I found it very hurtful to be in a four-bedded ward with other women who had their babies with them while mine was all bruised and awful looking in SCBU.' There is demanding pace on ward which some writers found difficult to cope with. They also said heat in unit was overpowering and there was no air conditioning. Fathers can visit any time. Food 'excellent', but steer clear of salads: 'lettuce brown at edges, eggs like rubber, tomatoes soft, a greenfly discovered!'

SNO writes, 'We continue to review our practice and to seek the opinions of our clients . . . we liaise with all the local pressure groups and voluntary help groups. Where possible, we attempt to accommodate individual's requests and wishes with regard to a particular aspect of care.'

Forty-eight-hour discharge can be arranged.

Suggestions Antenatal patients, especially those in a long time, should be able to wear their own clothes ('my memories of pregnancy are all nighties and dressing-gowns'). When baby is in special care mother should be offered single room.

Warneford, Radford, Leamington Spa, Warwickshire   MO

Antenatal Women describe great deal of duplication of investigations done at GP's. Waiting area cramped, line of chairs in corridor, but no long waits. Consultants prepared to discuss wishes and note requests on record. Some writers who went a week overdue felt under pressure to be induced.

Labour Mini-shave. Examinations by midwives 'carried out with sensitivity'. Writers say care was 'personal' and midwives encouraging: 'Genuine partnership with midwives' who showed 'real desire to do what we wanted'. In first stage side wards containing four beds near labour ward are used. Electronic fetal monitoring seems to be frequent. Midwives will dim lights in delivery room if asked. 'Midwife was encouraging and congratulated me profusely for pushing gently and in a controlled fashion.' Skilled at avoiding episiotomy. And writers said that episiotomy rate was 'less than 50%'. Modified Leboyer birth possible. Baby can be delivered on to mother's abdomen and cord left to finish pulsating before clamped. Couples left for extended time to get to know their babies. Baby can go to breast on delivery table. Father can go to ward with mother. One writer who had emergency Caesarean section said consultant came and talked to her and left ultimate decision to her and her husband. But father not allowed to be present and done under general anaesthesia.

Postnatal Demand-feeding; staff supportive and pupil midwives especially enthusiastic about breast-feeding; but 'plethora of conflicting advice'. Some writers said it was policy to give baby sterilized water. Baby can stay on ward all time, including through night, but writers advise asking for amenity bed so that you do not disturb other women who do not want their babies with them. Staff bring cup of tea if mother is feeding.

Suggestions Ward put aside for women wishing to have their babies with them all the time.

Leeds Maternity, Hyde Terrace, Leeds, Yorks   M O

SNO suggests that parents with special requests about treatment they hope to receive make them known to her in writing prior to admission.

Antenatal 'A cattle market.' Long waiting times, occasionally 4 hours, on average 45 minutes, without clothes according to writers. 'Production line'; 'terrible'; 'a degrading experience'; 'far too clinical'. The clinic was so crowded sometimes that 'you had to stand around for half an hour till a seat was vacant' . . . 'everything stops from 10 till 10.30 a.m. while the doctors have their coffee break'. 'The same tests were done in the hospital as at the GP's clinic. I only saw the doctor for 2 minutes.' 'Approximately six women are booked at 15-minute intervals. Averages out at 2½ minutes per patient.' 'Throughout my pregnancy I never saw a midwife except at the local health clinic relaxation classes,' wrote a 'high-risk mother'. One woman who attended eight times saw a different doctor each time. No continuity in care. Waiting-room cold. Hospital gown that doesn't meet. Some writers said there was no time to ask questions, others said they were encouraged to ask questions and discuss worries and that breast-feeding was encouraged. Most writers would have liked more information: 'Your file seems totally secret and is not for your eyes.' One woman who tried to see what her blood pressure was was told to lie down. Visitors had to sit separately in visitors' area, including husbands. A woman whose first baby had been stillborn wrote: 'Medical staff were more concerned with my emotional care than the nursing staff.'

Parentcraft and relaxation classes include tour of unit and seeing 'very off-putting' delivery rooms. Antenatal wards 'superb'. Full explanations are given of all treatment, including scans and oestriol checks.

Labour Staff 'kind', 'efficient'. Partner can often stay throughout labour, but this depends on staff on duty: 'The fact that he wasn't packed off for any reason made a great difference to my morale.' Prep room stark and functional. Several women described enema. Can request partial shave. Partner may not be allowed in for this. Foam wedges available, but you have to ask for them. Continuous electronic monitoring seems to be used frequently, but some women who said they hoped it wouldn't stop them moving about said that it had not been used. Amniotomy seems to be routinely done. A good deal of technology used, but it seems possible not to have things you don't want. Let your midwife know your wishes. Epidurals available. Sounds as if acceleration with oxytocin drip is frequent. Partner may be sent out during vaginal examination – 'I hated being alone' – and maybe for forceps delivery, but woman can ask for him to stay. One woman whose baby was delivered by Kielland's rotation forceps wrote: 'I haven't the faintest idea why and no one would tell me . . . no one explained anything then or later . . . it seems nobody tells the staff anything either.' Delivery rooms 'pretty daunting places'.

Several writers said they were told to put their hands under their knees in second stage, and partner can hold woman up. 'My midwife put my hands down on the baby's head that was beginning to come out; I had no idea it was that far along.' Midwives do not do routine episiotomies but may suggest anaesthetizing perineum in case they need to. Cord cut immediately and baby given to mother. Couple have short time together with baby. After being cleaned up one writer was left in delivery room from 6.30 to 10 p.m. with saline drip, unable to do anything to empty her bladder.

Postnatal Baby is removed first night and fed in nursery. Otherwise beside mother's bed in Perspex cot. Mother who had baby in SCBU said when he came up to ward no one showed her how to feed him. Discharge after 12 hours or more can be arranged in advance. One first-time mother said consultant asked her, 'Will you know what to do at night if it screams?'

Suggestions Booking clinic should be held at different time from ordinary antenatal clinics. Women should not have to undress before necessary. Smaller wards needed, constructed with soundproof partition. Some staff need 'more awareness of mothers' feelings'. Some writers suggested that communication between staff themselves and between staff and mothers could be improved.

★ **Saint James', Beckett Street, Leeds, Yorks**

Very modern/clean/tidy, 'friendly', 'warm atmosphere'.

Antenatal Spacious, plenty of comfortable chairs. Separate booking clinic with long waiting time. Routine scan. No smoking. Usual visits waiting only about ½ hour. Nursery available. Doctors 'helpful', always introduce themselves, and talk to couples together.

Antenatal Ward Partner and children allowed to visit any time. 'I was told exactly what was wrong.' Staff 'helpful'. Partner can stay throughout.

Labour Choice of enema and shave. Woman is never left alone. Can change position when she wishes. Woman can choose whether or not to have drugs for pain relief, but may need to be firm. Pethidine and epidurals available. Electronic fetal monitoring may be done. Midwives 'kind', 'efficient'. Woman can sit up for delivery. Given the baby, cord still attached, to hold. Can breast-feed on delivery table. Baby is cared for and examined in front of mother. Writers say 'speak up and say you don't want this and that' or 'why are you doing this?'

Postnatal Baby is beside mother's bed. Demand-feeding encouraged. Breast-feed right after delivery sometimes discouraged, 'but I insisted so she made a note "Mum wants to be woken" and placed it on the cot'. Mother goes to nursery to feed at night, is given cup of tea. Baby checked over by paediatrician in presence of mother. She is asked if she has any questions. Mother fills in chart of baby's progress. Bidets. 'You are left to do as you wish' with your baby, no rigid routine. A woman who decided she wanted to breast-feed after 2 days was helped by nurse who sat with her for over an hour. Non-smokers say day rooms very unpleasant. Meals are taken there and TV is there.

Meals: 'delicious', 'very good!' 'great' and choices available.

Visiting 3–8 p.m. every day and arrangements can be made for visitors at other times too. Own children 'most welcome'.

Forty-eight-hour discharge can be arranged.

Suggestions More education of women antenatally to teach them to ask questions, share in decision-making, be active birth-givers rather than passive patients. Two day rooms – one smoking and one non-smoking – needed. Less noise on postnatal wards so that it is easier to sleep.

Leicester Royal Infirmary, Leicester

Large, modern, 'impersonal', 'sterile', 'hot', 'unfriendly', 'like airport lounge', 'like car park'. Consultant and GP unit where 24-hour admission is allowed.

Antenatal Well organized but 'production-line atmosphere'. Very busy. No appointment system; may wait 5 minutes or 2½ hours: 'poor, harassed mothers waiting for hours'. Some writers say staff 'cold'. Scans done frequently. Some women offered package deal of induction/epidural/forceps. If woman refuses induction may be asked to sign statement indemnifying hospital against baby or herself dying. A woman who was admitted to antenatal ward with very high blood pressure, having refused to go in before, says she was greeted by senior member of staff with 'And about time too, you stupid woman!'

Labour No shave but other automatic procedures. 'You don't feel you have individual care because staff appear to have no authority to alter any procedure.' Writers had enema. One asked what was point of this since had had several bowel movements: 'No answer, they just got on with it.' Partner is sent out during prepping. Some writers said they were told that over 50% of labours were either induced or accelerated. Some women said that they had been given pethidine without feeling it was necessary. Epidurals available. Some writers complained of heat, but doors into corridor from labour rooms can be left open and corridor windows opened. *Ask* if too hot. Woman who 'did not have the strength of mind to ask for my husband', was happy when obstetrician popped his head through door and 'asked if I wanted him back'. One woman who did not want invasive electronic monitoring asked for Doppler (sonic aid) instead and this was provided. In transition woman may be told to use Entonox and stop breathing learned beforehand, though some midwives encourage breathing learnt in antenatal classes. Some writers critical of 'factory production line', 'technological management' and 'institutional rules'. Obstetricians and midwives, students and auxiliaries described as 'very kind' and 'gentle'. Staff shortages mean that they are 'hard pressed' and several writers describe being left during labour with drip and monitor for periods of about ½ hour. One writer said, 'My husband went to find someone when my blood was being sucked up the tube that the drip was supposed to be flowing down. Whenever the fetal heart seemed to have stopped no check was made by listening to the baby. Instead the machine would be examined, thumped, or changed. Sometimes it would be 5–10 minutes before heartbeats registered again. This I felt was wrong. If the child was in danger the time factor would be crucial.' Woman with hypertension said that when she was in transition an obstetrician came in with 'a dozen or so students' and told her that if anything was wrong with the baby he and the paediatrician would sue the couple.

Second stage: some writers said midwife wanted them to lie down to push; 'I had to argue to be allowed to sit propped up.' This woman said she was allowed to have 'a couple of blankets under the pillow . . . it was easier to cooperate then'. Some writers asked for lights to be turned off before delivery and this was done. One woman said midwife was about to do episiotomy without telling her. When she protested midwife told her accusingly, 'You have been reading *books*.' Most writers said they had episiotomies. But one asked midwife to 'have a go without'. She said she was told she would tear badly but in fact had an intact perineum. Woman who asked for Leboyer-style delivery said midwife told her she would wait for cord to stop pulsating before cutting it and would give baby to her immediately, but did not. Baby was handed to her 'wrapped in horrible green paper, like paper in public lavatories for drying one's hands' . . . 'I was reprimanded when I unwrapped her and covered her with a soft towel.' Baby may be handed to father while mother stitched. Some writers waited for over an hour for doctor to come to stitch. Couple usually had about an hour with baby after delivery, though some writers said baby was taken away and brought back wrapped up and put in cot. If this happens father could pick baby up and give to mother. It was not always easy for mothers to suckle babies after delivery: 'I tried to put her to the breast while they tried to take her for a wash.' Baby is usually tucked in beside mother when she is wheeled down to postnatal ward. But if it is night-time the baby is then taken away to nursery. 'There was no one else in the ward so I was not disturbing anyone. I was very upset and cried. They relented and brought him back for about ¼ hour and helped me put him to the breast before taking him away again.' Baby is taken to nursery first night so that mothers can sleep, but one woman who said that in that case she preferred to go home was given private room and the baby was with her and her husband also till midnight: 'I felt really well and exhilarated but was obviously expected to lie down, sleep and be quiet.'

Postnatal Help available with breast-feeding seems to vary on different wards. A woman on one ward had 'lots of help' but on another women described 'offhand approach' and one woman said it was 1½ days before she was offered any help. It is possible to demand-feed, but in words of nursery nurse at hospital mother may have to 'stick to her guns'. Encouragement given generously is not always of right kind. Many different views on right ways to breast-feed. Some writers who wanted to breast-feed said bottle was given to baby at night (1980) for first 2–3 nights 'to allow the mother rest'. Many writers enjoyed postnatal stay in general and most said nurses were 'kind', 'sympathetic', 'encouraging', but 'most staff dare not be flexible because they lack experience and are rushing around because there is staff shortage'. Two writers thought it was particularly difficult in this hospital for women coming from other cultures: 'I am strong, fit, relatively intelligent and gave birth in my mother country. I pitied the uninformed who could not understand the language.'

For first meal after delivery following a long, difficult labour, one mother, while in delivery room, was offered fish and chips. She said she was vegetarian and melted strawberry icecream was provided instead. Others described food as 'oxtail soup, sausages, mashed potatoes, soggy carrots all covered in gravy, and icecream. Everything except the icecream was cold.' They suggest get fruit brought in.

Roundhill Maternity Home, Forest Drive, Kirby Muxloe, Leicester

MO

GP unit.

Antenatal Care with GP. Booking visit only at hospital: long wait, given briefing on hospital policy but some women said there was no opportunity to ask questions or see wards.

Labour Attended by community midwife; partner can be present. Midwives allow births to be as natural as possible, but some sceptical about women's ideas of natural childbirth. Are skilled and sensitive to mother's wishes and needs. Freedom to walk about and no electronic monitoring, though some writers said that amniotomy was done to speed up the contractions. Woman can labour without drugs if she wishes. Midwife explains everything she does. Supportive of mother's way of coping with contractions with relaxation/breathing/massage. Some midwives insist on full light for delivery as they are anxious that they cannot assess state of baby otherwise. You can ask for extra pillows to deliver in semi-sitting position. Some writers described a great deal of enthusiastic encouragement in the second stage, but others were able to push in own rhythm and time. One writer says she was disappointed she was not able to touch her baby until it was sucked out and she did not think it was necessary to do this. But midwife sometimes unwilling to alter usual practice. Mother can hold baby and suckle on delivery bed. Parents left with baby for extended period.

Postnatal Breast-feeding encouraged but may be on schedule with complementary bottles; writers who were determined to do so fed on demand. Mothers can go to nursery to feed baby in night; one woman says she was told there was no point as there was no milk yet and her baby was hungry and needed a bottle. Mothers may be discouraged from picking their babies up: 'I didn't feel he was mine until I got home.' Staff 'well-meaning' but did not always respond to mothers' requests. 'Their idea is to look after babies so that mothers get rest and they tend to be bossy.' Can book for 24 hours and some writers think this is best if you want to care for your baby in your own way.

Suggestions A woman should always be able to touch her baby immediately on delivery. Staff could be more sensitive to individual mother's needs postpartum.

Victoria Hospital, Lichfield, Staffs   MO

Small cottage hospital; modern in outlook; very clean. Emergencies to Burton General or Good Hope, Sutton Coldfield. Lovely views from all windows.

Antenatal Waiting no longer than ½ hour; see own GP at every visit; midwives 'lovely', 'friendly', 'helpful'. Children welcome in clinic and consultation rooms. If scan advised go to Burton for it. Can see round and 'made very welcome'.

Labour Writers described full shave/enema; husband gets cup of tea while waiting outside. One writer says pethidine was 'forced' on her – 'You need to be very firm if you don't want it' – and there was not always discussion before giving it. Partner told to leave during examinations, but otherwise can take active part. No epidurals here. Woman has to move to another room for delivery unless hospital busy, when she can deliver in labour room. Episiotomies not done routinely. Baby wrapped before being given to parents while afterbirth delivered. Couple have about ½ hour together with baby.

Postnatal 'Very friendly, considerate staff'; 'pleased to help with anything'. Woman has 6 hours in bed and is then encouraged to move around. GP visits every day. Good help with breast-feeding, but top-ups used at most feeds until breast-feeding is established (1980), and baby may be given bottle at night. Baby with mother 5.30 a.m. until evening visiting. Visiting 7–8 p.m., but other times can be arranged if partner on shifts. 'Not much help for 3-day blues.' Helpful auxiliary nurses. Relaxed atmosphere and 'you got to know all other women and staff well'; 'your baby was yours'; 'as near to home as possible'.

Suggestions More support for mothers who wish to feed their babies at night. Mothers should not have to be in bed for visiting. Early afternoon visiting too. Quieter night staff.

Liverpool Maternity Hospital, Liverpool

Antenatal Some long waits (up to 2 hours) in overcrowded clinic. Women stand in queues and may see different doctor each time. Clinic can be confusing. But fairly relaxed atmosphere; clerical staff often 'abrupt and busy'; nurses helpful but staff shortages. Writers say same tests and examinations done as at GPs clinic. Though doctors may not volunteer explanations, they will tell you if you ask. Writers say they did not feel hurried. Some obstetricians recommend epidurals, 'seemed vaguely amused and patronizing about my whims – no epidural, shaving or fetal scalp monitor *unless* necessary', but all requests noted on record card and several writers had letter with requests pinned to case notes with consultant's agreement. One woman was told by senior member of staff that obstetricians had become much more flexible over last few years. Writers were sometimes required to fill in kick chart from 30 weeks on. Inductions: 22% (1980). Prostaglandin pessary may be given overnight.

Labour Most women not shaved. No enema if bowels emptied that day. Some women said they did not want continuous monitoring and found support from midwives. Large bean-bags instead of pillows. Epidurals and acupuncture available. Gas and oxygen also offered. Partners encouraged to be present and can stay for forceps delivery. Midwives 'competent', 'friendly', 'understanding', 'helpful', 'considerate', though some also described as 'quick', 'clinical', perhaps because large proportion abnormal obstetrics. Medical students 'helpful', 'obliging'. Some doctors 'extremely brusque with examinations' and information has to be 'prised' from them. It is worth asking questions because writers say that when information *is* forthcoming it is comprehensive, but 'no feeling of sympathy or understanding'. 16% labours augmented; some writers say they were delivered on the side, but midwife may be willing to deliver in any position in which mother comfortable; 46% episiotomies including forceps deliveries; 25% normal deliveries; 20% forceps deliveries; 15% Caesarean sections. Modified Leboyer delivery possible. Baby delivered on to mother's abdomen and cord left until it stops pulsating. Couples have about 20 minutes with their babies. Chairman of Medical Board says husbands are welcome to be present at Caesarean sections done under epidural.

Postnatal Facilities 'old', 'obsolete', 'overcrowded'. Friendly atmosphere and well-run wards. Nurses and auxiliaries 'friendly', 'efficient', 'helpful', 'nothing too much trouble', and fully committed to breast-feeding. Give advice, emotional support and practical help at any time of day or night. Breast-feeding mothers are together in one ward. Baby goes to nursery first night, but is beside mother all day. Is given plain boiled water if wakes. By mother's bed from then on. Staff will sit with mother during entire feed if necessary. Policy of demand-feeding, including during visiting, if curtains drawn. Food 'abominable'. Flexible visiting hours. Very active neonatal intensive care unit catering for babies born from 26 weeks onwards. Chairman of Medical Board writes that to put figures in perspective it must be remembered that 'hospital is a referral hospital for such complications of obstetrics as rhesus incompatibility' and women who have gone into premature labour. 'These babies are transferred *in utero* and this results in a high proportion of operative deliveries.' 'The Area Health Authority . . . closed two obstetric units and as a result the two remaining units . . . have a more concentrated and heavier workload, and this may account for some deficiencies which we recognize in our service' (and he mentions overcrowding). 'Lack of finance prevents us from doing anything about this.'

Suggestions Simple notices in antenatal clinics so that women do not inadvertently become queue-jumpers. Those having shared care should not have to attend hospital so often. It should be a woman's right to refuse pethidine in labour. Simplify and clarify 'baffling' routines on postnatal wards.

British Hospital for Mothers and Babies,
Samuel Street, Woolwich, London SE18

Small, friendly, very caring consultant unit where women say 'you feel you matter as an individual'. Building old but additions 10 years or so ago. Pleasant surroundings, including garden to sit in in summer. National training school for midwives. Part of hospital used to be isolation ward and is separate from main building. Transfer to this ward can be very cold, since mother and baby are put in wheel-chair, wrapped in blanket and taken across open courtyard in all weathers. Hospital is under threat of closure. Obstetricians 'keen on technology'. Domino scheme in operation and community midwife takes her patient in, delivers her there and takes her home 6 hours after.

Antenatal Appointments system but women booked in batches for the same time – first come, first served. Long waits with no facilities for children; 'gruesome'. Queues build up for blood samples/urine analysis. Clinic sister 'very caring' and 'remembers people individually'; 'spends a lot of time with individuals and gives plenty of explanations'. Obstetricians 'helpful' and 'kind' but when seeing consultant must undress in communal changing room. Dressing-gown supplied is skimpy and women wait 'humiliated and embarrassed', their tummies protruding. Cramped conditions, military rows of hard chairs closely packed. 'Fecund women overflow into the corridor'; seldom see same midwife or doctor twice, though all staff friendly and willing to discuss problems. AFP testing now routine and scans done. High induction rate, 30% (1980), though SNO says induction rate is going down. Four parentcraft classes, two at beginning of pregnancy and two at 30+ weeks for couples, but do not include relaxation. Childbirth film and tour of delivery suite. Shared care – woman attends hospital clinic only at beginning and end of pregnancy.

Labour All staff 'very kind' and 'helpful'. Woman stays in same room throughout. Mini-shave/enema/supervised bath. Ambulation encouraged in early labour. Drugs offered but can be declined. Epidurals available if anaesthetist there and epidural Caesareans possible. Doctors seem to have preference for quick labours and 'will persuade people with the technology if not challenged'. Partner may be able to stay all the time, including for forceps delivery, and can take photos of birth, but some midwives send partner out when doing examination or when doctor comes in. Couples who have said they want to stay together have usually been able to. Electronic monitoring often used. Some women ask for strict monitoring at beginning of labour, using external belt, and then had it taken off if everything was straightforward. Writers say do be firm if you do not want invasive monitoring; 'they are very amenable'. Midwife will dim light for delivery. Episiotomy is not done routinely, but some long waits for stitching; 10% forceps deliveries, 10% Caesarean sections, but SNO says this has been reduced. Missionary nuns train here and prayers may be said at delivery. Mother can suckle baby on delivery table and couple have time together with baby.

Postnatal Baby in nursery at night, on ward during day. Demand-feeding encouraged from the start. Staff ask mother if she wishes to feed at night and bring baby to her, but often there are agency nurses and auxiliary staff at night so 'be sure you tell them if you want to be woken to feed'. Own children can visit in delivery suite to see new baby and can come at any time convenient for family. Fathers encouraged to handle baby. Women who have had Caesarean births say they get lots of help with breast-feeding. Dextrose may be encouraged but mothers who refuse to give it met with no opposition.

Asian mothers can have food brought in by family at any hour convenient. Food 'very stodgy' and 'tasteless'; no choice of menu. Vegetarian and other special diets not catered for. Unimaginative salads at almost every meal. But woman who feeds in night is given hot drink of tea or Ovaltine. No smoking on wards.

Visiting limited 3–4 p.m. and 7–8 p.m. partners only.

Forty-eight-hour discharge possible but state early in pregnancy if you would like early discharge.

Suggestions More continuity of care. Though writers say staff explain what they are doing and why, some hoped for more encouragement for natural birth from doctors.

City of London, 65 Hanley Road, London N4   MO

Old hospital; 'use of drips, monitors and other equipment belies first appearance'. All letters received about this hospital have been critical of fairly high rating it was given in first edition.

Antenatal Sister 'lovely', 'kind', 'helpful', but some staff 'sharp-tongued'. One senior member of staff 'like sergeant major, barking out orders' and does not put women at their ease. Some married nurses with children of their own 'sympathetic'. Long waits, hot and sticky atmosphere because heating turned up high. Woman sees consultant once or twice at beginning and end of pregnancy. Those who have asked to see consultant have been told they are 'making a fuss'. One woman says she was told by senior member of staff, '*I* decide when you should see the consultant.' Registrars usually willing to answer questions. But women find it inhibiting to have entourage of student nurses, nurses and other staff when discussing personal matters with consultant. Apparently doctors do not always read notes before asking women questions. Two writers had been distressed by questions, the answers to which were already written in their notes. Tend to see different doctor each time. 'Disconcerting' as matters are not always followed up as they should be.

Antenatal ward – large numbers of women seem to be admitted for observation from clinic and many writers had had labour induced. One woman said that eight out of ten patients in clinic she attended were admitted and then induced and this may be described as 'helping things along' and be treated so lightly that woman has no chance to give informed consent.

Labour Mini-shave/enema. Sounds as if there is a high rate of intervention and readiness to set up oxytocin drip and do forceps deliveries and Caesarean sections, though it may be chance that nearly all women who wrote had various forms of intervention. Electronic fetal monitoring may be used. Writers did not think that they were always given accurate or honest information; one couple told it would probably be Caesarean section as 'the fetal heart is dangerously slow'. (It did not dip below 120.) Forceps delivery was done instead and parents believed that this was unnecessary. Room is not sound-proofed and writers say women can be heard screaming. Pethidine offered but not pressed when refused. It is often suggested that woman sits up to help descent of baby's head, but there is not enough support for her head and pillows only reach her shoulders. Writers who tried to turn on their sides sometimes said that they dislodged apparatus. Some doctors especially mentioned as 'understanding' and 'gentle'. Many members of staff examined mother without warning or asking permission. One father who summoned sister when his wife went into second stage was told to wait outside and baby was delivered in his absence though he had wanted to be there. Baby put on mother's abdomen, but for very short time. Most writers said it was for a matter of seconds. Baby was not brought back even if mother asked, until she had been stitched. One writer became distressed at not having her baby; she was told room was too cold, but says temperature was high. Some writers were concerned that as parents they were not considered to have a right to know about their own babies and treatment proposed. Father may be asked to leave after delivery and come back next visiting time which may not be till next day.

Postnatal Not enough staff; second-time mothers helped first-time mothers. Women from ethnic minorities and other religions 'come in for criticism' and 'many have hard time'. Several writers who asked questions or declined procedures said they were told they were fussing; 'I have found that it is easier to get on by saying "yes nurse, no nurse" . . . I suppose they call it "cooperation".' Some day staff praised for being 'cheerful' and comforting to unhappy mothers. Rules about picking baby up and feeding much more relaxed than a few years ago.

Postnatal check-up One writer says she waited 2 hours before staff started seeing mother and baby and points out that with 6-week-old baby this is too long. An anxious woman who had a serious obstetric condition asked questions of registrar who refused to answer and said it was a matter for GP (who had not been involved in her obstetric care).

Suggestions Better staff/patient ratio. Clinic receptionists with warmth and understanding. Investigation on how to improve staff/patient relationships.

This should examine ways of 'getting new view of patients, not simply as people who do what they are told' and are passive. Woman should never be 'told off' by staff in front of other patients. Recognition of importance of time for bonding of both parents with baby after delivery and opportunity to be together for extended period without interruptions.

Dulwich, East Dulwich Drive, London SE22   MO

'Old', 'cramped' hospital and 'general lack of privacy'. GPs deliver here, give their own antenatal care except for booking visit at about 20 weeks and another at 36 weeks.

Antenatal 'Sister treated me as an intelligent woman'; doctors are pleasant. Relaxation and breathing classes taught well.

Labour Mini-shave/enema. Partner may be asked to leave during doctor's examination, though otherwise welcome. Epidurals may be recommended. Midwives 'pleasant . . . but tell you what they are doing rather than entering into discussion'. Understand what is taught in antenatal classes and what women using breathing and relaxation techniques are trying to do. Student midwives 'lovely'. Some male doctors described as 'chauvinistic', 'soulless'.

Postnatal Two wards, one for smokers, other for non-smokers. Medical and nursing staff very busy and 'you have to ask twice if you want help'. Women who deliver in evening may get no food till breakfast time and one said she was 'ravenously hungry'. Some writers said they came out exhausted. Visiting strict 2–4 and 7–8 p.m.

Suggestions Membranes should never be artificially ruptured without woman's consent. More bathrooms on postnatal wards. Some writers would like longer with their husbands in the evening.

Greenwich District, Vanbrugh Hill, London SE10

Progressive hospital; good relations with Community Health Council and NCT. Senior midwifery officer writes, 'many grateful patients have expressed their pleasure and surprise at the individual care and approach to their needs, which have been given despite the size and modern clinical appearance of the building and the heavy workload'.

Antenatal Waiting around 2 hours. Women say they see different doctor each time 'and they quite often contradict each other'. Some writers were particularly anxious that doctors did not agree on date baby due. Waiting area always crowded; 'sometimes about 100 people were waiting;' 'I realized what people meant when they referred to clinics as like cattle markets'; 'I felt as though it was a sausage factory.' Senior midwifery officer says clinic waiting times are improving 'but are not good enough yet . . . much effort is being put in to providing midwives' clinics and two of these are now taking place weekly.'

London

Large parentcraft classes take place in evening; 'mothers or friends are invited and welcomed to them,' says senior midwifery officer. Induction rarely done and only for clear medical reasons; approximately 10% (1980). Prostin is applied to cervix overnight, with ARM later. An additional 3% of women have Prostin only.

Labour Women have choice in and influence on the way they are cared for. Senior midwifery officer states that they are cautious on approach to idea of active management and use of machinery. Doctors 'kindness itself'. Midwives 'very helpful', 'supportive', 'informative'. Electronic fetal monitoring used for high-risk babies. 100 mg pethidine may be offered. Senior midwifery officer says 'only the patient who *wants* to be is machine-monitored'. Epidurals available. Partner can be present but, say writers, is not allowed in theatre. Some writers were critical of procedures employed while partner was out of room. One woman had a failed forceps delivery while her husband had gone to the lavatory and when he came back he was asked to wait and the next thing he saw was his wife being wheeled to theatre for Caesarean section. 5% of labours are augmented; high rates for operative delivery: forceps 13%, vacuum extraction 3% and Caesarean section 15% (1980).

Some midwifery staff open to children coming in immediately after delivery and, in principle, even to being present at birth.

Postnatal Senior midwifery officer writes, 'There is still room for further improvement, especially in the postnatal area.' One woman who had epidural and 4½ l sodium chloride intravenously during labour thought that aftercare was not good enough; she had to be catheterized until tenth day. Mother has baby with her. One writer was grateful that after difficult labour obstetrician came to ward and 'sat and talked for ages'. Some night staff criticized as 'unsympathetic'.

SCBU Communication between SCBU and postnatal wards sometimes inadequate. Some mothers felt out of contact with what was going on in SCBU. One woman said she did not see paediatrician until 2 days after delivery and then had to sit in SCBU and wait until he had finished rounds in order to catch him. She was given no encouragement to breast-feed, expressed her milk and took it down to SCBU but was 'mostly ignored' and felt she was a nuisance. Milk bank helped with supplies of expressed breast milk from local NCT.

Suggestions Better communication between delivery suite and postnatal wards so that staff know exactly what kind of labour and delivery a woman has had and care for her accordingly. More understanding night staff. If baby is in SCBU paediatrician should visit mother and report on condition of baby as soon as possible.

★ **Guy's Hospital, St Thomas Street, London SE1**   MO

Staff 'approachable', 'friendly'.

Antenatal In McNie Centre (new block), busy clinic but has been reorganized to cut down long waiting times. Partners welcome. Two scans given routinely during pregnancy, one at booking and another at 32–40 weeks. Long waits for these. Genetic counselling service available. AFP testing done. Parentcraft classes.

Labour Prostaglandin pessaries often used to induce and majority of writers describe electronic fetal monitoring and actively managed labours. Staff give great encouragement and are 'extremely sensitive'. Partner welcome, including during admission procedures. Cassette and tape recorders in some rooms and you can bring your own tapes to play. Epidural service on request. Woman can discuss dose of pethidine if she wishes and indicate what type of delivery she would prefer: 'I had no drugs or hassles.' Student midwives, medical students and obstetric nurses may observe or do delivery. Writer was told by member of staff episiotomy rate 50%. Baby delivered on to mother's tummy and she is helped to put it to breast almost immediately. One writer said she was able to be with her husband and baby for 2 hours after birth.

Postnatal Demand-feeding practised. Bottled water also encouraged. Staff always willing to help with feeding. Babies room-in with mothers day and night, and are only taken to nursery during ward cleaning. Apparently life on wards is exhausting and it is difficult to get sleep. Babies who need phototherapy usually treated on ward and need not go to SCBU. Scheduled feeding for bottle-feeders. Baby weighed routinely on third, fifth and seventh days. Nursery nurses 'good' and 'helpful with practical breast-feeding problems'. Staff as a whole 'very committed'. Agency staff at night not so good. Clocks buzz loudly every hour on the hour day and night – one reason why many writers said they got very little sleep. Day/dining-room for main meals. Food 'fair' but plentiful. Ample and good baths/showers/lavatories/bidets. Visiting 3.30–5.30 p.m. and 7.30–8.30 p.m. Own children may come in afternoons.

Hammersmith Hospital, Du Cane Road, London W12

Large number of high-risk women attend this hospital.

Antenatal SNO writes that 'a constant effort is being made to keep waiting times to a minimum' but writers say waits very long, rarely in and out 'in less than 2½ hours'. Scans are done and entail extra queuing. Midwives' booking clinic, however, has more relaxed atmosphere and opportunity for discussion. Some antenatal clinic care done at Acton clinic Wednesday mornings. Writers say 'not told much unless you ask'. SNO says that 'as far as possible, women are seen by the same doctor at each visit . . . Sister with special responsibility for parentcraft, health education and relaxation classes with obstetric physiotherapist are in attendance at antenatal clinics to give advice.' Antenatal classes 'good' though 'pain relief pushed a lot' by midwife. Physiotherapist 'very good, similar to NCT'. Short refresher courses for second-time mothers. Shared care can be arranged.

Labour Partner encouraged to stay all the time, except in admissions room, including for VEs, forceps, stitching; given many cups of tea. Midwives 'very pleasant' but some are 'not *au fait* with breathing learned in classes', though encouraging and interested. DNO emphasizes that there is a 'policy of flexibility' during labour. 'Mothers are ambulant for as long as possible and fetal monitoring can be arranged by remote control if the membranes are ruptured and the mother wishes to be up and about.' To ensure the comfort of our mothers . . . wedges, cushions and bean bags are available. Taped music with individual volume control is in every delivery room; mothers can bring their own cassettes and records if they prefer. Photographs may be taken. 18% of women have ARM. Some writers said electronic monitoring was 'irritating'; 'I longed to pull them out'; 'an encumbrance'. Doctors do not always stop doing VEs during contractions. Some writers said they found it hard to get information about progress and so did not know where they were in labour. This made it difficult to make informed decisions about drugs for pain relief. There is a 24-hour epidural service; one is free to decline drugs if not needed. Medical student may be present, but asks first. Some writers enjoyed being able to sit up, with legs over side of bed or on stool and being upright in first stage. Women can also squat for delivery if they wish. 42% episiotomy rate; one writer said episiotomy done before head was on perineum – 'I had a student midwife who had been 40 weeks on the labour ward and had not yet seen a normal delivery' – 15% forceps; 13% Caesarean sections (1980). One woman writes that she was told forceps delivery was usually done for pre-term baby; she said she would much prefer not to have forceps for her baby born at 34 weeks and did not. Modified (*very* modified) Leboyer-style delivery can be done. Staff 'not too well informed' if you want baby put naked on you immediately and it is as well to state this. 'We said that we especially didn't want the baby's spine straightened suddenly.' Blinds can be down, light dimmed and quiet. Mother cuddles baby on delivery table after the mucus has been sucked out. Father can go with midwife to measure, wash, weigh baby while woman stitched; 'the registrar was instructing the house-man. I felt like a sampler. They were discussing various stitches and their advantages.' Both parents can then cuddle baby and baby can be put to breast. System whereby community midwife delivers woman in hospital and continues her postnatal care at home after minimum period in hospital.

Postnatal Women get up after 6 hours. Breast-feeding help variable; some women said they were given hours of help, others said they were told to give up after just a few minutes' help. Writers say that hospital routines interfere with sleep. Food 'excellent'.

SCBU Parents allowed in whenever they like, but mother is dependent on porter service to get there at first since it is a long way from ward; 'felt guilty wanting to see my child because of the palaver involved'. Nurses/paediatricians explain everything and answer all questions. Mothers and fathers encouraged to handle, feed, change babies. Hours of help to establish breast-feeding. Electric pumps available in SCBU and on ward (though not enough sets for all). After discharge mother can come back to feed her baby, 'a facility not mentioned until the day I asked to be discharged'.

Suggestions Better organization of antenatal clinic appointments. Improved communication between staff. There should be some way of suggesting changes and improvements and it ought to be taken for granted that mothers do this. Better liaison between SCBU and postnatal ward. When baby is in SCBU brief introduction for parents on principles of care, what is going on, how long baby may be there. Mothers of babies in SCBU should be grouped together so that they can act as a support group for each other.

★ King's College, Denmark Hill, London SE5

Antenatal Clinic always crowded, frequent delays, but 'relaxed atmosphere'. Writers said they never saw same doctor twice. Doctors 'pleased to discuss every aspect of pregnancy' and tell mother how her baby is lying. Ultrasound scans standard. Writers said staff were alert to minor problems and perspicacious about anxiety and tiredness. Shared care possible.

Labour Midwives 'friendly', 'cheerful', 'kind', answer questions and 'tell exactly what they are doing'. Writers described mini-shave and sometimes had suppository. 'Very high rate of acceleration of labour with oxytocin drip for first-time mothers.' Father made very welcome, 'not made to feel in the way' when epidural put in. Woman is never once left alone. Writers said they did not feel pushed to have pain-relieving drugs of any kind. Record-player in theatre and father can choose and change records. Partner may be asked to hold one leg while midwife holds other for pushing, but medieval-style birth stools available if you ask. Leboyer delivery can be arranged: 'marvellous'. Baby delivered on to mother's abdomen and midwife helps her suckle baby on delivery table. Episiotomy is not routinely done. Rate has been 90% for first-time mothers, but may be going down. Couple have extended time together with baby in delivery room; while woman is stitched baby is either in her or partner's arms.

Postnatal Single rooms 'very comfortable'. When student midwife delivers may visit on postnatal ward several times. Nurses 'pleasant', 'kind', 'helpful', give mother support with start of breast-feeding. 'Could not have been friendlier'; 'inspires self-confidence'. Suggested routine for feeding, but any woman who wants to demand-feed can go ahead and do so; policy to offer advice, not to take over. Baby goes to nursery first night 'so that mother can rest'. Baby is brought to her to feed. Otherwise baby with mother whole time. Never taken for tests unless mother told and invited to go too. Writers advise ask questions if there is anything you need to know. Staff 'terribly busy'. Food 'quite good'.

Suggestions One writer who found it difficult to relate to her baby could have done with more active help. Staff on duty should make their rules about visiting known to mothers and not leave them to 'break the rules' by mistake and then get 'told off'.

Lewisham, Lewisham High Street, London SE13 MO

Old building, long corridors.

Antenatal If woman has shared care she sees her own GP and goes to hospital only at beginning of pregnancy and a couple of times towards end. Long waits in clinic, up to 2 hours; 'boring'; 'impersonal care'. 'Sometimes sitting in a tiny booth or worse, lying prostrate on a hospital bed waiting for the doctor for ½ hour, wearing only a light dressing gown and getting cold.' Chairs placed back to back in long row; nurses 'treat everyone briskly'; doctors pleasant, helpful, willing to spend time explaining things and write requests in notes. Relaxation classes useful and run by young, dynamic physiotherapist who comes to see mother after birth on ward, but room where they are held is too small; 'breathing becomes a problem'. Each class only ½ hour by time teacher 'has laboured through the register and settled everyone'. Mothercraft classes overcrowded; 'some mothers have to stand and some fainted as it was very stuffy'. Eight-week course held at end of clinic time, so, as clinic often over-runs by up to ½ hour, long waits incurred. They are said to be 'perfunctory'. Topics include 'sales talk by Milton, who give free samples and sell Milton units cheaply'. Talk on pain relief including epidurals, pethidine, gas and oxygen. 'Side-effects of epidurals are minimized.' Trip round labour ward, delivery room and postnatal ward.

Labour Partner can be present throughout. If you don't want shave, say so. Enema routine. 'Efficient', 'pleasant' staff, 'excellent for difficult deliveries'. Apparently lots of VEs, which some writers said they found painful, by midwife, pupil midwives, doctor on duty. No lavatory which father can use. First-stage bed is in delivery room; 'plain, tiled, bare' and 'clinical'; 'off-putting'; 'I could have done without hearing women in labour screaming in the other rooms.' No pressure to have drugs for pain relief. If you do not want continuous electronic monitoring, say so, sonicals available. Nursing staff take great deal of trouble to do things mothers ask for. Some writers said that midwives did not realize how far advanced they were in labour and did not seem to know when they were having contractions unless they showed distress. As a result one woman found that everyone went off for coffee just as she had urgent desire to push. She rang bell and 'after several minutes' they returned and baby was born a few minutes later. Writers said they were not helped to sit up for second stage, which they would have liked, and some found great difficulty pushing lying down. Most writers had episiotomies. Some also felt this could have been avoided if they had been sitting and could do what they wanted. Episiotomies sometimes done without local anaesthetic. Cord cut immediately, though mother can lift baby out herself and up on to her tummy, 'but the gown made it impossible for me to feed her' (put it on other way round). Baby taken away while mother stitched and washed (some writers said for about an hour); 'my husband had to ask eventually if we could have her back again'. (Be ready to ask earlier.) Father does not seem to be able to go up to postnatal ward with mother and baby but only to come at visiting times.

Postnatal 'Light', 'airy', 'warm' wards. One writer who asked to be in a single room was told she would be less lonely on the ward. 'Strict military discipline ruled the ward'; some nurses on night duty said to be 'particularly bossy' and 'unpleasant'. Writers said they felt a lack of information, even that they were treated as if they could not be trusted with it. One writer said she was puzzled by secrecy surrounding patients' and babies' files and that even 3 months after birth when she went to hospital with baby for check-up nothing was disclosed to her though she asked for details. These writers felt they were not treated as adults. Lactation sister very helpful with breast-feeding. Two electric pumps, one in SCBU and other circulates on ward. But other help with feeding, especially first feeds, seems to be patchy and some writers felt 'helpless', 'confused'. Nurses not always accessible, as nursing station is at one end of ward and women in beds at other end have to wait to call nurse when she is around, and 'felt neglected'. Washing area at both ends of wards used by some women as smoking rooms; 'filthy at the end of the day' and at weekends, when no cleaners. Food bland, varied, 'like invalid diet'. One writer was critical of conditions at postnatal check-up with baby. Baby weighed on scales not even covered by paper and had to be kept almost naked until doctor free, 'waiting in a rather sordid corridor'. Visiting restricted; evenings only on weekdays and afternoons as well at weekends.

SCBU One writer was distressed that her baby was fed artificial milk. On the other hand, writers say they are impressed with kindness of nurses and their devotion to babies: 'They are immensely patient with mothers under stress too, are efficient and helpful.' Unit well run.

Suggestions Should be able to see same doctor each time in antenatal clinic. More lavatories, bathrooms, showers. Treat mothers as capable of understanding and they are more likely to be able to understand. Smaller wards, not more than six beds, would be quieter; women could get to know each other more easily than in large wards in which they tend to talk only to those in next bed.

★★ London Hospital, Mile End, Bancroft Road, London E1

Signs outside warn 'beware of falling masonry'. This is small, very friendly, but old and tatty hospital. Though externally 'a dump', it is surprisingly progressive. Caring, considerate staff who treat women as individuals with minds of their own, though there are variations in attitudes and practice between different consultants. 30% of women Asian. DNO writes, 'We have put a lot of effort into understanding and meeting their particular needs.' GPs deliver in this hospital and Domino scheme is in operation.

Antenatal Appointments system. Questions answered willingly. Staff 'helpful', 'considerate', 'reassuring'. Visits last up to 2 hours. But clientele very varied. May see only two doctors throughout. This, say writers, 'made it more personal'. Hospital has clinic run by midwives, shared care can also be arranged, with woman seeing her GP up to 7 months. Helpful antenatal classes but only run for 5 weeks. Breathing and relaxation taught similar to that taught by NCT. 'Very pro breast-feeding'. Tour of hospital included. Husband, relative or friend encouraged to attend too. Special classes for Asian women who do not speak English.

Labour Staff aim to support natural birth, with no drugs unless necessary; machinery and drugs available but not routinely used. Midwives encourage women to use relaxation and breathing. Hypnosis sometimes used. Midwife may encourage woman to remain at home in early labour and not to come in too soon. One consultant likes women to have mini-shave, others no shave. Enema not done if labour advanced. Partner (any support person welcome) is sent out for this. Labour rooms have comfortable mattresses and pictures on walls. One midwife assigned to woman in labour and stays throughout, joined by student midwives and doctors. Students praised for getting 'really involved'. Midwives 'very pleasant', 'extremely helpful' and do gentle vaginal examinations. Continuous monitoring not routinely used and DNO say; 'we encourage women to move around in the first stage of labour if they wish, and in the absence of complications'. Pethidine, gas and oxygen may be offered but can be refused. Woman is given water regularly. Doctors vary, e.g. one registrar 'would have been better in a cow-shed' and was 'rough, abrupt and rude'; but after a doctor's examination woman is usually left 'to get on with it' with help of midwife. Only 8% of labours augmented with oxytocin (1980). Woman has to change room for delivery, but it is close. She can walk there if she likes. Breathing for pushing is similar to that taught by many NCT teachers. If second stage continues long time may put monitor on baby's head, but unlikely to suggest intervention. 7% forceps rate (very low), 10% Caesarean section rate. Episiotomies only done when needed, 25% (very low). One woman who 'pleaded for an episiotomy' was glad that she was 'talked out of it' by her midwife and baby was born shortly after with no cut or tears. DNO writes, 'there has been generally an increasingly liberal attitude about position for delivery'. Student midwives and medical students present at birth 'are not obtrusive'. Baby delivered on to mother's abdomen and can be suckled on delivery table. Is checked by paediatrician beside mother, cleaned and dressed beside her, not taken away. Father can photograph labour/delivery and after, if couple want this, and can hold baby. Parents have extended time with their baby alone afterwards; one couple said staff kept the champagne they provided ready in fridge.

Postnatal Baby is with mother all the time. Staff shortages; nurses are overwhelmed with work when wards full. Demand-feeding. At times when staff

285

under greatest pressure there is more likely to be strict ward routine, which irritated some writers. Older West Indian auxiliary praised and is reason why one woman did not switch to bottle-feeding. Writers say help available at all times; 'one sister stayed late to help me because I was losing heart'. Sister has personal interview with each mother after couple of days to discuss labour and anything else she wants to talk about; 'they know each patient individually and cater as far as possible for individual needs'. Paediatrician, who visits daily, is 'very helpful and willing to answer questions'. Writers are united in commenting on dirty bathrooms: 'unless you get in straight after the orderly has cleaned them' baths and lavatory seats may be dirty; bidets available but some women did not use them because not clean. Writers said there was shortage of lavatory paper and paper towels, 'one shower room permanently flooded'. Food 'so-so', 'appalling'. Writers advise taking in your own. Visiting 2.30–3.30 p.m. and 7–8 p.m. Almost 20% of women return home within 48 hours.

Suggestions Cleaner postnatal wards and bathrooms. Put cleaning materials in bathrooms. Keep larger stocks of lavatory paper. Improve food. Two writers felt that appointments system in antenatal clinic should be reviewed. A number of writers would have liked more support with breathing and relaxation learnt in antenatal classes.

★ **The Middlesex Hospital, Mortimer Street, London W1**   MO

'Rather grim' Victorian buildings. Annexes and clinics hard to find. Out-patients 'unwelcoming' but 'light and airy' inside. No agency nurses.

Antenatal 'In dreary building'; 'many problem cases'; 'depressing', but kind staff except for some 'overworked' and 'unfriendly' receptionists who 'treat non-English-speaking women like idiots'. No interpreters. Writers say they waited for from 25 minutes to 2 hours. System of queues may not be explained by receptionist. Brief examinations almost always, but by different doctors. Some writers find it difficult to get information, e.g. about rhesus problems. 'Notes incorrectly made re dates on one occasion.' Not enough chairs. No facilities for children. 'All through my pregnancy I was nagged about not putting on enough weight'; oestriol tests may be performed if baby seems small for dates. Blood test may be done if woman goes past date. Scans at 16 and 30 weeks 'exciting'; 'images on screen were explained to me'. Induction rate according to writers who have discussed it with doctors is 20%. One woman who discussed induction when 9 days overdue said she was not happy about it and it was left, though she added, 'God help the anxious and inarticulate.' Doctors 'thorough', 'efficient' but 'impersonal'; 'midwives seemed to care about me as a person'. Shared care possible with GP. Classes good, and relevant to labour. Parentcraft classes 'oversimplified'.

Antenatal ward: 'kindly care.'

Labour No shave/enema or suppository. Any special requests noted. Great flexibility. One woman said her husband bathed her and was with her throughout. Partner can be present during examinations, epidural, forceps and stitching. Women without labour companions said they were left on their own during labour. Can walk up and down corridors and spend time in nursery with babies. Membranes not automatically ruptured on admission. Though some writers said they were put on electronic fetal monitor without discussion from early labour and were expected to stay in bed, 'a lot of messing around as clip would not stay on and abdominal strap method did not work well'. Some women had monitoring for 1–2 hours and if all was well it was discontinued. You can ask for this. One writer said monitor was not removed when she asked. Two writers said they were told monitor would be used when *asked* if they wished it. Dextrose drip followed by acceleration seemed to be frequent: 'I was in no position to argue.' Understaffed by midwives; well-staffed by doctors. Some writers felt that doctors intervened without watching women closely or in any way sharing in labour experience and that nearly qualified doctors were eager to do forceps. Women can have their own flowers in labour room and play cassette tapes – bring in equipment. (Hospital has its own, but not always in working order.) Medical student may sit with woman. Midwives described as 'extremely helpful' and give 'marvellous encouragement', and are 'friendly', 'give good emotional support' and 'personal' care. Some not so understanding: 'the midwife only looked at the monitor all day, not at me'. Another 'kept asking me if I wanted pethidine'. Epidurals available on request. Anaesthetist on call 24 hours. Choice of top-up of epidural before second stage, but also told of difficulty this may cause (not being able to push baby out). Writers report monitors not working properly, sometimes errors pointed out to staff by husbands. Say they prevent women getting into position they want. 'Both my husband and I were totally ignored from the moment the obstetrician came in.' In the second stage 'everyone shouts "push!"'. Midwife may hold up one leg, partner the other. 'Kept on telling me that I was not trying.' Some women were given episiotomies immediately after they started pushing. Others said midwife tried to manage without. Induction rate, according to women who have discussed it with doctors, is 20%, which is low. Leboyer-style delivery if requested; all lights turned down after delivery. Baby can be delivered on to mother's abdomen and put to breast immediately *if she asks*. Is weighed, wiped and then mother can hold baby while being stitched. Baby goes to nursery if night. Some parents asked to be left alone with baby after birth and this was allowed.

Postnatal Sounds as if there is a very festive atmosphere on postnatal wards! No rules; very relaxed; very social; 'easy-going but efficient'. Nursing attention 'tremendous', and nurses 'very helpful', 'caring', 'friendly'. Kindly, quiet atmosphere. Multiracial, very sensitive to individual needs and everything done to facilitate bonding. Baby is in nursery first 2 nights except by special request. Women appreciate lack of interference, insistence on afternoon rest time, when 'everything goes quiet – marvellous!' and flexibility of visiting. Psychological help excellent. Staff wish to support the family unit and babies can be in bed with mothers at all times. Feeding entirely on demand, though recommend not more than 7 minutes a side at first. Patient help is given. Very good help to get baby fixed. Boiled water is suggested, but mother does not have to give it. She takes over responsibility for her baby as and when she feels able. If baby noisy at night woman can go to nursery and feed there: 'No question of allowing or not allowing what mothers want to do.' When nurses not busy, 'instead of hiding away, several used to come and say "Anyone's baby want a cuddle?"' Ward sisters very highly praised. Understaffed at weekends. Visiting any time except 1.30–3 p.m. 'Bliss!' Some fathers come to breakfast, many stay very late. Beds often curtained off for privacy or parties; 'My husband often stayed until 11 p.m. and with curtains pulled, a take-away kebab and a bottle of champagne it was almost like being at home.' Baby is wheeled out 7.30–9 a.m. for ward cleaning/breakfast and to be weighed. Food 'lousy'. Mothers say 10-day stay is usually advised.

Suggestions Parentcraft classes should deal more fully with problems after mother gets home, e.g. feeding, exhaustion. Appointment system in ante-natal clinic needs to be made to work more efficiently and better facilities provided, including toys for toddlers, more personal care from staff. Women should not have to wait in corridor. Stop commanding women to push harder in second stage – let them find their own pace. Some writers felt there was too much interference in progress of labour. More 'domestic' things, e.g. pictures in delivery room to create relaxing atmosphere. Food should have more roughage, be served hot and less institutionalized.

★★ Newham Maternity, Forest Lane, London E7

Consultant unit and GP unit which is separate wing of hospital. Divisional nursing officer writes: 'My ideas in providing a midwifery service are to have the hospital as much like a home as possible and to be as flexible as possible.' Understaffed.

Antenatal Sonar scan may be done. Women having babies in GP unit have antenatal care with own GP. Can be shown round unit beforehand. Evening and afternoon parentcraft sessions most days in week; husbands encouraged to come. When labour is induced usually done with Prostin E pessaries, not syntocinon infusion, so allowing the mother, writes DNO, 'much more freedom of movement and it is much more comfortable for her'. Induction rate only 7 per cent.

Labour Enema or suppositories may be used, but can be refused. Hospital description of midwifery services states: 'Admission routine with patient's wishes taken into full consideration'. Women can walk about if they like unless drip set up. No sedation or drugs for pain relief unless woman wants them. Full epidural service available; 13% of women choose to have epidurals. Some labours actively managed, i.e. fetal monitoring with either scalp electrodes or external cardiograph. Episiotomies 27%; forceps deliveries 10%;

Caesarean sections 7%. Modified Leboyer births can be arranged if asked for. Fathers encouraged to be present during labour. All questions answered and much encouragement.

Labour: GP unit Sparklingly fresh, with homely wallpapered bedrooms and two armchairs; delivery room but if in use baby delivered in bedroom. First babies can be born in this unit. Community midwife delivers. Midwives described as 'deeply kind', 'comforting', 'caring', 'kind beyond belief: the midwife told me how and when to breathe'. At no time is woman left alone in labour and 'no strangers wandering in and out'. One or two companions can be present throughout, e.g. one woman had her mother and husband. A close friend came through for a chat at end of first stage. Partner does not have to wear gown or overshoes. One writer says that in transition pupil midwife held her hands and did breathing with her. Full explanations given. Midwives give back massage, roll up pillows to make wedges and even 'wedged herself against pillow and me'. Extra pillows provided willingly and woman can be in any position she likes. No electronic fetal monitoring: 'no machinery or gadgets were used at any time'. No examination during contractions. Second stage: 'midwife and doctor on each side of bed put my feet on their hips and said to push against them'. Baby usually put straight on mother's abdomen, cord uncut. Writers say baby is treated gently. Placenta allowed to come naturally and if mother is interested, shown and explained to her. After any stitching, which writers said took place immediately, mother suckles baby. Own family can visit in delivery room. Mother goes back to her bedroom with baby in 'plastic tank affair' by bed.

Postnatal Full rooming-in with mother looking after her own baby, with help from staff, immediately after deliveries; 85% of mothers leave hospital breast-feeding. Supervised extra fluids given by spoon only. Demand-feeding; no time restrictions at all. Conflicting advice avoided. Mother is encouraged to talk to and watch baby. Visiting 2–4 p.m. and 7–8 p.m. for fathers and own children. Hospital tried open visiting but mothers preferred it restricted. Forty-eight-hour discharge can be arranged.

Postnatal: GP unit Writers value most sense of security and continuity of having same people caring for them right through. Own doctor does examination of baby same day. Woman can go home with her midwife in ambulance 5–6 hours after delivery. Community midwifery service also offers home births.

SCBU Open visiting for parents and other siblings. Breast-feeding encouraged.

Suggestions Omit shave entirely. Offer full Leboyer- and Odent-style childbirth for those wishing it.

London

★ **Queen Charlotte's, Goldhawk Road, London W6**

Large, pioneering, obstetrics-only research and teaching hospital with excellent intensive care facilities and progressive methods. Large number of high-risk women come here. Cheerful atmosphere, up-to-date, 'welcoming', 'on the ball'.

Antenatal High standards of care. Waits may be 1½ hours. Receptionists 'friendly', 'efficient'. High technology, and some writers say they are 'left feeling insignificant'. Midwives 'friendly'; doctors 'attentive' and 'well-meaning' but sometimes 'patronizing'. Help given willingly by staff at all levels, especially, it seems, to women with problems. Those with straightforward pregnancies may feel of less interest to the staff. Writers suggest asking doctors and midwives for their names and writing down questions beforehand: 'I realized at my first appointment that if I behaved like a sheep I would be treated like one.' If you ask you can often see the same doctor at most appointments because you know the name; otherwise there tends to be no continuity. Personal requests are entered into notes and several writers read their own notes 'without raising eyebrows'. Ultrasound scans done; husband can be present and is welcomed; can also come to appointment with consultant. Genetic counsellor available. Induction rate 19%, majority with prostaglandin pessaries.

Antenatal ward: 'On a snowbound New Year's Eve I went in with a threatened miscarriage. Despite overworked staff, I was treated with the utmost care, sympathy and sensitivity . . . one feels in the best hands.' Another woman writes: 'Malaysian midwives were superb, explained everything, had good sense of humour.' But not so all nurses: one writer described a disturbing conversation which took place in her room. A nurse was complaining about a woman with cracked nipple: 'Stupid woman! I *told* her to use the other one. She wouldn't bloody listen.' The other nurse looked upwards and said, 'Oh God!' as though it was all too tedious for words. One writer said single rooms are 'ghastly: there had been no attempt to make it look anything other than a prison cell'.

Parentcraft classes; 'informative', 'comprehensive'. Partners welcome; 'much enjoyed by fathers who attend them'. One extra class for men only. 'Extremely good' relaxation breathing classes available. Tour of hospital 'invaluable'.

Labour Some writers described induction a few days past EDD for reasons that were not made clear to them. Some thought 'emotional blackmail' was used. One woman who said 'no thank you' said she was supported by midwives in her refusals. No enema, suppositories or shave. But amniotomy seems to be done frequently. Electronic fetal monitoring used routinely; 'I agreed to internal fetal heart monitoring when my consultant told me that perinatal deaths had been reduced from 15 per thousand, the national average, to 8 per thousand, on a par with Finland, the lowest figure in the world, and this in a hospital which specializes in high-risk cases.' Epidurals available on request and 73% of first-time mothers and 46% having subsequent babies chose epidural. Drugs for pain relief are not pushed but a woman who asked for less than 100 mg of pethidine says she was told this was impossible. Labour ward 'friendly', 'welcoming', 'often very busy'. Woman in early labour may be able to walk around or sit with partner in TV room. Writers say doctors often do not explain much, believing in action, not waiting around; 'I am going to do X or you will be here all day.' Although figures are not available, it seems that drips are set up frequently and many women described accelerated labour. Some said this was carefully explained first. Midwives 'great', 'exude confidence', 'wonderful', 'much more supportive than last time' according to writer who had a baby there some years ago. But women who have been to NCT classes sometimes say midwives do not understand breathing learned there. Husband's or other partner's presence taken for granted and he is encouraged to take active role. Given tea/coffee. Some women have more than one companion. He is no longer sent out for VEs. Students may be present, but woman is asked first. Community midwives are also delivering at Charlotte's. Woman often pushes with one foot on midwife's and one on her partner's hip. Can sit well up for delivery: 'The midwife put him straight on my tummy and left the cord to stop pulsing before she cut it.' Baby can be put to breast. Some midwives and pupil midwives very interested in Leboyer approach. Baby can be born in 'reverent silence' and father and mother can rest their hands on baby as she/he is emerging. Baby is then checked/weighed/wrapped; handed to father if mother needs stitching. Couple can have a long time together with baby in quiet room. Combined forceps delivery and vacuum extraction rate 26%; father can be present if he wishes. Caesarean section rate 13%; half of all Caesareans done under epidural with, consultant obstetrician says; 'the father and mother both being able to have and appreciate the baby within a few moments of birth'.

Postnatal Relaxed atmosphere; writers say they are given good care, but 'utterly hectic'; 'hardly a moment in which to relax'. Noise (banging of doors, delivery of goods) makes it difficult to get proper sleep and rest. There are so many interruptions that day is exhausting and writers say that they are 'constantly pestered by well-intentioned bodies e.g. physio/family planning/church/student groups/demonstrations of this or that'.

This is one woman's record of her day:

6.15	? number of feeds	11.15	empty bins
6.30	? all OK – night sister	11.20	? pain killers required
7.30	breakfast	12.00	lunch
8.00	breakfast tray and	12.30	collect lunch tray
	water jug collected	12.45	? all OK – administrator
9.00	bed making	1.00	? all OK – doctor
9.30	Hoovering	2.15–3.00	bath baby demo
9.50	papers	3.00	tea
11.00	coffee	3.30–4.30	visiting
11.05	? last feed	5.00	stores stock-up
11.10	clean wash basin	6.00–8.00	visiting

6.15	supper	9.30	? all OK
8.10	empty bins	sometime in the middle of the	
8.30	last feed	night ?	all OK
9.00	medicine round	6.00	bins emptied!

PS forgot post delivery and menu chart delivered and collected. *Plus* somehow fitting in feeding, changing, taking to nursery for (a) daily check and (b) heel prick, and then trying to do some exercises, top and tail myself bath, water flowers, etc. I had an amenity bed – so dread to think of the level of activity in the wards.

At least no one is going to get lonely!

Shortage of staff. One writer wanted to keep her baby with her immediately after birth but could not because of staff shortage; 'they were genuinely sorry'. Some writers said baby was usually with mother after third night. Otherwise policy of rooming-in. Baby can be in bed with mother much of the time. Writers said they got worried that their babies would wake other people and some discharged themselves early because they thought they were better at home for that reason. Staff nurses 'kindest people you could meet anywhere'; 'particularly impressive with their personal interest in you'. Some nursery night staff criticized as 'aggressive', 'intimidating'. Others 'very kind' and one night sister especially praised. Sometimes as many as thirty babies in nursery; 'I felt as if I was abandoning my baby', one writer said. Policy of demand-feeding; one writer who had baby there before says it 'really is being practised there now, instead of pretence'. Good breast-feeding counsellor sits with mother at every feed if necessary and teaches how to cope with problems 'with infinite patience, sympathy and expertise'. But conflicting advice and some mothers confused (1980). Some writers said their babies who were in nursery first couple of nights were given water when they woke. Electric breast pump available. Meals not kept hot for mother who is breast-feeding. Good pain relief after Caesarean section. Less good pain relief after episiotomy and suturing of perineum apparently. Psychiatrist specializes in helping women with postnatal depression. Staff, 'so busy that you feel like getting out of bed to give them a hand', have 'a knack of making you feel you're the only person giving birth that week' and 'everything is done with a smile'. Clean, modern bathrooms/lavatories, 'with bidets, thank God'. Good physiotherapy. Some writers said older children were not allowed to see baby first day, which saddened them. Visiting 7.30–8.30 p.m., but flexible. Five-day or earlier discharge possible.

Suggestions Antenatal clinic appointments system that works better. See same doctor at antenatal visits. Reduce noise: 'Is it really necessary to empty rubbish bins in wards at 6.20 a.m.?' Nursery staff should not insist that mothers have babies with them no matter how they feel (this from woman who had Caesarean section after difficult labour). Though it is 'only gently suggested' that mother should have baby in nursery first 3 nights, some did not really like this and ask 'why not let each mother decide what *she* wants?' 'Do not disturb' notices to put on door or clip to curtains round bed. Free out-visiting for fathers. Writers welcome research projects to achieve greater continuity of care from midwives and hope this continuity will be further extended. Greater publicity given to fact that family birth room is available, and that all members of family can be at birth there.

Queen Mary's Hospital, Roehampton, Roehampton Lane, London SW15   MO

Modern, 'friendly', 'relaxed', 'helpful', 'concerned to have good public image'. Pleasant grounds. 'Feels like cottage hospital.' Long, winding corridors. SNO highly spoken of.

Antenatal Writers say that they never waited less than 1 hour. 'Particularly slow after 10 a.m.'; 'once there were thirty people ahead of me in the queue when I arrived on time.' One writer asks 'Why do they give so many women appointments at the same time?' Booking clinic separate from ordinary clinic and this is great improvement. Doctors 'pleasant and willing to answer questions' and all staff 'kind', 'efficient', 'informative'. But women rarely see same doctor successive weeks. Small chairs for children; rocking horse; play group held in waiting room: 'Pity there is not another room free as children's screams make reading impossible and it can be quite wearing after an hour or so.' Most women have shared care, only going to hospital for booking and at end of pregnancy. Antenatal classes available including excellent fathers' evenings with slides and tour of labour room, breathing techniques taught, 'lots of encouragement given and plenty of humour injected'.

Labour Some writers say professor's patients less likely to have induction and do not have shave. Drip seemed to be set up readily. They say contractions it produces are violent and some would have preferred to take things much more slowly. Ask for it to be slowed down if contractions are long and come frequently from start. Consultant came round and asked permission to put up drip, saying that drip 'would not cause pain, only strengthen contractions'. Staff 'kind'; midwife who admitted woman turned up to see her on postnatal ward. May be asked if medical student can sit with you. Electronic fetal monitoring used. Drugs for pain relief offered at regular intervals. 'Friendly' and 'encouraging' midwives take pains to explain monitoring to couples. Labour and delivery take place in same room; ample supply of pillows. Partner excluded during enema and giving of epidural but present for rest of time, including internal examinations and catheterizing and stitching. Cups of tea provided for him. Epidurals often suggested. 'Bliss' said one woman who had oxytocin drip. Episiotomies seem to be done frequently. Baby is put straight on mother's breast. If straightforward delivery couple left with baby for ½ hour or so before baby is taken to be cleaned up.

Postnatal 'Relaxed atmosphere'; all staff 'very friendly', 'kind', 'helpful', 'always there to help' but leave mother to get on with things her way when she wants to. Baby can stay with mother day and night, though for first two nights she is encouraged to put baby in nursery. Baby has to go to nursery only when

293

cleaning done. Nursery nurses 'kind'. 'No pains are spared in encouraging breast-feeding.' Mothers complain of heat; say wards kept at 85°, no fresh air allowed. Babies wear no clothes, just wrapped in sheets and blanket. Several writers said their babies came out in rashes. All writers found it difficult to rest. They describe 'far too many visits by domestic staff, cleaning, bringing drinks'. Here is one woman's diary of her day:

Lights on 5.30–6 a.m. and mothers woken with morning tea. If mother is asleep when beds made at 7 a.m. she is not disturbed. Tell staff and it is made later on. 8 a.m. breakfast. Tea arrives at 8.30. Coffee not available. 9–10 a.m. doctors' rounds, but often doctors do not arrive till 11–11.30, so mothers do not know whether to go for bath or not. 10.30 coffee. 10.30–11.30 a.m. ward cleaning, mothers who are feeding go to nursery. Physiotherapist comes for postnatal exercises. Lunch is supposed to come at 12 midday but is usually half an hour late: 'inefficient serving system'. 12.30–2 p.m. rest. 2.45 p.m. cup of tea. 3.15–4.15 p.m. visiting, own children can come. Visitors with children can be seen in reception area. Only near relations allowed to handle baby and all must wash hands first. 4.30 p.m. temperature taking. Some writers would have liked cup of tea then. 6.30 p.m. supper. 7.30–8.30 visiting. 11 p.m. evening drinks.

At times other than visiting times you can see people in reception area.

Food 'absolutely inedible', 'dull', 'ordered 24 hours in advance; it is impossible to breast-feed when you yourself are starving'. One writer said she was weak with hunger by end of week. Fathers visit 'laden down with Chinese take-aways'.

Forty-eight-hour discharge possible.

Suggestions Changes in antenatal clinic 'so you feel less like a number'. Serving hatch on postnatal ward so women can help themselves to tea when they are ready. Make beds at same time as cleaning wards so women can get some rest. Provide evening drinks while mother gives last feed of evening so that she does not lie awake till 11 p.m. waiting for her drink.

Royal Free Hospital, Pond Street, Hampstead, London NW3

Enormous, clean, very comfortable wards. A high-tech hospital and care tends to be authoritarian.

Antenatal 'Very impersonal, crowded clinic'. 'Little consideration is given to the individual'; 'no opportunity to discuss the birth'; 'insufficient contact between different departments'. Shortest wait reported 1½ hours, some 3½-hour waits: 'One receives an appointment for 1 p.m. and along with thirty or forty other women with the same appointment wait like battery hens.' Other people, e.g. husbands, may occupy chairs while pregnant women stand, leaning against walls for support. 'I used to dread my antenatal appointments.' Writers said they rarely saw same midwife or same doctor twice. One obstetrician examining woman who was tense said, 'I hope you will do better than this when you are in labour.' 'Doctors just prod and grunt at you.' Shared care possible. Excellent teaching of relaxation and good fathers' evenings.

Antenatal ward: woman admitted at 37 weeks for diabetes tests said she was put in ward with women who had had their babies. Sitting beside a friend's bed giving her baby a bottle of dextrose while she ate her dinner a nurse 'Told me off in front of the entire ward: "You have no business interfering with other women's babies and giving them infections" . . . I was so upset that I burst into tears' and she begged to be induced. ('A constant stream of visitors had been picking up this baby anyway.')

Labour Partner made to feel welcome and encouraged to help, but not allowed in for prepping – mini-shave, enema (one writer had two), even, with one woman, when she was 7 cm dilated. (She said enema worked on delivery table.) Shower, sometimes cold. Midwives 'kind', 'wonderful', 'really sweet', and 'chatty'. Induction by prostaglandin pessaries. One writer says senior obstetrician doing labour ward round said 'Why is this woman lying here doing nothing, rupture her membranes!' She had amniotomy and oxytocin drip, but cervix did not dilate and the result was an emergency Caesarean section. She was distressed that she had not been allowed to start her labour with prostaglandin pessaries alone and amniotomy only when cervix was ready. Some writers thought that induced labours had been accelerated too fast. Woman may not be allowed to drink – is given wet cloth to put against her lips if thirsty. Electronic fetal heart monitoring standard practice and used in all but quickest labours. Pethidine offered and epidurals available. Women say they would like facts made available so that they can make considered decisions for themselves about treatment. Emphasis on modern medical technology entails frequent use of acceleration. 'One is very easily panicked by the "Well, if you want to risk the life of your baby."' Some writers had long and painful contractions with syntocin drip; one baby registered immediate distress with first prolonged contraction and an injection of salbutomol was given; the mother says, 'They all act in the belief that the course they are taking was the right one. They undoubtedly saved my baby's life after endangering it in the first place.' Woman having rapid labour, more than half dilated, said, 'Someone wielding a drip and without even bothering to explain why began to set it up.' She was drowsy at end of first stage and asked her husband to tell them to take it away, which was done. Inadequate soundproofing. In fathers' waiting room women can be heard 'screaming away down the corridor'. Medical students may be present. One woman said this was 'a pain'. It appears that nearly everyone has episiotomies. Women are not consulted about this, told 'We're going to cut you, dear.' Midwives are often happy to deliver women standing, squatting or on all fours. But you need to *ask*. Baby is usually placed on mother's abdomen as soon as born and given to her to suckle. Cord need not be cut straight away. Suctioning not done routinely. But some writers say that baby was 'whisked away'. Couple have extended time alone with their baby after it is washed and wrapped up.

Postnatal Baby with mother and writers say there is 'peace and quiet much of the time'. Sometimes shortage of clean baby linen 'and when I went into nursery to collect more I was shouted at'. Smoking in day room only. Cleaners sometimes criticized for unpleasantness and 'banging into babies' cots' and 'slamming doors'.

One writer remarked on poor communication with GP. Some mothers say things are done to their babies without consulting them first, such as giving dextrose solution, and that there are delays in calling a mother to breast-feed when a baby wakes and cries.

Food very good but lacks roughage. Choice of about five dishes at lunch and supper. Breakfasts 'drearily repetitive': hard boiled egg, cereal and 'stewed tea'. As much fresh milk from kitchen as wished.

Almost unlimited visiting for fathers, nurses sympathetic to visits of friends and relatives who have travelled long distance. Own children can visit, have cuddle on bed. Visiting 2.30–4.30 p.m. 'could be tiring', and 7–8.30 p.m. Children can come in evening if more convenient. 8–8.30 p.m. husbands only.

Postnatal clinic One mother was told she could not breast-feed while waiting for appointment.

St Bartholomew's, West Smithfield, London EC1   MO

Large, old, 'not particularly clean', very busy but everybody 'friendly' and 'gives impression that they are efficient and know exactly what they are doing'. 40% of women have operative deliveries here (i.e. forceps or Caesarean section).

Antenatal Clinics overcrowded; may have long waits (up to 3 hours), though usually it is 1 hour or less. Tests take longer. Too hot in summer. Staff 'helpful', 'friendly', 'take time to answer all questions' and 'deal with worries'; 'I was made to feel as though I were the only patient'. Examinations are unhurried, though may see at least six doctors in thirteen visits. No facilities for fathers. Scans done. Students work here, take blood pressure for practice. Inductions appear to be frequent for post-maturity of 1 week and other reasons, though woman's point of view is considered. Antenatal classes are 'not good', according to writers.

Labour Atmosphere relaxed, 'caring', 'intimate'. Partner can be present throughout, including preparation and suturing of perineum. One writer said midwife stayed throughout labour. Pethidine available and choice of pain relief is up to woman herself. Woman who had Caesarean birth said obstetrician explained simply and sympathetically why she needed it and what was going to be done. She was frightened and asked if her husband could be with her, but he was 'hustled out of the way' when she was taken to theatre and not allowed to be with her when she received general anaesthesia. 90% episiotomy rate, 22% forceps, 18% Caesarean sections. Mother helped to put baby to breast after delivery, but this is sometimes inexpertly done. One senior member of staff 'pinched the nipple so hard that it remained black and bruised for a week'. When her husband complained 'she threatened to take the baby away'.

Postnatal 'I have never experienced such kindness, encouragement and help in hospital in my life,' says mother of third baby. 'Terrific' nurses; 'nothing too much trouble'. Staff always available to advise and help; demand-feeding encouraged. Mother cares for own baby completely and some writers praise staff for help with breast-feeding when they thought of giving up. But though majority of nurses considerate, occasional one 'dictatorial' and 'rude' and agency night staff sometimes criticized for being 'unhelpful' and 'rude'. Babies kept in very hot nursery at night. Generous visiting hours.

Suggestions Antenatal clinic needs larger waiting room and better appointments system. Wards should be smaller. There should be study of ways in which postnatal stay could be less tiring for mothers. Babies should be allowed by mother's bed at night.

★ St Mary's, Praed Street, Paddington, London W2

Old hospital, 'looks like public lavatory' inside, but is clean, well run and 'most important of all, they treat you as an individual'. Main building done 1981. Midwifery training school. Staff 'caring'. At time when some reports on this hospital were coming in Alec Bourne Obstetric Unit was closed for major upgrading and moved to Harrow Road. But re-opened in 1982 and Harrow Road unit closed except for antenatal care. DNO writes; 'Midwives and obstetricians aim to give the woman and her baby an informed choice in the management of their pregnancy, while giving a high standard of technical care.'

Antenatal 'A major review of clinic premises, facilities and methods of offering care and education to pregnant women is being undertaken,' according to DNO. All staff 'kind', 'helpful', 'answer questions'. Sister in charge always ready to answer queries and sort out problems. Doctors and nurses 'take pains to remember people'. Women said they rarely had to wait more than quarter of an hour, though occasionally one hour plus when very busy; 'always impressed at how smoothly clinic ran'; 'shortest waits at start of clinic'. Separate cubicles for changing and waiting for doctor; privacy is appreciated. One woman ('I never felt just a number') wrote that apart from first two visits she always saw same registrar, who also delivered baby, 'but he said I had been lucky'. There are some midwives' clinics and you can ask to attend one of these if you like midwifery care.

Harrow Road clinic 'Big class divide between these two clinics.' Clinic is about twice as large and waiting twice as long. No facilities for children. 'No time to ask questions' and writers say women tend to be passive and take what comes.
   Antenatal ward: one woman, in room of her own, brightened it up with paintings, rug, photographs, books, which 'was a source of great pleasure to everyone from the cleaners to the consultants'.
   Writers said they enjoyed classes and fathers' evening was good; can see round wards. Low induction rate, 9% (1980).

Labour No shave necessary but suppository may be given for which partner asked to leave. Short-staffed but calm atmosphere. 'All help and support with breathing I could wish for' and 'my husband was helped to feel involved'. Couple can usually be together throughout labour and can spend early labour phase in TV room if they wish. Woman is given food and drink, husband nothing; 'he would have liked tea when I had a cup'. One father had nothing to eat or drink for 15½ hours. Continuous electronic monitoring used routinely, 'very reassuring as that was a busy night and they were drastically short of staff'; 'fascinating', 'I loved to hear the baby's heart beat and see the contractions on the chart'. 26% of women have epidurals, available on request; 'superb'; 'anaesthetist very friendly'. Topped up on request, well timed so that woman can feel to push. Checks every 30 minutes to see if further topping up needed. Women who did not want drugs for pain relief said they could labour without any; but 'if you do not want electronic monitoring, do not go in until you feel second stage is about to start'. Gas and oxygen available. Labour with lights dimmed. Some midwives very much praised, though occasional writers said they did not get enough emotional support and expert encouragement because midwives were too busy; 'no one looked at me to tell me if I was fully dilated and it was safe to push'. Blood samples may be taken from baby's head. Father sent out for this. Woman is well propped up in second stage, may push against midwife's hips. Some women say there was a time limit on pushing of 30 minutes. Father can be present for forceps delivery. Fairly high rate of operative delivery here; 15% forceps and 13% Caesarean section. Episiotomy rate 70% for women having first babies and 40% for those having subsequent babies. Baby is handed to mother straight away before cord cut and can be suckled immediately. Though one couple had 2 hours with their baby they thought that this was 'our good luck' and another woman wrote 'after about 10 minutes they took her away'. Woman may have to wait to be sutured. One woman said she spent ½ hour waiting – 'most uncomfortable . . . exhausting'. One woman's mother who arrived ½ hour after birth was also welcome in delivery suite.

Postnatal DNO writes, 'Mothers are encouraged to develop a natural feeding pattern and to have their babies with them all the time.' 'Lovely, friendly atmosphere'. Nurses 'kind', 'helpful', 'considerate', 'sweet', but some auxiliaries described as 'positively demonic', 'utterly unsympathetic', 'cruel to girls unable to speak English'. Emotional support and help with breast-feeding. Rooming-in practised and policy of breast-feeding on demand; 'staff act as if you are very important'; 'everyone is made to feel someone who is cared about, a person who matters'. Some women thought there was unnecessary weighing and worrying; 'my baby lost 4 oz on her first day of life'. This mother became anxious because senior member of staff asked her why she thought it had happened and expressed great concern. On the whole the mother is left to care for her baby in her own way, so if you want help, *ask*. Wards very tidy. Plenty of baths and showers. Staff very pleasant, keep mother informed, do tests with her present, and go to ward to give results of tests as soon as possible. Ice-packs provided for sore perineum but some women said there were not enough foam or rubber rings to sit on. Opinion about food varies. Visiting times 'fairly easy-going'.

SCBU SNO writes that 'particular care is taken to establish family relationships in a friendly, supportive atmosphere, though the stress of the situation is acknowledged'. Women say SCBU is 'marvellous' and staff help a lot with breast-feeding. If baby is having phototherapy mother can spend all day next to light box, touch baby whenever she wishes and take baby out when she wants to. Father allowed in nursery, no one else in theory, but writers say that other family members come too, 'discreetly'. One mother of jaundiced baby being given phototherapy in nursery says she felt very sad to see other women with their babies and not have hers. Could not gear be next to mother's bed?

Suggestions Tea for fathers during labour. Self-service system for food and linen, freeing nurses for important jobs and reducing need for 'obnoxious orderlies'. If nipples flat and baby can't get fixed use Natural Nursing Shield (rubber ones), not ordinary nipple shields. Provide tea on waking at 6.15 a.m.

St Mary's Wing, Whittington, Highgate, London N19   MO

High-tech hospital, old-fashioned exterior. 'Friendly staff compensate for nineteenth-century atmosphere.' Patients of Elizabeth Garrett Anderson deliver at Whittington and EGA doctors attend them.

Antenatal 'Institutional'; 'little room for any individuality'; 'felt like second-class citizen'. Sounds as if induction is done frequently. Sometimes woman is delayed because too many inductions taking place at one time: 'I was extremely upset, prepped the night before and had a sleepless night'. 'I feel that postponing induction from day to day is psychologically unendurable.' It also makes one wonder how necessary some of these inductions were! One woman was told that her induction was to be put off till next day as they were running behind and 'You wouldn't want your baby to be born in the middle of the night.' Classes 'not exactly encouraging'. Double attendance at hospital and NCT classes discouraged. One writer said teacher said she did not expect mothers to remember anything and that, frankly, breathing exercises do not prove helpful to most. 'Schoolmarmish' teacher 'always asks in front of everyone why a mother missed the week before'. One woman did not go back after such an incident. Room airless and not enough mats for all women. Three evening films and lectures for couples together, better than day sessions.

Labour A woman who refused a scalp monitor had it put on a few hours later, since doctor insisted. Partner told to leave while it was inserted. 'Drip was in my hand, monitors and blood pressure wrap on my arm; it was nearly impossible to move. I got bad leg cramp. These pains were nearly as bad as the contractions.' Monitors sometimes 'run out of ink' and various accounts of them breaking down. 'The lady in the next bed's machine broke down and a student nurse wheeled it away. Unfortunately it was plugged into the same board that my drip was and my arm was suddenly, in the middle of a contraction, yanked across the bed . . . my husband prevented injury to me by leaping up and grabbing the drip and holding it.' Pethidine and epidurals available. Staff 'very encouraging' and 'cheery' at delivery, but some writers could have done with encouragement earlier on.

Information on postnatal ward has come in from too few women to be made use of.

St Teresa's, The Downs, Wimbledon, London SW20 MO

High standard of comfort and nursing. Well decorated; very clean. Flower arrangements in passages. 'Calm', 'relaxed', 'friendly' atmosphere. Staff, including tea-ladies and cleaners, stay here a long time.

Antenatal Considerable criticism of antenatal care by writers, though longest wait 30 minutes. GPs deliver here and care can be shared with GP or woman can have private consultant. Partner can come and stay all the time. Most writers said there was plenty of time to talk and discuss worries and that staff were 'helpful'. Ultrasound done at hospital. Those writers who had consultant care often seem to have had labour induced, though it may be chance that these women wrote.

Labour Shave normally done but can be refused. No enema. Woman can walk around. Some writers did not have electronic monitoring though many did have it and some said it gave them confidence. Partner can be present throughout and staff welcome him, explain things to both and encourage him to take part. Woman can labour without pain-relieving drugs if she wishes, but hospital is noted for its epidurals. Caesareans done under epidural. Midwives 'helpful'. Woman who had Caesarean said she enjoyed seeing trees through theatre window. After delivery baby was laid beside her head on delivery table so she could kiss and cuddle her. But husband could not be present. Some writers had baby in cot beside them after Caesarean, and others said baby was taken up to father. In second stage woman can sit up for pushing, but some writers were on their backs with legs in stirrups. 'Midwife had scissors ready for episiotomy,' said couple who had asked not to have one. On request midwife put scissors down and baby was delivered without cutting or tearing. Baby handed to mother before being wrapped. Father can also hold baby. But looking back at labour one said his wife was treated as if she was suffering from a disease that only medical experts with modern machinery and drugs could cure.

Postnatal Happy atmosphere, very comfortable single rooms 'bright', 'quiet', and writers describe rooms with own bathroom, dressing room, french windows on to balcony. Rooming-in during day but 'women are strongly discouraged from having their babies with them at night'. 'Drugs were offered left, right and centre to make mothers sleep through the night.' One writer who asked to have her baby with her day and night says she was told this could not be done and felt she was labelled as a 'trouble-maker'. 'Do things the way the hospital wants and you will be OK. Rebel and you've had it.' Though writers in 1979 said they were told 'we will feed the baby' at night, since that time reports suggest that baby is given nothing without permission, no top-ups and no sugared water. Some women thought they did not get enough help with breast-feeding. Some said they were urged to keep to feeding routines. Reports of conflicting advice. Nurses are 'friendly' and give individual care. If mother gets tired of having baby with her or wants to snooze baby is 'greedily' wheeled away by nursery staff. The nuns are totally warm-hearted and amusing. The matron and Sister Bernadine especially. 'The bedside manner is thriving here and is held in as great esteem as equipment and medicine.' 'Marvellous' Catholic chaplain and 'Womie the paper man, great for morale'. Food good and plentiful. Visiting 2–4 p.m. and 6–10 p.m.; free for fathers. Own children welcome in afternoons. Women normally stay 1 week.

Suggestions Less emphasis on drugs. More flexible routine. More freedom of choice. Delivery rooms less 'bleak'. Better advice on breast-feeding.

St Thomas's, Lambeth Palace Road, London SE1   MO

'Friendly', very busy. Luxury of new wing contrasts with postnatal wards in old wing. Views either 'fantastic' or 'awful'. Mary Ward (antenatal ward) overlooks Big Ben and the Thames. Postnatal wards overlook powerhouse.

Antenatal Care may be handled entirely by GP practice. Consultants come to practice. Given own notes to keep. Encouraged to ask about tests. Midwife from practice goes into hospital and delivers. 'I prefer community-based system to centralized "chicken-run".' Before this system was started it was discovered that women saw on average 7.4 doctors while pregnant. Now woman sees just one doctor and consultant: 'All women come back for postnatal check-ups.' For those having antenatal care at St Thomas's there are long waits (1½ hours). May see consultant several times and can ask to see him or other consultant if you would like to. 'Impersonal structure', effort made to give care and attention, but staff sometimes too busy for this. Students work here, examine and question, but always ask first if they may. Doctors and midwives 'understanding', 'friendly'; woman say they feel they have time to ask what they want to and all questions are answered fully, 'without reservation'. Waiting area bright. Ultrasound may be done. Some women felt they had insufficient information about this. Several writers would have liked to have had their partners with them to see too: 'It was such a moving experience.' They often have to wait for appointment and with full bladders get very uncomfortable. Excellent cafeteria.

Antenatal classes 'good', but 'elementary', 'slow and over-simplified'. Senior physiotherapist 'very good'. Enjoyable tour of maternity unit. One class for fathers to become familiar with hospital and its procedures. 'Very friendly', but writers say preparation for labour 'scanty compared with NCT classes'. 'Breathing techniques inadequate', 'importance of relaxation under-emphasized and presented in hazy way, unrelated to nature of contractions'. 'Groups too large and time wasted on repetitive advice by different lecturers.'

Antenatal ward: relaxing atmosphere. Some women found close proximity of TV set disturbing.

Labour Staff 'very welcoming', 'friendly', 'supportive', 'sensitive', 'kind', 'chatted', though one midwife described as 'sharp', 'snappy'. One writer delivered by her community midwife said it was 'wonderful to see a familiar face'. Mini-shave/enema. Some writers felt coerced into induction at or soon after term for safety of baby and thought inductions were done too readily. Prostaglandin pessaries used first. Amniotomy seems to be done more or less routinely. One writer who asked whether it was necessary said she was told, 'It'll speed things up' and it was done promptly. Women given no food in early labour. One who had no food for 24 hours felt this was far too long. Some writers described acceleration of labour; 'was fully explained'. Partner can be present throughout except for induction, and is given meals. Woman may be encouraged to walk about if she feels like it. Helped to breathe through contractions and praised for doing so, but some discouraged from breathing lightly and told to take deep breaths. Some writers had very 'mechanized' labour and said they hated to think how they would have coped if they had not had encouragement from labour companions: 'A battery of doctors and nurses kept coming in and the monitoring equipment kept going wrong.' One woman who had vaginal and abdominal monitors at once said the pressure caused pain. Pethidine offered. Epidurals available and epidural Caesarean sections done: 'A thrilling experience! I was very well prepared and supported by staff.' Husband can be present and hold baby immediately. One woman said anaesthetist helped put baby to breast: 'A measure of just how personal the staff tried to make it for all three of us in clinical surroundings.' Tape-recorder available in delivery ward but rooms not soundproofed. Women would have liked more pillows. Labour room 'clinical' with high, narrow bed and 'masses of gear'. Some writers said they were on the table far too long and 'ached all over' but were not allowed to get off it. It is so uncomfortable 'that I didn't know how to lie'. Several writers wanted to sit or kneel up. 'I felt it could have been calmer; less urgent "open up" would have been sufficient.' Enthusiastic encouragement given in second stage and some writers felt unnecessarily hurried. Forceps delivery was sometimes suggested after 40 minutes, but this was fully explained and father could remain. No routine episiotomies. One writer described second stage of 1-hour 50 minutes and delivered naturally with intact perineum. Modified Leboyer-style delivery done on request, but *very* modified. Baby given to mother immediately and can be put to breast. But one partner said: 'They whipped the baby off to a brightly lit room to check and wipe her down. So much for modified Leboyer! I think they only do it to pacify the mothers.' Mother can hold the baby while being stitched. Only person who objected to partner's presence was nervous student. Several writers tell of medical students with shaky hands stitching without supervision and taking a very long time (up to 2 hours!). This should not happen. Parents have time with baby after delivery. If you want a single room ask at this stage. Most writers much prefer them to general ward.

Postnatal Very busy: 'a valiant attempt to create a happy atmosphere'. Mothers completely free to care for their babies and feed them as they wish. 'We practically prescribed our own pain-killers and laxatives.' But some women feel 'lost' and 'helpless', though staff very friendly. Baby goes to nursery first night and most writers asked to have babies with them from then on, but some said this was 'strongly disapproved of by the night staff'. Very noisy and difficult to sleep at night. Women discharge themselves early to get sleep. TV set in ward noisy, on almost continuously and disturbing for some mothers: 'a huge television dominates the ward'. Ward 'congested', 'draughty', 'uncomfortable', 'noisy'. 'My bed was in passage *en route* for bathroom.' Some staff have not caught up with modern research on breast-feeding and, writers say, 'bully' mothers suckling babies as long and as often as they want. Encourage them to give boiled water and 'wind' baby. Told they will get sore nipples. Mothers falsify feeding charts to keep staff happy. 'Well-meaning but contradictory advice.' 'Caesarean ladies' are not supposed to have babies with them until fifth night, but one writer insisted and had hers on third. Delightful nursery nurses 'who clearly loved babies'. Constant pressure of people offering cups of tea, meals, painkillers, and checks of baby/stitches/uterus. Single rooms more peaceful, partner allowed any time. Messages from day to night staff often not passed on. Relaxed visiting times. Visitors can hold baby. Officially partners only from 7.45 to 8.30 p.m., but not in practice. Food 'not bad', 'somewhat plastic': can order small, medium, large portions. Breast-feeding mothers can go to kitchen any time for glass of milk. Writers advise taking in some extra baby clothes. If you want early discharge start process to get out before weekend. Labs close over weekend and no blood tests can be done. Writers advise if you have help at home, arrange to leave as soon as possible to get rest.

SCBU Paediatrician comes to explain everything to mother and answers all questions. Mother can see her baby any time she likes, can hold baby through incubator portholes, feed and care for baby. 'I spent long hours in the nursery just watching my baby or cuddling him through the portholes. Sometimes I cried a little. Members of staff chatted to me and made me feel better. Paediatrician kept me informed of tests and rephrased anything I did not understand . . . One day I was having a rest on my bed when the nursery nurse wheeled my baby into the ward, followed by all the staff from sister downwards. Their delight equalled mine . . . It was almost like a party, everyone laughing.'

Suggestions More staff. Ideally, single room for everyone at night, communal area for day. More bathing facilities on postnatal wards. Women who left to recover from exhaustion suggested early discharge should be more readily available. Mother with baby in SCBU suggested that baby should be able to be in incubator beside mother's bed.

South London Hospital for Women, Clapham Common South, London SW4 MO

Badly understaffed. Some writers say 'crowded', and 'dirty': 'staff rushing around' and some writers found them apparently uncaring.

Antenatal Long waits, up to 3 hours, usually 1½–2 hours, followed by 'extremely swift' examination, 'with no time or encouragement to ask questions'. See different doctor each time. Some doctors 'have difficulty speaking and understanding English', which makes discussion even more unlikely and, one writer said 'embarrassing': 'When I asked him to repeat the things he'd said, he replied, "Nothing for you to worry about", which obviously made me worry.' Mothers with toddlers have to cope with bored, fretful children. Broken rocking-horse. 'Makes waiting harder for everyone.' Several writers said that breast-feeding was not mentioned at clinic. For scan must go to St James, SW12. Some writers asked what scan was for and said doctor would not tell them. 'Friendly', 'enjoyable' antenatal classes include discussion on breast-feeding.

Labour Some writers described being induced when a few days overdue, apparently for no other reason: 'No one told me what they were going to do or how they were going to do it.' Partner encouraged to be present throughout. Everybody 'kind', 'helpful'. Epidurals available and some writers were given epidurals without asking for them: 'I was told to sit up and given an epidural.' One husband was told, 'Your wife needs help.' He asked, 'What help?' but doctor refused to say and asked him to leave. She asked, 'Why can't he stay' but 'they threw him out' for forceps delivery. She says she was not told it was going to be a forceps delivery: 'I guessed when I saw what appeared to be enormous forceps taken out.' One writer said no one talked to her except her husband during the 7½ hours her labour lasted after induction, except for an auxiliary who told her to read. This, she said was 'pretty difficult lying flat on your back with a drip in your hand and a tube in your back'. Some women with drips set up said they were warned not to move the hand, and this was completely immobilizing. Some writers said babies were not given to them after delivery but were put in corner of room out of sight. 'After being stitched, the doctor and a midwife walked out leaving me completely helpless' with the baby across the room. This writer says an hour later the nurse came in to wash her and take her back to ward. Her husband was only informed of birth then.

Postnatal Mothers look after their babies themselves from the beginning: 'Marvellous'. Baby is with mother all the time except for a couple of hours 'rest' in mornings. Nurses usually described as pleasant, but understaffed and too busy to offer much help: 'I enjoyed that as I preferred to be left alone.' Women who spoke no English suffered under this system. An Asian woman stopped breast-feeding because she had no 'encouragement or reassurance from staff'. Some writers say staff are occasionally 'indifferent', or even 'callous' to Asian women. Postnatal wards tend to be 'very noisy' and one writer says 'no attempt to keep noise down'. A woman who took baby to nursery because she was tired was turned away and told that there were too many babies in there already, though she was obviously distressed. Mothers have babies with them during night whether they like it or not. One woman who could not move easily after epidural asked for a drink when she got to ward and told there was a water jug on her locker, but she could not reach it. She asked to see her baby, as she had not yet had a chance, but says she was told she must wait till morning. She insisted and nurse got baby, but mother not allowed to hold him. One mother was perplexed some hours after delivery when told to go to nursery, get baby and 'top and tail' him. She had no idea what this term meant and had never held a baby before. Facilities 'appalling'; baths and lavatories 'dirty', 'always a queue'. Easy-going about visiting. Especially fathers.

Suggestions More space and staff in antenatal clinic. Some doctors should be less abrupt. Less noise. More lavatories and bathrooms.

University College, Huntley St, London WC1

'Friendly', 'welcoming', high tech hospital, 'enthusiastic', 'kind', 'interested', staff.

Antenatal Very busy clinic, long waits of up to 2½ hours despite appointments system, though SNO writes that clinic now 'looks very attractive and much lighter, there are toys for the children and I do not think that the waiting time is very lengthy'. Sister in charge goes round asking how everyone is while they wait and talks to children. Even so writers say it is 'boring' and 'exhausting'. Doctors 'not hurried', 'helpful', 'friendly', 'will answer questions'. 'Made to feel that my baby was very special', 'felt like a person, not a lump of meat'. Some older mothers said that clinic emphasized risks; 'I was often reminded that I was 38', and they became anxious as a result. One writer, anxious about having a baby with Down's syndrome, said consultant spent 10 minutes discussing her fears with her and 'didn't act as if he didn't have the time or I was silly'. One writer was relieved that when she asked about episiotomy 'a very reasonable doctor said it would only be done if necessary'. Shared care possible and arrangements can be made for home deliveries. Domino deliveries can also be arranged with very early discharge from hospital and planned 48-hour discharges. Good antenatal classes and teaching of relaxation 'excellent'. But fears about episiotomy raised in classes were 'made light of' by physiotherapist; 'episiotomy is regarded as almost inevitable'. All questions treated seriously and reasons explained. Some women said they were told there was a 45-minute time-limit on pushing. Women are firmly warned about dangers of NCT and 'unqualified people'. Some writers said they were told that women attending NCT classes are 'neurotics' and 'tend to have more difficult labours than those who attend UCH classes'; 'nearly everyone I spoke to went to NCT classes but kept it secret'; midwives and health visitors running local-authority classes in area have been told by obstetrician at UCH they must not accept UCH patients and that all first-time mothers will have episiotomy and all second-time mothers who have already had previous episiotomy. Tour of hospital.

Labour SNO writes that husbands or consorts are welcomed in the labour ward; 'we encourage patients to air their anxieties'. There is 20% induction rate (including augmentation). SNO emphasizes that these statistics reflect the large proportion of high-risk cases dealt with here. Partner may be told to wait outside while woman is being admitted; shave/enema. One writer, admitted when having contractions every 3 minutes, still had shave/enema and midwife did not pause when she had contraction; 'I called for my husband and burst into tears and she then let me alone.' Even so, her husband was not allowed in. While in labour room, partner is usually with woman from then on, though one writer did not have her husband with her in transition because no one would get him and says she 'felt desperate'. Midwives 'wonderful', 'very friendly', 'unbelievably caring'; 'I wanted to stand up and the midwife got me a step ladder to lean against'. Supportive care from midwives and students who 'unlike antenatal teacher do not mind NCT mums at all'. Pethidine may be offered but woman can refuse it. 29% of women have epidurals. Partner can help with breathing, give water to drink and is made very welcome. Some writers felt that staff were 'obsessed with high technology'. One woman described internal monitor breaking down and external monitor used instead. Woman is moved to another room for delivery. One writer said she wanted to sit upright to push but it was strongly recommended that she did not do so. But another said she was allowed to get on all fours. Episiotomy is 'just about routine here. For reasons all explained very rationally at antenatal classes by the professor.' Every writer but one (26) had episiotomies. One woman said; 'it is difficult to avoid having episiotomy whatever one's preference is' and she 'felt violated'. Others said episiotomy was done routinely 'before I or my husband knew what was going on'; 'I was told to stop pushing and wait for the episiotomy'. Writer who had Caesarean section under general anaesthesia said her daughter was with her husband in waiting room and beside her bed as she woke up. High rates for operative delivery; forceps rate 18%, Caesarean section rate 20%. Baby given to mother immediately and can be put to breast straight away. A few writers described long waits to be stitched. One said she waited 1½ hours. But most were stitched immediately; 'the doctor explained what she was doing and was very gentle. A medical student was with her consoling me – two great, warm women.' Partner not encouraged to stay during stitching.

Postnatal Most women breast-feed; policy of demand-feeding. Help given is 'remarkable'; 'delightful', 'friendly' nurses and nursery nurses. No artificial milk given, but first night babies given water and mother is not woken, though some women ask to be wakened. Most writers said baby was in nursery adjoining ward first night and whenever they wished baby to go to nursery, but after this were with them all the time. If baby is in nursery mother is called when baby cries. Some night agency nurses were 'awful', 'lazy', and 'unsympathetic'. One senior member of staff was described as 'very officious'; 'I was very briskly treated in the midst of breast-feeding and was told to move as they wanted to make the bed.' But on the whole mothers agree that 'attention given could not have been beaten'; 'it is a very relaxed, friendly atmosphere'. Some writers thought that atmosphere could have been more restful if strict routines could have been more flexible, e.g. keeping meals hot for breast-feeding mothers. Couple can have evening out on last night and staff will babysit. Food 'appalling' and 'not enough of it'. Generous visiting. Fathers-only visiting times 'lovely'. Visitors also allowed outside visiting hours.

Suggestions Reduce antenatal clinic waits. Better agency nurses. One woman said hospital needed 'more midwives who are sympathetic, understanding, and speak English'. Improved food.

★★ West London, Hammersmith Road, London W6   MO

Decrepit, antiquated, off-putting building: 'dreary', 'depressing', 'tatty', 'in bad shape', 'very run down', but full of 'super', 'friendly' people, who are extremely caring and pay particular attention to individual wishes and needs; 'humane', 'civilized' policies.

Antenatal 'A very caring place'. Pleasant, bright, airy space; doctors, receptionists, midwives all helpful. 'Relaxed', 'friendly', 'informal', 'sociable' atmosphere. Staff 'all smile'. 'Cheerful'. Wait on average ½ hour though sometimes only 20 minutes. Modern reception area with carpet, has play space; there used to be toys, but they were 'nicked'. Some writers had seen a variety of different doctors and students 'some of whom didn't seem to have a clue'; 'In ten visits I saw seven different doctors', but recently writers have said they saw same one each time. Obstetricians give opportunity to ask questions and are 'patient', usually willing to discuss things at length, including feelings, and are 'good humoured'. Everything is 'explained and I was left to make my own decisions'. Wishes are noted down. 'I never felt I was being fobbed off though each individual doctor obviously interprets hospital policy differently.' Occasionally a woman found a doctor 'brusque' and because visits were so hurried found it difficult to ask questions or get information. The great advantage in this clinic is that woman usually stays put and *staff* move from place to place. Results of blood tests not always available in notes when they should have been. Scan at 16 weeks but can opt out. Operators pleasant and friendly. Few complaints of general reassurance in place of accurate information. Partner and children can attend, encouraged to come in to examination too; 'I was always left feeling very happy and looking forward to next visit.' One woman with breech baby thought options for delivery should have been discussed with her. Some writers were not convinced of need to induce labour, but were anyway. Induction with prostaglandin pessaries and drip may not be used. One writer had 8-hour gap between pessaries and oxytocin drip. One writer was upset that drip was set up without anyone examining her first: 'I was shattered.' Eight excellent, informative and friendly antenatal classes 'give great confidence'; breathing and relaxation taught; partner can attend all classes. Anaesthetist and obstetrician visit and discuss breech and other complicated deliveries. Some writers got impression that induction and acceleration rates were high.

Labour No shave/enema. Staff 'kind', 'helpful', 'informed', 'informal', 'marvellous', 'lovely', 'courteous'. Women encouraged to move around as much as they wished and try different positions. They were able to control their own labours, if not entirely, at least as long as possible. Hospital does not provide food in first stage. Writers advise having meal before you leave home, some feel they became ketonic unnecessarily. Feed your partner too, though he will be given cup of tea. Couple can bring their own plants/posters, play their own music. But some writers describe amniotomy done without warning and were surprised how technological the hospital was, e.g. doctor said: 'We have 12-hour labours here.' One writer said they had to cope with pressure from doctors immediately they went in to 'speed things up'. One writer said her husband was sent out before oxytocin augmentation was discussed and when he came in she was 'all wired up and in tears with no chance of consulting with the doctor'. Epidurals are available and are often advised. Some women offered package deal of induction/epidural/possible forceps. Midwives tend to be 'strict but very helpful' in second stage. Some 'do not go along with the new physiological birth model'. Some writers said their backs were 'put up' when they seemed to be 'demanding' things. Woman may be able to squat in delivery but it depends on midwife. Midwives keen to avoid unnecessary episiotomy. 'Even when they introduced forceps the doctors explained what they were doing in such a gentle, respectful way that it was as if they were *suggesting* what they would do. This made me feel cared for.' Anaesthetist 'most gentle', is 'tower of strength', 'reassuring and explains exactly what he is doing'. Some writers said they were given time limit of 1 hour in second stage and found this 'frightening'. Others had well over an hour. Forceps delivery, 'for which partner can stay', may be done simply with local anaesthetic if mother wishes: 'Somebody helped me put my hands on the little body and pull it on to my stomach . . . she lay quite calmly looking at me. I felt very glad that no drugs dulled the perception for either of us.' Research has been done in 'exploring methods to increase the probability of a labour that progresses to delivery within a reasonable time scale'. Exactly what does this entail? In spite of good experience some women hated being monitored: 'Oh, that beastly monitor that was not working properly!' One woman said 'external monitor nearly drove me mad, as baby moved a lot and midwife was continually moving it'. Leboyer-style delivery can be arranged, blinds drawn, baby given straight to mother, blanket put over mother and baby: baby stays with mother while she is stitched. Both are taken to ward. Hospital policy is that couple have extended time alone together with their baby if all is well after delivery. If anyone tries to hurry you through this or neglects to offer it, say you need time together. Some writers disliked being stitched, sometimes for very long time, by an unsupervised medical student, but these are in older reports and this is no longer done. Birth chairs available.

Postnatal Very understaffed. Breast-feeding on demand and nurses help with it though women who do not know what they want and are lacking in confidence may get conflicting advice. On Annie Zunz ward, which women describe as 'fabulous', 'fantastic', mothers look after babies themselves from the beginning and staff are there only as advisers. Baby is on ward day and night. Some writers were surprised at how quiet it was. Twenty-eight, however, were desperate, describing it as 'a form of torture'. Some said they got not more than 3 hours sleep at night. This may not be the ward for you if you are feeling ill. Nurses are reluctant to take baby to nursery and one writer said she had to 'plead' with them and gave up because she did not have enough energy. On the other hand, many women seek the environment this ward has to offer, to be able to care for baby without any interference and sleep with baby in bed, and even one who had a difficult delivery and was in pain said: 'Being forced to learn how to care for her from the start meant that I had some idea of what to do when I got home,' and that it was 'wonderful to lie with my baby in my arms at night'. The other ward, Baker Forrester, has nursery. Staff 'extremely kind', 'helpful'. But here, too, women complain of sleep deprivation and come out exhausted. Agency nurses may be out of tune with hospital policy and attitudes, are sometimes described as 'rude', 'unhelpful', and 'made us all dread nightfall'. Nurse told one mother of crying baby who had not got baby 'fixed' on breast that what baby needed was 'real food', and bottle-fed the baby. Lack of continuity and commitment. Conflicting information, especially on Baker Forrester. At night on that ward babies may be quietened by large amounts of dextrose when they cry and are sometimes given Cow and Gate. Mothers say they were reduced to tears. One woman, brought baby by auxiliary at 4 a.m. after it had been in nursery because she wanted to get to sleep, says she was 'told off' by agency nurse for breast-feeding because she said she had already given baby bottle of milk. Bathrooms 'grotty', 'freezing cold', 'dirty'. Lavatories which do not always flush, 'like the worst kind of public lavatory'. 'On two occasions I was interrupted behind the curtains using bidet/bath by male visitors using sink.' 'If these conditions existed in my own home I am sure I would be refused a domiciliary delivery.' Couples have evening out together night before discharge while staff babysit. Very free visiting for fathers and they can be there practically all day.

Food 'good' and plenty of it, but vegetarians not catered for. Daily salads excellent though they may be 'draped with dead flesh'. Some vegetarians went hungry. Breakfasts good: cereals/porridge/boiled eggs/white or brown rolls/butter/jam/tea.

Sometimes confusion about day and time of discharge and women sit around waiting for permission to leave. Forty-eight-hour discharge possible.

SCBU Staff 'very kind', 'understanding'.

Suggestions Give building good clean and redecoration. Less emphasis on 'managing' of births: 'Doctors lower down hierarchy should put more of the professors' humane theories into practice'. Monitors should be kept in working order and only used when really necessary. A woman who objects to monitor should not have to have it. Quiet clock in labour room. Some women who had complicated labours and deliveries wanted a chance to talk these over with staff who knew what had happened shortly after – could this opportunity be provided? More nursing staff on postnatal wards. More preparation for breast-feeding in antenatal classes. Groups to discuss breast-feeding with breast-feeding counsellor after birth. Stop waking up all mothers at 6 a.m. When baby is taken to SCBU full explanation to mother at the time. Mother of baby in SCBU tends to miss out on mothercare talks and demonstrations and needs extra 'clueing up' by nurses. Lower beds so that more comfortable after stitches. 'Occupied' notice on bidet/bathroom doors. Provide vegetarian food and when serving a salad to vegetarians, hot, cooked vegetables should not be piled on top of lettuce, producing 'warm and soggy mess'.

Westminster Hospital, London SW1

High-tech hospital, very large, extremely busy. High proportion of immigrant mothers attend. Antenatal clinics separate from hospital at Marsham Street and St Stephen's, like 'Nissen huts'.

Antenatal Longest wait ½ hour but generally 15 minutes. Same two midwives always present who 'treated us like old friends', but women tend to feel there is not much chance to air worries and get answers to questions because everyone is so busy; *ask* for what you want. Most writers said they saw same doctor most visits: 'He never talked over me to students present'; 'made me feel important'. Breast-feeding counsellor available. If you would like Leboyer-style delivery discuss this with obstetrician and it will be written in your notes. Domino delivery possible, with discharge after 6 hours, but you may have to be very keen to get it. Community midwives seem not entirely happy with this since doctors intervene and urge that labour should be speeded up. They find they are questioned as to methods and that their decisions may be overruled. All women have ultrasound at 17 and 34 weeks, either at hospital or at St Stephen's. Marsham Street has toys for children if you ask, St Stephen's a voluntary helper who runs a playgroup. Classes available and obstetricians encouraging about women attending NCT classes.

Labour 'Cheerful', 'fresh' rooms and labour and delivery take place in same room. Induction rate high – 33%. Method is fully explained. Writers said that labour was induced routinely when 2 weeks past EDD, but obstetrician explains why. 'I would have liked to wait a bit longer but didn't feel in a position to argue.' Most writers described enemas. A student doctor and midwife are assigned to each woman in labour and usually stay with her throughout. One writer appreciated student doctor massaging her through contractions. Woman allowed to be in position she likes, though since every writer was put on dextrose drip movement was necessarily restricted. Partner can be present throughout, except may be asked to go out while woman uses bedpan. There is nowhere on same floor where he can get anything to eat or drink. Most writers said their husbands were made to feel very welcome and part of a team; if the man was asked to go out, and the woman was firm, nobody was likely to bother about it after that. Electronic fetal monitoring used. Epidurals available, are fully explained by anaesthetist and Caesarean section can be done under epidural. 'I got the impression that everyone enjoyed their work.' Women well propped with pillows for second stage. When forceps delivery procedures carefully explained and partner can be present. If woman chooses Leboyer-style delivery lights are dimmed, there is complete silence and baby is delivered on to her abdomen, cord still attached. Writers say cord was not cut till it stopped throbbing and mother was told before cord cut. This was done even if she had a forceps delivery. Midwife suctions mucus while baby held by mother. Baby given to father to hold while mother is cleaned up and then back to her. Baby can be put to breast on delivery table. One woman described being given pethidine *after* forceps delivery for pain relief. 21% of deliveries are by Caesarean section, a very high rate.

Postnatal Two wards seem to have rather different policies. Baby in nursery first three nights and some mothers who asked to have their babies with them were not allowed to: 'Silly really, as you are woken up by other babies, so no extra rest gained.' After this baby can be with mother night and day and if you want your baby at night you will be on Chadwick ward. If you would prefer baby in nursery, on Helland ward. Some staff advise scheduled feeding and there is conflicting advice on feeding times. But when women feed on demand, 'nobody says anything'. No topping up, though babies in nursery given water at night. Woman with inverted nipples said that midwife or nursery nurse sat with her for every feed for over an hour sometimes. Otherwise women left to 'do their own thing', 'with knowledge that there is good help always in background'. Most nurses 'kind', 'funny', 'treat mothers like people'. But severe staff shortages and 'terribly tight routine'. Day after delivery mother may be visited by consultant and all staff connected with delivery: 'Made me feel as if I had done something terribly important', 'a very personal touch'. Paediatrician examines baby in mother's presence. Though women say they are 'treated as individuals', agency staff are sometimes used at night and are criticized for being 'brusque', and 'insensitive'. Bathrooms 'pretty awful' sometimes. Food 'all right provided you choose carefully'. Rest period, 3.30–5 p.m., curtains drawn. Women who do not want to sleep can go to day room. Visiting 2.30–3.30 p.m. 'a bit mean' and 7–8 p.m. fathers only. 'Sometimes very strict, depending on staff.' Visitors can be taken to day room.

Suggestions One writer who felt there was 'intense dislike sometimes' between day and night staff felt that something should be done to eliminate conflict between them on postnatal ward. More sympathy to members of racial minorities and more understanding of their dietary customs. More bathrooms.

London

Whipps Cross, Leytonstone, London E11   MO

Modern, bright, clean; spacious, comfortable wards. Understaffed; 'busy', 'efficient'. *Short-stay unit where own children can be at birth.

Antenatal All staff friendly and helpful but not enough midwives, so often do not have time to talk. If you want accurate answers ask sister or doctor. Longest wait seems to be about 1½ hours and an average of about 1 hour. Not enough chairs when full, and writers say husbands and friends occupy chairs needed by mothers. Children underfoot and unoccupied. Waiting and refreshment areas 'not well designed'. Conveyor-belt system. 'Doctors seem rushed and have little time to explain.' One writer says doctor 'only speaks to you if he absolutely has to', but other writers said doctors explained what they were doing. Some women only saw two different doctors throughout pregnancy. Separate booking clinic. NCT adviser and Asian interpreter present. Partner welcome in examination room. Ultrasound and AFP testing done routinely unless refused. Explanatory leaflets given at booking. 'Very helpful' relaxation and parentcraft classes. Writers said they were told that induction was done routinely at 42 weeks. Some of them would like to have known what indications were for induction in their cases, as they were not convinced by rudimentary information given. Writers thought induction done rather frequently. Vaginal prostaglandin used.

Labour Mini-shave/no enema. Partner asked to wait outside. Then woman can walk around and sit in day room. Couples may have some hours more-or-less alone together in labour. Student midwife may sit with them for all or part of this time. Partner made to feel 'completely welcome' and 'needed'. Some women, trying to use breathing learned in classes, said they were unable to do it because of numbers of people wandering in and out of room. Amniotomy may be done very early; one woman had waters broken when 1½ cm dilated and was then put on drip and monitor: 'All this distressed me greatly.' Woman is allowed to be in any position she likes until onset second stage. Midwives 'patient'. Lots of young midwives who have 'infectious enthusiasm for their job' and 'treat patients as individuals'. Pethidine available but no pain relief forced on woman. Epidurals done when considered necessary by medical staff e.g. when baby posterior, and may be advised 'to help you relax'. One woman said her husband was not allowed to be present for her epidural Caesarean section. Electronic monitoring used: 'fascinating to watch'. One woman writing about amniotomy said doctor was 'calm, sympathetic and answered questions'. It sounds as if labour is frequently accelerated with oxytocin drip. Some women refused this or delayed having it. One writer said: 'If your baby literally dropped out before they can interfere, you'd be OK'. Some doctors allow fathers to be present at forceps deliveries; others do not. One woman, told her husband could be with her by own doctor, was upset when another came in 'and very rudely told my husband to get out as the consultant did not like husbands there . . . it made me feel very cheated'. Baby can be delivered straight on mother's abdomen, even with forceps delivery. Modified Leboyer delivery done. Midwives skilled at avoiding episiotomy. Father can hold baby.

312

Writers describe babies being put to breast in delivery room after stitching. Parents have time alone together with their baby after spontaneous delivery: 'lovely'. Forceps-delivered babies can be touched by mother but may then be 'whisked away' without explanation by paediatrician, which some writers found disturbing as they thought something must be wrong. Father can go up to ward with wife and baby. Some writers say Caesarean section rate high.

Postnatal 'Lovely', 'calm', 'friendly' atmosphere in postnatal wards. 'Very relaxed', 'not all authoritarian'. Most staff 'helpful', 'kind', 'always answer questions'. Wards have lovely views. Often very full. Mother can cuddle baby when she likes, choose whether baby stays with her at night or goes to nursery. Modified feeding on demand. If in nursery mother can be woken when baby cries or staff will feed water or artificial milk. One special nursing auxiliary helps to breast-feed and will sit with mother for hours 'and stay on if there is a problem when she should be off duty'. One mother who wanted her baby with her during the night met with disapproval from staff nurse who thought baby should be in nursery for the first few nights. One woman said night nurses were irritable and non-caring 'and scoffed at us for keeping our babies with us'. Most mothers breast-feed. Much help given, but no interference and it is not 'pushed'. Though babies are given water, complements rarely given, and when they are either SMA or, if mother wishes, complements from breast-milk bank. Each mother interviewed every morning by midwife and any problems discussed; all senior staff regularly in ward contact with mothers and make it their job to be briefed about each individual. Writer who was depressed said everyone was understanding and she was *not* told to pull herself together: 'Staff are sensitive to women's needs.' Women comment on very peaceful atmosphere and how little babies cried. 'Most staff really do seem to care about helping to form the best possible relationship between mother, father and baby.' Fathers are encouraged to hold and care for baby. Visiting 2–3 p.m. and 7–8 p.m. fathers only; fathers can visit at other times too by prior arrangement. Postnatal exercise classes on Wednesday evenings 'great fun'. Baths, showers, bidets 'all very clean' but bidets do not all work correctly. Food sometimes 'appalling', sometimes 'good': alternatives available. Breakfast often starts at 7 a.m., second course at 8.30 a.m. Day room heavily smoke-filled. Forty-eight-hour discharge possible.

Suggestions Better communication between doctors and midwives and antenatal, intrapartum and postnatal teams: 'I was told one thing at parentcraft classes and then doctors did the opposite.' One writer who felt she was induced unnecessarily suggested 'chance to discuss induction with doctor, rather than merely being told doctor's decision by junior doctor'. Play area or creche in clinic for children. Labour ward should have sound-proofed rooms. One writer who said husbands had 'good view of women running to lavatories after enemas', said that partners' waiting room should not be next to lavatories. Visiting hours for fathers and own children longer but visiting time for other people shorter.

Loughborough Hospital, Loughborough, Leicestershire   MO

GP unit. If complications woman is moved to Leicester Royal Infirmary. Transfers well organized. Only four reports received; all are very good.

Antenatal Care from GP and local midwife at health centre, except for one visit during sixth month.

Labour 'Everything explained'; 'friendly atmosphere'.

Postnatal 'Fantastic! Nothing too much trouble.' 'Good atmosphere.'

Luton and Dunstable, 770 Dunstable Road, Luton, Beds

Acting DNO writes, 'We welcome constructive comments which might help future mothers.'

Antenatal Waiting area has been doubled in size and there are toys for children to play with. But writers say there is conveyor-belt atmosphere: one auxiliary weighs, another checks urine, sister takes blood. Between each exercise women return to waiting room. 'Then marched off to cubicle to strip.' 'I had a number of questions I wanted answered but all the nurses kept telling me to "ask the doctor",' says woman who had forceps delivery previously. She saw consultant but 'was only time for a couple of questions' which 'he answered with grunts' before disappearing through the curtains, 'leaving most of my questions unanswered'. Writers say they saw different doctor at each visit. Complain of 'cattle queue' and being 'processed'. Advise using interview with midwife booking you in as 'is only occasion on which you do not feel hurried and can ask questions sitting upright with clothes on'; 'I always felt I was just a number on a list.' Women advised to take packed lunches when going to booking clinic. Woman whose baby was breech said she could not get discussion; 'finally I became so depressed and so desperate that I paid for a private appointment with the consultant'. Acting DNO says induction only undertaken for medical reasons. There are still home deliveries within the district.

Labour Acting DNO says, 'New labour wards are far less clinical, with wallpaper', and writes 'We hope that mothers will take the opportunity to discuss with the sister or nursing officers any queries or anxieties they may have when they are in the unit'. Not enough reports from mothers about labour ward to warrant including impressions from them. But from the way the eleven women describe care in labour the suggestion is that they felt pretty anonymous. 'Midwives very kind and try to answer questions if they can and if you ask, but nobody seems to have much time.' 9% forceps deliveries; 7% Caesarean section.

Postnatal Flexible feeding. A woman whose baby died said she felt as if she was sitting on a platform at Euston station afterwards. Baby died at night and mother not given news till morning, so had no time alone to grieve. 'I had nine people in and out of my room before lunch after being told, five medical staff and four cleaners. I desperately needed to talk to someone, but no one came.'

Visiting 3.15–3.45 p.m. and 7.30–8.30 p.m.; baby's brothers and sisters welcome.

Over 50% of mothers discharged within 48 hours of delivery and another 37% by the sixth day.

SCBU Staff 'kind', 'helpful', 'answer questions'. Paediatrician fully explains baby's condition. Mother is encouraged to touch and hold baby. Father can visit as often as he likes and for as long as possible.

Suggestions Midwifery should become mother-centred rather than task-centred. Cleaning staff should be told when there is a grieving mother, perhaps with notice on door that would convey nothing to outsider but inform all staff. At postnatal examination woman should not have to try to ask questions lying flat on her back with no pants on while staring up the doctor's nose.

West Kent General, Marsham Street, Maidstone, Kent

Antenatal No long queues, but chairs arranged in long line in narrow corridor, so everyone sits facing blank wall. Some writers say they had long wait in examining room on couch, without clothes, for doctor to come in. 'Doctor said little, examined me and started to walk out. I asked a couple of questions, but replies were brisk and she stood with door open to answer me.' Tour round unit possible.

Labour Midwives encourage woman to walk around as much as she likes. May be left alone if partner sent home. 'Midwife came in and said she would just give me something to relax me. I ask what and she says pethidine. I say no thanks. Great fuss. She calls doctor. Another midwife comes in to tell me off for listening to "stories" about pethidine. I refuse to make decision until my husband is allowed back in. Doctor suggests half dose.' This woman agreed and then was given full dose. Midwives help with back massage, very good at it. Some described as 'very brisk', others chat. Writers advise asking early in labour, or before, for things you want. Woman has to be moved to 'austere' delivery room and partner may be sent out then and is only allowed back in when insists. Electronic monitoring available. Writers describe holding leg by ankle with someone else on other side in second stage. 'Midwife wanted me to push all the time. Other student doctors and midwives came in. I felt very surrounded . . . I reached down to touch the baby but he was pulled away from me.' Mother said that he was sucked out, checked, given 'a jab' and wrapped 'in rough towel' before being given to her. Advises saying *beforehand* what you want done at birth. One writer who asked to feed baby on delivery table was told 'yes, but only 2 minutes each side' and midwife went out of room: 'I hadn't a clue what to do and he did not feed.' Baby was then taken to nursery. Writers describe being sewn up by students who take a long time;

'over an hour'. One said she got 'bored', 'got cramp' and the student and doctor talked and ignored her even when she tried to ask questions. Her husband had to wait outside and baby was taken away just when she wanted him with her.

Postnatal Some writers consider postnatal care 'depressing', advise going home as soon as you feel fit enough to do so. One writer, whose baby was taken to nursery after delivery, said that this was a 'bad time'. She was moved to ward and left 'unable to remember where nursery was, unable to sleep and very hungry. It was night time and very noisy and I felt very, very alone.' Writers describe babies being kept in nursery and brought for 4-hourly feeds (1980). 'I asked to be woken to feed in the night and put jolly cartoon on cot saying "Demand-feeding – please wake me." No one does and when I ask one nurse says no and the other "Oh, I just gave him some dextrose."' You can insist on having baby by your bed and demand-feeding if you wish. Some women have great difficulty in breast-feeding. Nursery nurses help, check baby is properly fixed, but 'most helpful are part-timers who have breast-fed babies of their own'. One writer said baby was test weighed on third day: 'I was told off for letting him feed so much' and she says sister told her she would overfeed him and make him fat. 'Next feed I gave him one side only, then took him down to the nursery and weighed him, then back to the ward and gave him the other side. Everyone seemed happy!' 'Constantly asked had I opened my bowels, even on first morning, when I had not eaten for 36 hours.' Bathrooms and lavatories old and 'tatty'; no bidets. Lavatories just off ward and bathrooms down corridor, so difficult to wash after going to lavatories. Take extra sanitary towels.

Food 'dreadful' and insufficient in quantity. Writers advise getting wholemeal bread, fruit and salad brought in in sealed containers.

Flexible visiting. People who have travelled a long way allowed in outside visiting hours. Evening visiting for fathers only 'but not many people took much notice of this'.

NB. Some of these reports came in before Peter Huntingford moved from the London Hospital to the West Kent General.

Suggestions Getting the things you want in labour should not have to depend on which midwife you get. Partner should not be sent out during stitching if woman wants him there. Breast-feeding mothers should not be criticized for 'over-feeding' their baby. Hot drinks more generously available on postnatal wards.

St Peter's, Maldon, Essex   MO

Small GP unit in separate wing of larger geriatric hospital. Only alternative to St John's, Chelmsford, in large area of Essex. Usually second-time mothers after straightforward first births.

Antenatal Care is with own GP, with two brief visits at about 20 and 36 weeks to hospital. Midwives 'friendly'. Can ask for quick tour of labour and delivery rooms.

Labour Beds divided by curtain in labour room. At night may be only one midwife on duty. One writer said her midwife was 'tired and harassed'. Routine shave/enema/shower. Partner can be with woman throughout. One woman who asked for pethidine was told that midwife was busy delivering another baby and could not give it to her and had pethidine at end first stage. Baby given to mother to hold after delivery. Midwife may do stitching herself. One woman waited 2 hours to be stitched while midwife tried to get hold of duty doctor who was too busy to come.

Postnatal Pleasant wards. No nursery, baby is never removed. Nurses and midwives 'friendly', 'helpful', 'cheerful'. Very relaxed atmosphere. 'Always someone on hand to help but no one tried to give unwanted advice.' 'I enjoyed it very much.' Women are not woken till 7 a.m. On the other hand sleep not easy as delivery rooms across corridor. Food plentiful.

Afternoon visiting for general visitors and hour in early evening for partner and own children. 'The one hour was not strictly enforced, but nor was the ban on visitors other than husbands, so I had to bear with my mother-in-law when I just wanted to see my husband and other child on their own.'

Suggestions More than one midwife on duty at night. Separate labour rooms. More bathrooms and installation of bidets.

Malmesbury Hospital, Malmesbury, Wilts   MO

'Friendly', 'informal' GP unit.

Antenatal 'Relaxed', though one writer says 'Senior member of staff has obsession with weight control.' See own GP at each visit. 'Can establish relationship, ask questions.' One writer said sister called her 'the lady with the medical shopping list'. Waits not long. Antenatal classes 'conscientious' with good physiotherapist.

Labour Met at door by midwife; 'friendly', 'casual', 'makes you feel at home'. Partner may be asked to go out before mini-shave/enema; otherwise there throughout and involved. 'Next best thing to home.' Woman has to be moved to another room for delivery, wheeled across in 'beautiful, antique wooden chair' but 'unnerving to have to go'. Few VEs. 'My midwife just knew by looking when I was ready to push.' Woman can push sitting upright. Episiotomy not routine and midwives skilled at avoiding damage to perineum. Baby put on mother's tummy after delivery. Cord not cut immediately. Father can cuddle baby and mother can put baby to breast.

Postnatal Staff 'very keen on breast-feeding'. Baby brought to mother to feed at night. Small, very quiet ward. But 'too much routine'; 'you have to insist on what you want to do'; 'staff talk of feeding time as at zoo'. 'I was told by one nurse "You can't nurse your baby all the time." When I asked why was told

"Matron will be after you. She doesn't like it." I said it was my baby, not matron's.' One writer said she had her baby at 3 a.m. and since the rule is that babies go to nursery at night, 'lay awake wondering what he was doing instead of being able to stare at him non-stop'. She found this upsetting. 'Mixture of stroppy and caring staff.' Food 'quite good' but 'why give constipated mothers white bread?' Short stay of about 30 hours can be arranged.

Suggestions Let mothers do as they like on postnatal ward. Cut routine. Women should be able to feed on demand. Staff ought to discuss feeding advice together so they do not confuse women with different advice. Stop 'bossing GPs around'.

★★ GP/Midwife Unit, The Park, Davyhulme, Manchester

Small, self-contained, independent unit run by midwives within larger hospital. SNO writes, 'An increasing number of women are rebelling against the interventionist policies of the last decade and are demanding a more sensitive approach to childbirth.' Here 'the mother delivers – is not "delivered". She retains control over the situation.'

Antenatal Care with own GP and midwife. Booking visit in early pregnancy; AFP estimation and scan; another visit at 36 weeks. Woman sees consultant twice during pregnancy. No induction. Midwives who work here also do home births.

Labour Non-clinical atmosphere. Midwives 'friendly', encourage natural birth, 'attentive', 'encouraging', 'good at back-rubbing'. Plants/pictures/curtains/flowered wallpaper/radio/cassette-player/easy chairs/carpet. Personal attention. Fathers welcome throughout. Some writers described having enema. Woman can walk around during labour; no drips or machines; no electronic monitoring; can relax in warm bath. Woman can choose whether or not to have analgesic drugs; pethidine offered; most women have Entonox only. Woman can deliver in position of her choice. SNO says, 'It's your baby and your experience. We are privileged to be able to assist you and share in the delivery of your child.' Birth stool available. Mother can lift baby out herself. Midwives skilled at avoiding episiotomy and encourage 'breathing out' of head.

Postnatal Peaceful, relaxed atmosphere; family-centred care; no rules. 'Fabulous!'; 'fantastic!'. Rooming-in, with nursery at night if mother wishes. 'I was soothed and cosseted more than I had ever been in my life.' Staff give time to talk informally: 'They are friends.' Father helps in caring for baby. Women supported in making their own decisions about baby. Own children can visit and hold baby. Visiting hours flexible. 'The best holiday I ever had.'

★★ St Mary's, Whitworth Park, Manchester   MO

Modern, 'efficient', 'caring' hospital with 'emotionally supportive', staff who are 'top calibre'. The hospital equipped to deal with any emergency, 'but machines do not detract from personal touch'; 'you really feel you matter'; 'air of caring efficiency'.

Antenatal Usually long waits; not always enough chairs. Sisters 'helpful', 'considerate' and will 'spend their time answering questions'; 'inspire confidence'. Pleasant atmosphere. Consultants described as 'very approachable', 'treated me as an articulate human being', 'went into great detail about tests available to detect abnormality and didn't try to influence me to have them when I knew termination was totally out of question for me'. One writer said, 'Consultant asked me if I was familiar with Leboyer technique and said I could have it if I wished.' Most doctors spend time with women, some consultants described as 'in a whirl'. Writers advise 'tell obstetrician your wishes about labour and ask if they can be written in your case notes'. Clinic well organized and having scan does not add time to wait. A card ensures you do not lose place in queue for doctor while having scan. Scans carefully explained. Care 'very thorough'. Information available on diet/relaxation; talks by midwives on care of newborn in 'relaxed, informal atmosphere'. Films for couple together.

Antenatal ward: 'friendly'; 'marvellous staff'; 'caring attention, with emphasis on emotional support'. Own children can visit regularly without special arrangements having to be made. Extended visiting hours for partners who cannot visit at normal times, and 'done without fuss'. Post- and antenatal patients share wards; one woman who had lost two previous babies could not face seeing babies – staff moved her to ward where she did not have to. 'At no time did any of them suggest that my attitude was strange or unnatural.' All rooms 'comfortable' and 'spotlessly clean'. Smoking allowed in day room, where women smoke heavily despite pressure from nurses.

Labour Shave can be declined. Some writers critical of conveyor-belt obstetrics, referring particularly to routine ARM and fetal monitoring, which some obstetricians and midwives think essential. Others say 'hospital doesn't force anything on you'; 'staff generally let me do my own thing', though even so some obstetricians insist on continuous monitoring. 'The electrodes somehow became detached and the monitor went dead and I had a fright.' Staff 'generate confidence'. 'Everything was explained.' No pressure to have pharmacological pain relief. When epidurals given (and they may be recommended) no top-up given before second stage so that woman more likely to be able to push baby out herself; 'the anaesthetist was constantly at hand with encouragement and reassurance and followed up his work with a postnatal questionnaire'. When registrar wanted to accelerate labour, midwife called consultant who agreed to give woman more time. Woman is in one room throughout labour and delivery 'friendly', 'attentive', midwives go out when they sense that couple want to be alone. Partner can usually be present throughout, though some have been sent out before VEs. Possible to arrange epidural Caesarean and anaesthetist has even come to hospital when off duty for a woman having an emergency section who 'desperately wanted to see my baby born' after previous baby's stillbirth. Delivery unit team 'exceptional', 'calm', 'very kind', 'friendly', 'put me at ease straight away'. Partner can stay throughout operation and is 'kindly treated'. Doctors explain operation carefully to couple. 'It was a fascinating and totally enjoyable birth . . . when she was born she was placed on my tummy *à la Leboyer*.' Several writers said everything was just as they wanted. Midwives give time to see if mothers can manage without episiotomy. Woman can put baby to breast after cord cut and baby is wrapped. Then couple left alone with their baby 'for a long time'. One couple had 3 hours together.

Postnatal 'Out of fourteen mothers on ward, only seven were breast-feeding and most of these were also giving bottles.' Some writers said artificial milk supplements were given freely. One writer who didn't want to said night nurse 'backed me and told me not to complement and feed him whenever I wanted to'. Woman who had emergency Caesarean said 'off-duty obstetrician who had given antenatal care called into ward to congratulate us'.

SCBU Meals on ward kept hot whenever mother visits SCBU. She can spend 24 hours in unit in special mother-and-baby room before baby discharged.

Postnatal clinic Long waits followed by speedy check-up; 'I feel that a postnatal should not be just a physical check, but on how well new mums are coping.'

Suggestions Avoid hold-ups in routine examinations in antenatal clinic by allowing some 'do-it-yourself', e.g. weighing. More preparation for student midwives before they work in antenatal clinic so they understand examinations before and they can be speeded up. More education about breast-feeding for nurses on postnatal wards. List of local support groups for new mothers should be supplied at 6-week check-up.

★ **Withington Hospital, West Didsbury, Manchester**   MO

Old building. Public relations top priority. 'Old workhouse tarted up.' 'All members of staff make an effort to be friendly and to treat one in a personal way.'

Antenatal Clinic friendly place: 'staff call you by name and try to make you feel recognized'. But wait usually 2–3 hours. Women do not usually see same doctor: 'I only saw the same doctor twice, but felt that the more people that examined me the better chance there was that what one missed another would pick up.' Usually a medical student present, but woman asked if she minds and can refuse. Doctors 'informative', 'considerate'. 'At no time did I feel I was being rushed through an assembly line.' Questions answered thoroughly. 'When I asked about the size of the baby in relation to the pelvis the doctor disappeared and returned with a bright blue rubber pelvis and a doll and delivered the child several times, this during a particularly busy afternoon.' Woman who had scan was given results to look at. Antenatal classes taught by physiotherapist who had children herself; well presented; questions encouraged. She visits wards and reports back on how women got on. She also asks those who have delivered if anything has happened that has not been discussed and what they found helpful or not. 'The emphasis was on respecting the wishes of the individual.' Breathing and other techniques taught. 'They are good fun and a way of meeting other expectant mothers.' Parentcraft classes follow them and done in informal way over cup of tea. Because classes are held during day fathers cannot attend, but encouraged to come to films in evening, including film of epidural.

Labour Staff 'supportive' and 'encouraging' in very institutional physical atmosphere. Epidurals available on request; no need to book ahead of time. Writers think labour often accelerated with oxytocin drip. Electronic monitoring frequently used, but woman's consent sought first. Father can stay throughout and is included in everything. 'Everything was explained carefully before it was done.' Those who like a high-tech hospital seem happy with care during labour here. After baby cleaned up and mucus extracted given to mother to put to breast.

Postnatal All babies room in; staff give 'a lot of support'. Mother can ask for her baby to be taken to nursery at night and this is encouraged on first night. Mother is free to make her own choice about method of feeding and bottle-feeders are 'not made to feel guilty'. Nurses 'sit with mothers tirelessly helping them establish feeding'. 'They seemed to care as much as I did that things should go well.' Baby can be fed on demand, picked up whenever mother wishes and is cared for by her. Rules flexible, e.g. regulation that mother is not to feed during visiting hours or in front of visitors, but some writers did this with no problem. 'Staff very protective and I was always asked if I cared to see visitors.' Any time of day mother can go with visitors to talk with them in visiting room. 'I never heard a sharp word spoken, and staff seemed to get on very well with one another.' 'Everyone keen to make the patients happy'; 'staff come in for chat'; 'I felt I was leaving real friends by the end of the week.' Woman chooses her menu the day before. Food 'not bad'.

Suggestions Improve interior decoration, which is 'pretty grim' and 'depressing'; 'no colour'. More baths.

Wythenshawe Hospital, University Hospital of South Manchester, Manchester
MO

Large, clean, efficiently run, 'impersonal', overworked midwives.

Antenatal Clinic 'appalling', 'cattle market'. Long waits unless arrive around 8 a.m. Lucky if see same doctor twice. Writers found visits very tiring at end of pregnancy. Say some obstetricians 'offhand'; 'do nothing to calm anxiety'. Others 'reassuring', 'helpful'. Most women have scans, but partner not admitted.

Labour Writers describe highly mechanized labours in which they tend to be 'the body in the bed' with tubes, electrodes and straps attached. They say policy is 100% fetal monitoring and some described distressing situations which made them anxious when they queried or said they did not wish to have it. 'They treat you like a nuisance if you do not toe the line exactly as you are told.' All those who wrote had electronic fetal monitoring. Epidurals favoured, 'but no one pushes you to have one'. Can arrange epidural Caesarean: 'Everyone explained what they were doing and how I would feel . . . plenty of opportunity to change mind and have general anaesthesia.' One woman who had elective Caesarean said there was ample time to discuss implications with consultant. Midwives usually 'marvellous', and couple can be together right through but midwife there immediately if needed, and is 'encouraging'. One writer found midwife unsympathetic and felt they battled against each other all the way. Mother not rushed, quiet atmosphere, though students may observe. Some writers wished they could have been more upright in second stage, and felt they were pushing against gravity when lying flat. Some writers felt they did not really need episiotomy. Couple have time alone together with their baby after delivery: 'very special time'. One writer who had epidural Caesarean said husband not allowed to be present but said 'my baby was given to me immediately to lie at my breast'.

Postnatal Mother can have baby with her whole time if she wishes. Very supportive staff give 'best of help' with breast-feeding, but in 1979 feeds were still every 4 hours. Little help or encouragement for demand-feeding then. 'Throughout my stay I was treated as an intelligent woman and every effort was made to give as much information as I wanted.' Not enough staff on duty at night; pleasant but overworked. Food ranges from 'adequate' to 'inedible'. Vegetarian food difficult to get and not enough vegetables anyway. Plenty of bathrooms/lavatories and 'marvellous' bidets. Flexible visiting.

Suggestions Are enemas really necessary? Partners should be able to be present during prepping. It should be possible to choose to have doses of pethidine smaller than 100 mg; internal examination should always be given before giving pethidine. Several writers felt their husbands were kept outside till they were 'all strapped up' and felt that their partners should have been able to be with them all the time. There should be an opportunity to meet all midwives who may attend mother before birth and to discuss hopes for birth. Does baby's cord have to be cut so soon, in one case blood spurted almost to ceiling? Although women having very complicated labours felt they were given full information, those having straightforward ones did not always feel this and would have liked to be kept much more in touch with progress. Less readiness to manage labour and intervene actively.

Edith Greaves Maternity Unit, Margaret General, St Peter's Margate Road, Margate, Kent

Antenatal Long waits, but comfortable chairs and canteen. One writer says she saw same doctor for most visits. Staff 'ever so cheerful when doing blood pressure'.

Labour Midwives 'not keen on pethidine', 'helpful with breathing'. Large delivery room. Partner present, except for examinations. 'It makes it seem less frightening when you've got someone you know near you.' Women encouraged to lie on side throughout labour. Mother holds baby immediately.

Postnatal 'You don't get pushed into breast-feeding.' 'You are your own boss with the baby.' Mother can have baby with her all the time. Baby not in nursery at visiting time. Demand-feeding. One hour's visiting in afternoon and evening. 'Warm friendly atmosphere.' Food 'good'. All rooms and lavatories 'lovely and clean'.

Savernake Hospital, Nr Marlborough, Wilts

Small, easy-going cottage hospital. Antenatal care with own GP. Midwives work both in unit and in surrounding community, and home births can be arranged.

Labour The District Management Team writes that 'patients' wishes regarding delivery are very much considered'. Midwife-style birth. But inductions are done here and a couple of writers describe being induced when 10 days overdue and for no other obvious reasons, with ARM and oxytocin drip later. Shave/enema. Encouraged to walk about at first, but may be flat on back through labour once drip set up. One woman said she was told 'when the contractions get too strong, tell me and I'll turn the drip down'. Gas and oxygen and pethidine offered. One writer said gas and oxygen mask was jammed over her face and held there while she was trying to fight it off and found midwife 'unsympathetic'. Writers comment on efficiency and quietness at delivery. Midwives skilled at avoiding episiotomy and keeping perineum intact. After mucus is extracted baby handed immediately to mother. Husband can stay for about 10 minutes and then baby taken to nursery.

Postnatal Breast-feeding mother could often be on ward by herself with baby beside her. One writer said her baby slept with her for most of first night. On subsequent nights, however, baby was removed and mothers who asked to have their babies with them were refused. 'One night when I was called to breast-feed there was another baby crying for about ¾ hour and no nurse came.' Theoretically demand-feeding but many conflicting ideas. First-time mothers get confused about how to do things. One writer said babies given continual top-ups if mother is not careful to let her wishes be known unequivocally. Others say sugar water offered. One midwife 'scared me out of my wits by looking at my baby and saying "was I the mother who insisted on no sugar water or top-ups because the baby looked a little jittery" which, of course, he wasn't'. At meal times all mothers must leave babies and sit down. Food 'average'. Almost always auxiliaries on duty at night who 'drink tea in kitchen' and 'chat'. These auxiliaries offer many conflicting opinions. But they are necessary because midwives are 'very overworked', though are 'friendly' and 'give personal care' as much as they can. Charts to fill in when baby fed and bowel movements. One woman gave up breast-feeding because auxiliaries gave bottles when they came in and found baby crying. She said she seemed much more contented after bottle-feed.

Visiting 3–5.15 p.m. and 6.15–8 p.m. and at other times by arrangement with ward sister. 7.15–8 p.m. fathers only (or next of kin). Own children can visit 10.30–11.15 Saturdays and Sundays, 4.30–5.15 p.m. weekdays; must be accompanied by an adult.

Suggestions Though some women said they could decide themselves when to feed their babies not all mothers seemed to have been encouraged to do so. Writers think they should be helped to make their own decisions. Night nurse should be in nursery all the time.

Middlesbrough Hospital, Park Road North, Middlesbrough, Cleveland

Consultant unit. SNO writes, 'We are very much aware of building's physical deficiencies.' Staff 'pleasant and helpful'.

Antenatal Travelling great problem. Consultants visit clinics in outlying parts of district. Women having shared care say they do not know who is responsible for what, hospital or GP. 'Hospitals do not seem to trust other doctors.' Antenatal clinic is 'cramped, overheated waiting room' with no provision for children's play; patient moves from one location to another: large waiting room to small waiting room to give urine; to Room 1 to be weighed and answer questions; to Room 2 for blood pressure check; back to small waiting room; to Room 3 for blood sample; back to large waiting room; to small waiting room, or if in last batch, to other small waiting room to transfer to small waiting room when seats are available; to changing cubicle and then to examination room: 'I found this quite bewildering.' 'At each stage overworked doctors, nurses, orderlies, receptionists are pleasant and attentive.' Full information given; 'they acknowledged that I had a brain'. One woman wrote that one to three doctors were trying to see over 200 women in course of morning and women were stationed in eight cubicles as doctors moved from one to another: 'This must be confusing for them too.' SNO writes, 'Time and motion study has been done.' She says inductions are 'done as necessary, but the patient's wishes are respected'. Classes, some of which are in evenings so fathers can attend. Domino scheme in operation here.

Labour SNO writes that: 'Patients are encouraged to have with them the baby's father or some other person of their choice.' Writers say 'staff go to any trouble to answer questions'. SNO writes, 'Drugs for the relief of pain are offered to our patients, but it is their privilege to accept or refuse. There is also a well-established epidural service which is used quite often at the patient's request.' She says that 'immediately after delivery the baby is placed on the mother's abdomen, and then put to the breast if the mother wishes. If she does not wish to breast-feed, she is encouraged to cuddle her babe.'

Postnatal Not enough letters from women to include their comments but the

SNO writes: 'Babies are in their cots at their mothers' bedsides at all times' if all is well. They are 'fed on demand whether they are breast- or artificially fed'. 'Patients are allowed to handle and pick up their babies whenever they wish. If a baby is particularly fractious, he/she is taken into the nursery, settled and then returned to the mother. During summer, when the weather permits, the patients are allowed to sit out on the lawn to enjoy the sunshine. Visiting is restricted to afternoons and evenings, but arrangements are made for visitors who are unable to visit during the times stated to visit at other times.'

SCBU 'Parents are allowed to visit their baby at any time during the day or night, but are encouraged to inform the nursery staff prior to their arrival. There is one bedroom for the use of mothers. Babies are put out on the lawn in the summer months, when their condition, and weather, allows it.'

Suggestions Reduce visits to hospital antenatal clinic and have more GP clinics. Hospitals and GPs should have copies of each other's records. Women having shared care should not have to repeat information at hospital clinic. Reduce shuttling around in antenatal clinic by rearranging partitions to provide only one waiting room, which would be 'less dislocating' for women. Provide creche, preferably with staff, and robust play equipment, adjacent to main waiting-room; mothers would inform receptionist so they could be called when their turn came; or combine this with creche for hospital staff.

New Milton – see Barton-on-Sea

Newcastle General, Newcastle-upon-Tyne, Northumberland   MO

Something of 'baby factory' according to writers but staff 'impressive'. Writers say there is no continuity of care.

Antenatal Women say they saw different doctor each time they went and some were seen by five different members of staff at each clinic. 'Credence not given to experienced mothers' own judgements.' It may be difficult to get time for discussion with consultant. One writer who thought clinic was 'awful' said that there were good midwives' clinics two afternoons a week for low-risk women. Domino delivery possible but rarely done. Then woman has antenatal care from GP and community midwife (who visits home) and 8–12 hours' stay in hospital following birth. Advantages: 'familiar faces'; community midwives 'friendly', 'helpful', 'efficient'.

Labour Father welcomed and present throughout, but must be masked for second stage. Labour rooms 'full of technical paraphernalia'. Electronic monitoring used routinely, sometimes without asking mother's permission, and scalp monitor may be attached without informing her first. Some writers said induction was done without explaining the reason and there was no time for discussion. One writer said she was simply told to come in because she was 'overdue'. Other writers say their wishes for normal birth were respected if they were articulate and made it quite clear what they wanted. Writers

325

suggested there was active management of labour for nearly everybody with ARM and drip. Most women could not move around in labour and lay 'like stranded whales'. Some excellent senior midwives and midwifery tutors, though some midwives seem subservient to consultants. All, however, are sympathetic. Writers say there is high epidural rate. Anyone who wants one can have it. Obstetric anaesthetist attached to unit. Most writers had had episiotomy (one says hers was 'horrendous'), though some midwives were concerned to maintain intact perineum. Sometimes delay of some minutes before mother given baby to hold. Woman who had general anaesthesia for a Caesarean section said she could breast-feed immediately she came round.

Postnatal Care 'excellent' and good help with breast-feeding. One ward apparently is particularly good; one is 'tyrannized' by senior member of staff. Writers say early discharge not often allowed. Postnatal check-up 'cursory' and some women wondered why they took trouble to attend.

Suggestions In antenatal clinic it should be possible to see same midwife each time and only see doctor if there are problems. Some writers suggested that intravenous oxytocin drip and fetal heart monitor should be used with more discretion.

Princess Mary, Newcastle-upon-Tyne, Northumberland

Busy university teaching hospital; many high-risk pregnancies. Old building but is being modernized on yearly basis. Atmosphere 'very friendly'.

Antenatal First visit takes about 2 hours. If there are special things you would like in labour, e.g. Leboyer-style delivery, write to consultant and ask if these can be put in your notes. Writers who did not do this tended to say that they had little choice and that decisions were made without consulting them: 'I was merely informed of decisions'; 'robbed of all sense of choice or control over the birth of my baby'. Partner can attend antenatal clinic and talk with doctor, though he may be asked to leave room before VE and one couple who protested 'got nowhere'. Some writers who had scans found that dates they were given were less accurate than their own dates. Some writers thought that inductions were frequent. Antenatal classes 'superb', taught by 'really lovely' sister who also gives 'marvellous postnatal support'. On antenatal ward staff are 'never too busy to chat' and a writer who was anxious said she was given good emotional support. 'They keep everyone cheerful.'

Labour DNO says, 'We keep a relaxed atmosphere in the delivery suite and there is no fixed policy regarding shaves or enemas on admission.' One woman who was induced at term plus 6 days for mild pre-eclampsia said she had long wait between being prepped at 6.30 a.m. and induced at 5.15 p.m. and only had a bowl of soup between. Her labour was long and difficult and she was exhausted. Partner or 'named friends' (DNO) encouraged to participate throughout but may not be allowed in admissions room. One writer who said she would not go in without him had her husband with her. Epidural rate

60% and probably increasing. Many writers had epidurals not because they wanted them but were told they must have them to bring down their blood pressure. Partner may be asked to leave while epidural given. Epidural Caesareans done, but writers said their husbands were not allowed to be present. Some writers suggested Caesarean rate was high. One consultant warned that his staff 'talked about all sorts of things during an operation'. (Need they?) Staff relations among doctors sound very hierarchical. Midwives 'very understanding' and some had read Leboyer, helped women feel confident and told them they were doing well. Many writers had forceps deliveries. DNO says, 'In a normal delivery the baby is delivered and placed on the mother's abdomen and after separation of the cord the mother is handed the baby and the first breast-feed is given.' Some writers said staff would give baby Leboyer-style bath if asked. Then couple are left with their baby. Occasionally, however, baby is taken to nursery after delivery and couple had no chance of time alone with their baby.

Postnatal DNO writes that 'full rooming-in is increasingly encouraged from birth and there is . . . a reduction in complementary bottle-feeds. Feeding is on demand.' Some writers felt there was not enough encouragement with breast-feeding if baby was sleepy. Writers said there was constantly conflicting advice given to get baby 'fixed' on breast and some writers were advised to put baby in nursery when crying 'as he can't be hungry'. 'An auxiliary advised me that my milk wasn't rich enough and to use top-up bottle feeds.' 'They are theoretically keen on breast-feeding, but have insufficient skills to give practical help' (1979). 'I felt a bit of a nuisance.' Some writers said father was not allowed to pick up baby while in hospital. Neither was mother allowed to carry baby out to car in case it was dropped on NHS premises! Bathrooms 'cramped' and much in demand. DNO writes there has been 'a significant change in visiting hours with the emphasis on flexibility'; now 4–8 p.m. Food 'poor', 'plentiful'. 'Poor' cooperation with GPs and community midwives. On discharge one woman said they did not know she had left and she had to get in touch with them herself afterwards.

SCBU DNO writes, 'mothers are involved in the care of their babies . . . and there are no restrictions on family visiting'.

Suggestions Encourage father to pick up and cuddle baby. Provide more bidets and showers.

New Obstetric Unit, St Mary's, Newport, Isle of Wight   MO

'Bright', 'compact', 'cheerful' building with modern amenities. Busy, but many staff helpful.

Antenatal Some women wrote down how they wished their labour to be and these notes were attached to their records. Shared care with GP can be arranged. Induction seems to be fairly common. One 'elderly primigravida' who was 4 days 'overdue' refused, as she had had no internal examination and 'no satisfactory explanation as to why it was necessary. This decision had been taken without any consultation with me!' Psychoprophylaxis classes 'excellent', taught by community midwife. Hospital does not always tell mothers about these classes.

Labour Some midwives highly praised for 'treating women as individuals and adults', but it is 'a matter of luck whether a woman gets one of these'. Some women said that amniotomy was done routinely and would like to have been asked about this first. Electronic fetal monitoring often used and woman may be strongly advised to have it. Writers comment on doctors' 'mechanical' approach to labour. It appears that labour is readily accelerated with oxytocin drip. Pethidine given in high doses (150 mg). 'I was informed that this was the lowest dosage given,' one mother said. This knocks women out. 'I felt that the whole labour process had been taken out of my hands completely as soon as I arrived at the hospital. Staff took control and emphasis was on speeding up delivery.'

Postnatal Most aftercare 'extremely good'. Sympathetic help with breast-feeding and 'a very positive attitude'. Some women said there was little understanding of pain from suturing and one says she was told 'you are making a fuss about nothing'. One writer said she was treated 'like a naughty child for not doing as I was told'.

Suggestions Less emphasis on speeding up labour and getting baby delivered as fast as possible. Less routine approach to labour and more awareness of individual women's needs. Encourage women to have confidence in their own physical functions. Less induction and other forms of intervention. More emphasis on continuity of care such as is provided by community midwives.

Newton Abbot Hospital, Newton Abbot, Devon   MO

Antenatal care with own GP.

Labour Staff 'supportive' and 'considerate'; 'they were happy to have our active participation in the birth' and 'took care to let my husband be involved'. Some writers wanted to try positions other than semi-sitting and one asked if she could get on all fours, but this was refused. Episiotomies not done routinely, but some writers who did have them would have liked to be able to see if their babies could have been born without and said that episiotomies were performed after 30–40 minutes in second stage. Baby can be delivered up on to tummy.

Postnatal 'I was rather bewildered and occasionally upset . . . because of conflicting advice and rules regarding sleeping, feeding and fluid intake.' One writer said senior member of staff told her, 'This baby needs to sleep as much as it needs to be fed. Leave her until she wakes,' and ½ hour later asked her what she was thinking of to leave baby for 4 hours without a feed. Several writers advise early discharge home.

The Mount, Northallerton, N Yorkshire   MO

Pleasant converted country house on outskirts of town; 'sunny and airy', 'quiet, leisured atmosphere'.

Antenatal Attend own GP and hospital clinic twice, once for booking and about 5 weeks before baby due. Waiting only about 10 minutes. Waiting-room has plenty of toys, and students (and sometimes SNO) play with toddlers. Guided tour of hospital can be arranged and opportunity to discuss any worries and ask questions. One writer said SNO told her she could 'do her own thing' and would not be 'managed'.

Labour Partner is asked to wait in entrance hall while woman changes, but can then be with her throughout, including for forceps deliveries. Shaving only done if obvious that episiotomy will be done, e.g. before forceps delivery. One writer said that doctor who stitched her was 'offhand . . . She disappeared somewhere and I was left hanging in stirrups for what seemed like ages.'

Postnatal No routine imposed. Mother is left to do things her own way if she seems to be coping. Attitudes 'easy-going'. On ward baby is with mother from 5.30 a.m. till night. Rooming-in in amenity beds. But there are not enough of these. Writers say temperature is at 'hothouse level'. One group of mothers switched off all the radiators and opened all the windows. Nurses have time to chat about babies even when hospital full. No pressure to breast- or bottle-feed. Night staff will wake mother for feeds once the milk comes in. 'A number of older nurses with children of their own and practical approach.' Mother whose baby had projectile vomiting said she got 'lots of unfussy, relaxed help'. A depressed woman was 'given cuddles'. 'Staff are closely knit team, sharing aim of making everything as informal and calm as possible.' 'I hate hospitals and felt really bolshy about having to have baby there but I enjoyed it, largely because I was treated as an intelligent adult capable of organizing myself.' Pressure on bathrooms when hospital full. Food 'superb'; 'real coffee'. Visiting in evenings for fathers only, but this is not enforced and visitors sometimes bring in other children.

Barratt Maternity Home, General Hospital, Northampton

Consultant and GP unit. Midwifery training school. Understaffed.

Antenatal DNO writes, 'Our previous substandard, overcrowded antenatal clinic has been resolved by conversion of other premises . . . to provide more spacious accommodation with privacy.' Midwives 'friendly', 'very kind' and 'helpful' and some writers said they looked forward to clinic visits. Advise discussing worries with staff. Say tests were explained. Some writers say doctors were often late for clinic and did not have time to stop and talk properly. 'The doctor was talking to the midwife about a party he had been to the night before. I wanted to ask him something but felt I was interrupting their conversation, so I didn't bother.' Some doctors 'impersonal', 'brusque'.

Northampton

But some young doctors particularly praised. Midwives in clinic encouraged breast-feeding. Weekly antenatal clinic at Stony Stratford Health Centre; twice-monthly consultant referral clinic at Daventry and also at Newport Pagnall. Ultrasound scans done and alpha-feta protein screening. Induction rate 18% (1980). Some women have home births in this area.

Labour Writers describe enema and part-shave. Partner can be present throughout and one writer suggests 'bring packed meals so he won't miss anything'. Augmentation of labour seems to be frequent. DNO states: 'Acceleration of labour is not our aim but augmentation by use of oxytocin drip or prostaglandin to reproduce normal uterine activity as closely as possible is practised.' Pethidine and epidurals available and 20% of women have epidurals. Staff described as 'kind', 'encouraging', 'friendly', 'relaxed', 'helpful', and 'human'. Some midwives 'keen on natural childbirth'. 65% of women have electronic fetal monitoring. It can be delayed if woman wants to move about. Two writers commented on how tired midwives seemed, 'so much so that they didn't have the energy to talk to mothers'. A single mother said, 'Various people kept popping in either to turn the drip up or give me an internal, but really I was left totally on my own.' Wedges available if woman wants to sit up and can be used in second stage. Woman is often asked to push with her feet on midwife's and partner's hips. Some writers felt there must have been a more comfortable position. 10% forceps deliveries, 12% Caesarean section. Baby usually given to mother after cord cut and can be put to breast on delivery table, but some mothers had to ask for this. After baby is washed and weighed couple may have about 10 minutes with their baby, but some were not left alone at all. Some writers were perturbed that there was routine paediatric examination passing fine tube down baby's gullet to check no obstruction.

Labour: GP unit Women who had babies there two or three years ago say it has much improved and emphasis is on natural birth. Staff are 'friendly', 'pleasant', 'gentle', 'explain what they are doing all along', and 'couldn't be nicer'. Mothers who have had babies in consultant unit as well as in GP unit say they prefer latter. Midwives let woman control her own labour and push whenever she feels she needs to; 'really super'. Wedges available but some midwives 'whip them away' during second stage 'and go in for legs-up technique'. Some writers say they touched their babies' heads when almost out, but midwife may ask mother to keep her hand out of the way. Woman is encouraged to put baby to breast straight away: 'a lovely experience'. Baby is left with parents.

Postnatal Policy of demand-feeding. Baby spends first night in nursery. Some mothers were happy with this, but others said nursery was too far from ward. Some women said they could not sleep because they were worried about baby being away. Dextrose given to babies at night. Some babies given milk if mother omitted to say she didn't want this. Staff helpful with advice about breast-feeding and provide nipple shields, hand pumps, etc. Some mothers complain of conflicting advice.

330

SCBU 'Smashing!' Parents welcome and urged to cuddle baby and 'give lots of love'. No set visiting times. Nurses 'never too busy' and 'encouraging about breast-feeding'. Writers say ask the staff about any problems. Grandparents can come to see baby through window and brothers and sisters can look through window if accompanied by parents. But other family members not allowed in. 'Routines on postnatal ward clash with SCBU routines, so one day I had to see the doctor, breast-feed my baby and have my dinner *all* at 12 o'clock! Mealtimes were 'one long battle to get something if you weren't there to order when staff came round with menu'.

Suggestions Some writers objected strongly to routine test of newborn involving passing tube down oesophagus into stomach; they said it was not done in front of them and they only knew about it after the event; one woman whose baby was 'a bit mucousy' said baby was given stomach wash at same time and she thought this should not have happened without her permission. Improve communication between staff themselves. Provide ward for breast-feeding mothers next to SCBU to avoid long journey from postnatal ward to feed. Welcome siblings in SCBU and let them touch and cuddle babies.

Preston Maternity, North Shields, Tyne and Wear   MO

New hospital due to open January/February 1983. Improvements seem to be delayed until new unit in operation: 'not the happiest hospital'. But writers praise one enthusiastic consultant who is trying to change things.

Antenatal Vastly overcrowded. Some staff are described as having 'inflexible attitudes'. Two consultants ask women to ask questions, but many women do not want to discuss care. Consultant 'very approachable and pleasant'. Woman asked not to be monitored and asked if consultant would write this in notes, which he did. Writers say everybody has ultrasound scans. Booking-in visit can take up to 2 hours; subsequently appointments system. No room for toddlers. Hospital encourages shared care.

Labour No longer full pubic shave. Some writers had been put on drip and said they were not given a reason for it. One woman felt 'battered' by contractions after oxytocin drip set up and felt that 'other people and forces had affected the birth of my child more than I'. If you do not want your labour accelerated unless necessary, *say so*. One woman who went in with slow trickle of waters first noticed 20 minutes before, dilated to 5 cm in 3 hours, but still had drip set up. Electronic monitoring used frequently, but it depends who is on duty. Woman may simply be told: 'It's safer for your baby to put the monitor on.' Some writers say they were persuaded to have pethidine when they did not feel they needed it. One woman was recommended 100 mg to relax the cervix when 4–5 cm dilated and feeling that she was coping well. One writer said she asked for small dose of pethidine but was told she must have standard dose. There are staff here who 'bend over backwards' to give woman kind of birth she wants, and are 'very kind'. In the second stage woman may be flat on her back, except for head and shoulders slightly raised. One woman who asked to sit up more says she was told she could not. When she was pushing as taught in NCT classes with jaw relaxed, lips parted, she says she was told to shut her mouth and 'push properly' (1980). One writer said during delivery senior member of staff asked if she minded an external monitor, as it gave them 'added protection against future litigation'. Baby is given to mother to be cuddled immediately and parents and baby are left alone together.

Postnatal Smoking and non-smoking wards. Understaffed. No complementary feeds given to breast-fed babies. Partners are allowed to visit every afternoon. Writers describe long stays. Pressure to leave comes from mothers rather than staff.

Consultants here would appreciate having more information from mothers after the birth, apparently. There is weekly meeting at which problems are discussed. One writer who had an unhappy birth experience said her consultant talked to her for about an hour 'with honesty and concern' and asked her to send in typed account.

Suggestions Some doctors who 'love gadgetry' should learn more about physiological childbirth and be less anxious to intervene.

★★ Norfolk and Norwich, Brunswick Road, Norwich, Norfolk

Modern, busy unit, lots of staff, noise and bustle. Writers say that staff on both administrative and nursing sides are 'very helpful'. DNO writes; 'I have seen a growth of awareness in my staff to meeting parents' needs in a changing society, and an adaptability which bodes well for our future caring.'

Antenatal Though one writer thought treatment 'impersonal' and wanted more continuity (1979) others say, 'I wasn't just another bulge'; 'staff always have time to treat you as an individual however busy they are'; 'I always came away feeling as if I had been treated as a human being'. Long 'tiring' and 'tedious' waits, first visit may take 'up to 2 hours' says DNO (though some may have waited longer). On later visits woman may be 'on the premises for 1–1½ hours', according to DNO. She adds 'Attempts have been made and continue to be made to keep waiting in the very busy antenatal clinic to a minimum.' Woman whose baby was breech said 'everything was explained to me'. DNO points out that time spent discussing problems or answering queries is dependent on number of patients attending a clinic session but says that arrangements can be made when a woman particularly wants to discuss something. Writers say that though the odd nurse is 'bossy', staff are 'always willing to discuss any problems'. One problem which cropped up was that scans gave some women different dates which they found confusing. Some writers suggested that induction rate must be high. One writer said induction was proposed twice and if she had agreed to it baby would have been five weeks early. Parentcraft classes in evenings for couples together, for first-time mothers in daytime, with three shared evening sessions with partners, refresher sessions for second- or third-time mothers and daytime sessions for 'solo mums and their babies if they wished to keep coming'. DNO says 'people wishing to adopt are seen individually' . . . 'tours of our maternity unit are available and special family tours with older children are done on an individual basis. Toddlers have their own tour of the postnatal ward, where they can meet newborn babies and be prepared for their coming experience.' She comments on 'increasing sensitivity' of midwives teaching classes.

Antenatal ward: women are 'not kept in unnecessarily' according to woman whose blood pressure stabilized – she went home after 3 days. Everyone 'always very friendly and helpful'. Older children cannot visit in afternoon, can come in evenings.

Labour DNO writes that 'individualized attention' is offered. 'There is an increased awareness of enhancing endomorphine [the body's own pain-relief mechanism, see p. 65] levels by ensuring the mother's happiness in her labour. There is also an increase in mothers and fathers helping their babies deliver and this change is aided by the midwives enjoying such sharing; as well as the parents increasingly wishing to be active participants. We continue to enhance labours when necessary with cyntocinol infusion and prostaglandin pessaries.' Writers said they had shave and enema. Delivery staff are 'terrific'; 'they made us feel as though we were the only parents in the hospital'; 'the midwives made me feel very clever'. Couples appreciate having times when they are left alone during labour and midwives are sensitive to when they would like to be together like this. One writer was asked by obstetrician 'what I thought about the waters being broken to augment the labour', and said 'waters were broken very gently'. DNO writes, 'fathers actively share the experience of their child's birth and, on an individually considered basis, will sometimes share forceps deliveries and Caesarean section under epidural'. Epidurals used for breech births. Women who have had epidural Caesarean sections say staff are 'keen and sympathetic' to their wishes. Night before delivery anaesthetist comes to discuss procedure. During operation anaesthetist 'chatted and we laughed and joked . . . anaesthetist kept up running commentary on surgeon's progress: "He's got the head! Now the body's delivered! It's a girl!"' Mother can see and touch baby immediately and once weighed and wrapped can cuddle baby as operation proceeds. Writers say there is no nagging in second stage. Midwife explained to one mother delivering breech that she should not push till she had to as baby would need as much room as possible; 'I felt much better knowing this.' Women who found lithotomy position impossible asked to sit up and immediately several pillows and wedge brought. Baby delivered on to mother's tummy (including breech baby) and can be put to breast on delivery table. DNO writes, 'The father and mother are encouraged to have a period of getting to know their infant following delivery.'

Postnatal Writers say all midwives very 'into' breast-feeding. Baby rooms in 24 hours a day after first night (third for Caesareans, though one mother who asked for her baby to be brought in second night was able to feed her then).

DNO writes that postnatal wards are now 'more relaxed'. 'Our sisters . . . have made a concerted effort to read and inform their staff of the changes in knowledge of breast-feeding . . . they look at their wards with a view to helping the mothers adjust to their new role without hindrance from a hospital routine, though fluctuations in workload and staff make this a difficult area to meet everyone's needs.' Writers say there is 'non-interfering care' and staff are 'sympathetic', 'from sister to auxiliary keen to encourage breast-feeding and genuinely sorry if a woman decides it's not for her'. 'They try to persuade her to continue, but recognize that it is her decision.' Mother copes with baby in her own way, but help always available. Feeding is 'almost on demand' and mothers can feed in bed. Dextrose water available if required, but not forced on anyone, though 'it is so hot that babies sometimes appreciate a drink'. Attitudes are 'relaxed', 'informal'; 'they made you feel that you and your baby were of supreme importance, however busy they were'; 'one is kept completely in the picture'. When women first went to ward they said they sometimes had to ask if they could feed baby, but request was 'readily granted'. Ward orderlies, auxiliaries, midwives, nursery nurses and doctors are all praised. Bidets are 'very soothing'. Doctors examine stitches every day. Ice-packs for sore perineum. Rooms 'pleasant', 'clean'. Food 'substantial', 'fairly good'. A vegetarian said she was given vegetarian food with no hassle. Not enough warm drinks. Some very noisy domestic staff.

Suggestions Try to reduce long waits in antenatal clinic. If there must be waits, explain why. More baths and shower rooms. More steps to get into and out of bed. Mothers who want baby moved to nursery between 10 p.m. and 5 a.m. should be able to have this.

★ **City Maternity, Nottingham City, Nottingham, Notts**   M O

Hospital is described as 'being very concerned to make birth a very happy and exciting experience and to allay fear and anxieties, and is very good if women want to do their own thing'.

Antenatal Queues build up but staff always 'friendly' and 'helpful'. Partner can be present when scan done and both can see baby. Worries can be discussed with midwives. Woman with breech baby says she 'popped in on spec.' and was told to come back any time if she had further worries. Several writers described going two weeks past date without threat of induction (1980).

Antenatal classes: writers give these their approval. There is evening meeting for couples to discuss birth.

Labour Midwives 'very friendly'; 'sensitive to couple's wish to be left on their own'. Happy about women using breathing learnt in classes and respect women's own ideas of how they want their birth to be. On the other hand, one writer was asked if she attended NCT classes and from then on 'staff were very wary of us'. General agreement that midwives were very 'considerate', 'aware of our wishes', 'willing to leave us to get on with it'. 'The midwife was with us all the way.' Some doctors are described as 'insensitive'. Epidurals suggested as aid to relaxation. May be strongly recommended for breech deliveries. Writers describe labours 'wired up to numerous machines', but this seems to be changing because of the midwives' encouragement of natural labour. Continuous electronic monitoring available. Say if you do not want baby to have scalp clip on. Some midwives encourage women to be up and walking around. They obviously have different views about second stage. One woman said, 'I was not told when to push, but was encouraged when I felt the need to push', whereas other women say, 'I was required to push when I felt no urge', '40 minutes were allowed in second stage and then it was time for episiotomy'; attitude of midwife was that episiotomy was inevitable and that I was being "awkward" in wishing to avoid it'. Father can be present for forceps delivery, but may not be allowed in for VEs. Several writers criticized shift changes, 'There was a shift change 5 minutes before I gave birth.' Woman can put baby to breast on delivery table. One writer, finding suturing painful, told doctor, who simply said; 'I have to do it like this'; 'felt as if I was being sewn up like a football and treated like one'. Birth chair available.

Postnatal Woman is expected to look after her baby in her own way from the beginning; 'no dictatorial nurses'; staff 'sympathetic', 'caring'. Day staff mostly excellent: 'Gave help in getting baby to fix.' Encourage mother to cuddle baby whenever she wishes. But conflicting advice may be given about breast-feeding by different shifts. One woman who liked to feed her baby lying on her side was criticized by nurses for doing so but was given no reasons. Bidets appreciated.

SCBU Mother is asked if she would like to be in room on her own. She can be present while tests done and parents can visit any time. If woman misses meal when she is in SCBU staff provide food when she returns. Unit is several floors down but mother can go down to breast-feed during night 4-hourly.

Suggestions More understanding of physiology of breast-feeding.

Nuneaton Maternity, Heath End Road, Nuneaton, Warwickshire

Modern, bright and airy with 'pleasant and sympathetic' staff. Many changes since 1977 in this hospital.

Antenatal 'So many women attending clinics that one felt guilty of keeping the doctor too long asking questions.' Appointments system, but rarely kept to; 'usually ½ hour late'. Women say they didn't see same doctor on every occasion but that they did see consultant at least twice. Writers said inductions offered more frequently by one consultant than another. Women have asked for a few days' 'reprieve' and got them. One writer with leaking waters was given option of going on antenatal ward or having drip.

'Good' parentcraft classes in evenings for both parents; 'informative' and include a look round hospital, baby bath demonstration with newborn infant and visit to SCBU.

Labour DNO writes, 'women are individuals and are treated as such'. Partner can be present but is 'advised to go out when woman has bedpan and internal examination', according to DNO. 'It is a rare occurrence if they wish to stay in room.' Mini-shave only. Several writers described amniotomy. Pethidine offered, but can be refused. Electronic monitoring appears to be used frequently. DNO writes, 'we feel it would not be helpful to include statistics of induction, episiotomies, forceps delivery and Caesarean sections. We do not practice 9–5 midwifery, therefore all inductions are done purely for medical reasons. Episiotomies *are not* done routinely but if and when necessary. Instrumental deliveries too are a medical decision.' Some writers said labour suite was not well-manned at night and said staff were 'overworked', but 'extraordinarily relaxed'. Some writers said they would have felt more comfortable in second stage in sitting position but were expected to lie down. Writers say midwives are skilled at avoiding need for stitches, even with large babies. But some writers who had long second stages said repeated threats of forceps were made to make them push harder. One writer described with pleasure how her husband sat beside her holding the baby while she was washed and tidied up. When she had her previous baby, in same hospital, he had been sent out.

Postnatal Writers say there is a much more relaxed atmosphere than a few years back. DNO writes that 'breast-feeding is on demand and there are no restrictions on mothers handling their babies'. Mothers fill in charts with details of feeds and nappy changings. Some said they had conflicting advice about breast-feeding. Staff shortages; one writer said on 2 days there was only a sister with two auxiliaries, 'which meant that mothers' problems had to wait'. Mother can be present during examination by paediatrician if she asks. DNO writes, 'fit mothers look after their own babies from the second day onwards'. 'Baby is with mother from 6 a.m. until 10 p.m. except during ward cleaning.' General visiting of own children every afternoon 3–4.30 p.m. Husbands only, every evening 7.30–8.30 p.m. Fathers allowed to hold their babies. Women whose partners on night shifts can be visited in afternoons. In private rooms visitors can come in early as soon as room ready. Food 'good'.

SCBU DNO writes, 'there is open visiting for partners and mothers are encouraged to stay in the mother and baby room and look after their baby day and night prior to discharge. Mothers are encouraged to touch their babies if in incubators and help look after them, feed and cuddle them . . . siblings are allowed in at visiting time.'

Postnatal check-up.

'My consultant spent ½ hour discussing my labour, showed me my contraction sheet. He explained the extent of the episiotomy.'

Suggestions More staff on delivery suite so woman need never be left alone. Epidurals available 24 hours. Longer visiting hours on postnatal wards.

Couples should be able to sit in day room to 'eliminate that hospital bed feeling'. Bidets are lovely but salt should be provided. More staff on postnatal ward.

Oldham and District, Oldham, Lancs

Informal, 'friendly', 'smoothly efficient', 'personal care from midwives'. This is a hospital in which emphasis is on midwives' care.

Antenatal Writers describe waits of 1½–2 hours in 'crowded waiting room, pushed through on conveyer-belt system'. 'Weighed, blood pressure, sit again, see doctor, exchange a few words, out.' 'Staff too busy to answer questions.' Nowhere to leave children and many are in waiting room. 'I saw three different doctors, would have preferred one.' 'Only one explained what he was doing; others did *when asked*.' 'Impersonal, tiring, only interested in you medically'; 'as a person you don't count'. 'Doctors and other staff have teacher–pupil relationship with women'; '"we know, you don't. Therefore don't question our authority"'.' There are parenthood classes and fathers can go on tour of unit with mothers.

Labour Acting DNO writes, 'induction of labour/acceleration only if there is a medical or obstetric indication . . . continuous care of mother . . . antenatal, first stage, labour ward and postnatal beds . . . on each floor under the care of its consultant ward team. The mother is transferred in her own bed to and from the labour ward to remove the need for constantly getting on and off trollies.' Many women are in fact delivered in the first-stage rooms which are more 'homely' than the labour wards. Writers say admitted in labour with 'minimum of fuss'; enema or suppositories given. DNO writes that 'in most instances shaving of the perineal area only carried out prior to delivery'. Partner may be sent out during prep but is otherwise encouraged to be involved. Writers say they were told what was happening. Couple may be left alone together for time. No drugs pressed on women; ask for gas and oxygen if you want it. Midwives 'reassuring', 'friendly'. Woman who wanted to walk about was told she must get into bed; 'could not get into comfortable position in bed'. Continuous fetal monitoring available. Epidural analgesic available. Women can wear their own nightdresses during labour. They are usually wheeled to different room for delivery, partner masked and gowned. Women lie with partner holding shoulders, feet on midwives' hips. Episiotomy not done routinely and midwife tells woman before doing one. Mucus suctioned out before baby handed to mother; father can hold baby while mother stitched. Couple have short time alone with their baby. Writers described father leaving and baby being taken away so mother could sleep.

Postnatal DNO writes, 'there is considerable flexibility regarding feeding. Modified demand-feeding for both breast- and artificial feeding is practised and baby is put to breast as soon after delivery as possible for those mothers who wish.' Is brought to mother when she asks after delivery, but is taken to nursery first night; after that, by mother, who looks after her own baby. Some women said conflicting advice was given 'which can be very confusing'. Writers say they were not always sure who to ask for what. But 'everyone is ready to help' and it is all 'very homely' and 'intimate'. DNO writes, 'babies requiring intermittent phototherapy are nursed on the maternity unit with their mothers'. She says, 'there is a flexible approach to visiting and children are permitted to visit their mothers'.

SCBU DNO writes that 'there is a sensitive attitude towards the grieving process for those women who unfortunately may lose their baby'. Food 'in small amounts' but 'good'.

Suggestions Facilities for children in antenatal clinic. Reorganization of clinic so that mother can see same doctor throughout antenatal period. More time to discuss problems with midwives and doctors. Some women would appreciate support from midwives with breathing and using different positions to help progress of labour.

★ Orsett General, Orsett, Essex

'Fairly large, modern hospital', 'very clean and bright'. 'Welcoming', 'not antiseptic at all'. Staff 'pleasant and kind', 'seem happy in their jobs'.

Antenatal 'Efficient with a personal touch'; 'during my pregnancy at every visit staff were the same and we got to know each other'. Sometimes long wait to see doctor. 'Doctors happy to spend time explaining things and do not rush'; 'I got all the attention and reassurance I could possibly expect.' Questions always answered. Frequent scans. Helpful education for birth; four films and discussion on breast-feeding, what to expect in the hospital, caring for baby, contraception, etc. Three relaxation sessions.

Labour Inductions done with Prostin. Several writers said labour had been accelerated within couple of hours of membranes having ruptured. Partner there throughout, except for forceps delivery. One woman who wanted him there for forceps delivery said she was told it was 'hospital policy that he could not be there; I do feel, though, that had I not been exhausted and unable to insist he stay, they would have complied'. Midwives supportive, 'but know little of NCT techniques'; 'encouraging', 'helpful'. Everything is fully explained to partner. Pethidine offered – it seems that large doses are given; 'I remember very little about my labour'; 'I was too exhausted to push' after pethidine (so had forceps), but there is no persuasion to have pethidine. One writer said 'the shift delayed their lunch by almost an hour to stay with me till delivery'. Mother can hold baby immediately after delivery.

Postnatal Nurses 'kind', 'understanding', 'caring'. Baby is with mother all the time. Great support for and help with breast-feeding but bottle-feeders not made to 'feel inadequate'. Some writers said they were given contradictory advice, however, and felt they needed more time than nurses had to give, 'though staff do their best'. Writers said they were not 'patronized' and 'everything was done on an equal adult-to-adult basis'; 'I was never interfered with'. Those writers who wanted to be independent felt that nurses had time to give when necessary. It was more difficult for mothers who were not sure of themselves and who wanted reassurance. Life on wards is 'hectic'. Writers said they had to be in day room at specific times for their meals even if their babies were crying. Partners can visit 8 a.m.–8 p.m. and can feed, change and cuddle baby.

Suggestions Improve quality of food.

★★ John Radcliffe, Oxford

Very modern, 'bright', 'airy', 'cheerful', in attractive, impressive, but dauntingly spacious physical surroundings. Most staff 'pleasant' and 'helpful'. DNO writes, 'staff are continually discussing and considering how individual client requests can be best met within the present financial restrictions'.

Antenatal Efficient, very busy clinic. May see different doctor each time. But most writers say they were treated 'as a person' or words to that effect. Some women thought it was like 'a baby factory' and found it overwhelming 'with so many people to see and instructions to follow'. Long waiting times. Shared care with GP and community midwife can be arranged, but 'once the Junior Registrar got hold of me I seemed to be chasing up there for one spurious reason after another'. Hospital does not always keep GP informed. No continuity of care, which writers deplore. Doctors vary; 'nothing was discussed; I felt this was an insult to my intelligence" 'doctors always told you what they found on examination . . . did not treat me as an "object"'; women who found clinic visits depressing were those who experienced impersonal treatment. Sometimes encountered bad-tempered nurses; 'I came away from each visit more or less in tears.' 'It was extremely bureaucratic'; 'we were herded from one queue to another'. One couple who had unhappy experience in 1979 had 'marathon meeting' with professor to discuss problems. Some writers thought personal approach in special high-risk clinic made this clinic much better than normal clinic. See same doctors and midwives each time; questions encouraged and everything explained; students introduced to patients who may be asked if they may examine them; waits for this clinic are not long. Staff 'extremely enthusiastic' and 'I was treated as an intelligent individual in a relaxed, friendly manner'. In 1981 parentcraft classes were reviewed and evaluated by clients. There is now early preparation class and extra evening session. Two evening films for partners as well. Classes good for meeting other pregnant women and partners welcome. Varying induction rates between different consultants. Induction done with prostaglandin pessaries to ripen cervix. Many women induced without oxytocin drip. Overall induction rate 25% (13% with prostaglandin treatment, 10% with oxytocin).

Antenatal ward – staff take 'real personal interest' and questions are encouraged. Women who were on professorial unit said atmosphere is 'relaxed', 'friendly', 'with no rules'; longer-stay patients dressed, go out for short walks, for meals with husbands or home for weekends; 'morale-booster'.

Labour: consultant unit Partial shave at which partner can be present. Suppository; one woman had 'crack in rectum from one being forced in at wrong angle'. Asked when first arrives in labour room what feelings are about pain relief. No pressure put on woman to have pain-killers. Epidurals readily available; 'was fantastic'. Epidural rate 28%. Electronic fetal monitoring used often but midwives very understanding about women wanting natural labour. Woman can sit in chair. Staff introduce themselves. Are 'kind and encouraging'; 'they made me feel as if I was the only woman having a baby'; 'everything is explained'; 'my NCT breathing was welcomed by midwife who was in favour of mother doing as much as possible to help herself'; 'everything is relaxed'. Writers critical of membranes being artificially ruptured as soon as they go into delivery suite; 'apparently we have no choice'. Writers say partners were never asked to leave for any examination and were fully accepted by delivery team and encouraged to take active part. Can be present for forceps delivery. Meals may be offered from staff canteen. 'Doctor who gave epidural explained it all to me and my husband'; 'throughout the midwife treated me like a queen and my husband like the prince consort.' But writers mention lack of continuity of care by midwives. Acceleration frequent with some consultants. Total rate 19%. Some writers said they were not consulted about this. 'An oxytocin drip was prepared and although we said we preferred to let labour take its own course, we were told that Mr X doesn't like his patients to be in labour too long once membranes have ruptured. Again no real say in what was being done. I felt I was being taken over by staff and equipment.' Writers welcomed opportunities to make their own suggestions and said that these were welcomed. One woman whose labour was progressing slowly suggested it might be a good idea to get off the bed and walk around for a bit. 'I was unstrapped from the monitoring machine and left for half an hour to walk around and have a wash. This worked wonders with hastening up the labour.' Writers much preferred those labour rooms with window; others are like boxes, even though they have flowered wallpaper. Praise for atmosphere at delivery; 'quiet', 'relaxed', 'humorous'; 'I felt the staff were anxious to deliver my baby the way I wanted.' Some writers were told by midwife they would not be able to push longer than 1 hour as it was 'against hospital rules'. 'Not so, just ruling of some consultants.' They were told policy to do forceps delivery or vacuum extraction if woman has not delivered by then. This may have been why some writers were told to push harder and longer than they thought necessary. But most recent writers say that they were told to push only as hard as they wanted to. Rooms not adequately sound-proofed; 'I heard the woman in the next delivery room screaming.' DNO writes, 'staff continually strive to meet individual requests . . . staff are experimenting with various supports and extra bean-bags have been purchased . . . with the decrease in the use of oxytocin patients are more mobile and able to be up and about'. Medieval-style birth stool available if you ask. Physiotherapists now visit delivery suite to help mothers during labour and to show staff how to help women with breathing in labour. Forceps delivery 17%, Caésarean sections 10%, episiotomies 48% (includes instrumental delivery). Most recent writers say things like 'It's so nice not to have stitches. Last time nearly all the women were staggering round with pillows to sit on, preoccupied with stitch pain. This time, I've not heard much talk of stitches. It is remarkably different.' Baby placed immediately on mother's abdomen and baby handed to father if woman needs stitching. Mother encouraged to put baby to breast on delivery bed, couple have time alone with baby to feed and get to know their child. Some women described how they lifted their babies out of their own bodies; 'then she was on my tummy, all slippery'; 'a wonderful thing to put my hand on my hot, sticky daughter'. Writers who have Caesarean sections may be given option of general anaesthesia or epidural; several describe epidural Caesarean as 'an incredible experience', 'a natural Caesarean birth'. When birth is not straightforward atmosphere of delivery room may suddenly change, one said room suddenly filled with people and machines, but she was 'told nothing because they were too busy looking at machines'. She had 'very gentle and understanding midwife' who told staff crowding in, 'don't make so much noise'. Another, whose baby had an abnormal cord, asked if the baby was alright and was told 'just', rather than being given accurate information; 'there was a great deal of whispering going on and so naturally I expected the worst'. Her husband had left by the time she was told the problem; the baby was perfect but she could not accept this for several months and became very depressed. Writers suggest that sometimes midwives find it difficult to cope with insensitive individuals who destroy peaceful atmosphere for birth. One writer who said midwife was 'a friendly and confidence-making presence' and whose 'real delight at seeing a completely unaided delivery was a joy to see, was appalled at sudden change in atmosphere of delivery room as doctor arrived to suture perineum; 'clatter, bang, the door smashes open. "Why aren't these lights on?" addressed to nobody in particular by an irritated young man in jeans. Noisy talking between doctor and hand-maiden. Stirrups, smells of antiseptic, green sheets. The local anaesthetic hardly hurt but the "tailor" started stitching straight-away and that did. In desperation, got into conversation with tailor eventually saying something like "it must be rotten for you coming in after the event – people won't be grateful to you like they are to the midwives". The tailor replied, glancing at my husband, "the husbands are!" with a chuckle. I wish I could have told him to keep his junior common-room vulgarity to himself. I can understand that stitching up a perineum in the middle of the night is not fun, but couldn't they and their hardware enter the room quietly? Couldn't they stop and count to twenty before they open the door, just to remind themselves that the people inside have only minutes ago completed an enormous task? The contrast between the quiet, purposeful, warm thing of the birth and the harsh, strange stitching was very marked.' Writers also said stitching sometimes took a very long time. 'The stitching took almost an hour to complete. The medical student was trying very hard to suture correctly but was obviously very inexperienced.' Mother is wheeled to ward with baby beside her in cot. Staff shortages mean long delays between delivery suite and ward level.

Labour: GP unit GP unit is integral part of main hospital. Low-risk women do better in GP beds than in consultant beds and their babies do too. Lower and less frequent dose of pethidine, fewer forceps deliveries and fewer babies have breathing difficulties. In labour woman meets midwife at home when labour starts or in hospital when she arrives. Partner may be turned out during prepping but is otherwise made to feel welcome and is encouraged to help. Woman can walk up and down. Midwife or pupil with her almost continuously. No drugs 'pushed'. Most women manage with gas and oxygen only. 'The pupil reminded me of breathing techniques learnt in classes.' Can have low lights and gentle music. GP often comes for birth.

Postnatal DNO writes, 'demand-feeding is in operation – unlimited feeding time has been introduced according to individual needs. The routine use of nipple cream has been discontinued. To help overcome the conflicting feeding advice weekly feeding seminars have been introduced . . . an open meeting to which paediatric/obstetric nursing personnel of all grades are invited. Mothers with interesting feeding ideas or with particular problems also attend. Feeding-advice sister passes on her expertise and help, not only to members, but to all members of staff . . . To help overcome conflicting advice the emphasis is on the mother deciding on a postnatal routine to suit her individual needs. Only basic advice is now offered in writing.' Writers say that there is generous help with breast-feeding problems, but that, 'you were always made to feel that the baby was yours'. 'Sometimes difficult to find a nurse' – this can be worrying for mothers of first babies who feel they need more help. But another writer says, 'I was very much left alone to get on with things by myself, which suited me admirably.' Single rooms are in great demand. Babies now room in at night instead of being in nurseries. Sleeping can be difficult. One writer who was in bed next to nursery said she was woken by any of four babies crying and then had to wake other mothers. She went home 'exhausted'. Nurses were 'very rarely seen' at night, though they were supposed to wake mothers when babies cried. Acute shortage of midwives poses problems. Staff will make tea for mothers doing night feeds, 'just like a hotel'. But they complain of 'unbearable heat'; 'surely it is not necessary to keep babies at temperatures over 80°, when they are sure to be going to much cooler homes'. Cleaning staff sometimes 'short-tempered'. Plenty of showers/lavatories and 'blissful bidets', but broken shower roses. 'The hospital is very short of all sorts of goodies. The effect of economies is clear – no sterilized sanitary pads in the machines, and lots of routine maintenance not done. It is sad to see the place looking tatty round the edges.' One woman who said that doctor told her to use ice-packs to ease pain of perineal bruising says she was refused them by auxiliary and told she didn't need them. Baby with mild jaundice may be moved to window and mother to bed by window. Freezers with expressed breast milk at ward levels.

Food could be better, with more roughage. One writer said, 'I was so hungry after labour, but only offered a cup of tea . . . it would be lovely to have something on offer if only biscuits or a sandwich.' Writers advise taking chocolate bars in!

Visiting 11–12 noon partners only. 3.30–4.30 p.m. and 7 8.30 p.m. Own children can visit in afternoon. Can always see visitors in day room. Relatives can hold baby.

GP unit patients are looked after by their own midwife visiting twice a day for first 2 days and then once a day.

SCBU DNO writes, 'a parent dayroom with kitchenette facilities has been furnished by League of Friends. Creche facilities introduced for siblings. Mothers invited to stay overnight with their babies prior to discharge of baby from unit.'

Suggestions More nursing staff, especially on postnatal wards. Change antenatal care so that it is not so 'regimented' and 'consider the whole woman'. Seek continuity of care from midwives, especially between antenatal clinics and wards and delivery suite. Midwives should be able to do their own suturing. The many writers who complained about the postnatal wards being excessively hot – 'like a sauna' – suggested heat should be turned down. 'Somebody should take time to explain simple general baby care to first-time mothers.' One writer who says 'we did not seem to have long enough together to share our baby' suggests that husbands who cannot visit in morning should always be able to have longer with mother and baby in afternoons. Some writers felt they were kept in without being given adequate reasons and felt trapped, even if it was in the 'Headington Hilton'. They suggest; 'let those women who want to go home do so as soon as they feel fit enough'.

The hospital is open to suggestions for change. Write to Miss Kate Aletson, Divisional Nursing Officer.

DNO writes that immediate future aims are 'to work towards the introduction of midwives' clinics, to introduce health education programmes to the waiting area in the clinic. To work towards giving a more total client care, especially looking to more continuity of care in the postnatal night duty situation . . . and to review and discuss the current episiotomy rate.'

Pembury Hospital, Pembury, Kent   MO

Antenatal Clinic held in unprepossessing outbuilding, very long waits. Some writers described consultants as 'friendly' and 'kind' but other doctors are described as 'snide', 'sarcastic and dismissive', 'look for things going wrong but do not seem happy when things right' and 'show no pleasure when everything is normal'. One writer said consultant examined her at 32 weeks without addressing a word to her, turned to student and asked him why the baby felt smaller than date suggested . . . told him that it was in transverse position and "I'll probably have to do a Caesarean unless it moves".' This mother was very upset. Several writers said they were asked to come in for induction when 9–10 days past EDD and were not given an option. Writers describe large number of nurses in clinic who 'chat with each other and do not pay much attention to mothers'.

Labour Everyone 'extremely kind and attentive' though women may be examined frequently by 'polite, friendly but heavy-handed students'. Midwives and pupil midwives especially mentioned for the 'loving support' they give. Continuous electronic monitoring may be used; 'I was more or less forced to stay in one position . . . I would have liked to be able to move about'; 'there was something dehumanizing about having wires trailing out of my body to a machine and since everyone was at pains to reassure me that if the recording was erratic it was more likely to be the machine on the blink than anything wrong with the baby, I did wonder why they placed such faith in the procedure'. Pethidine offered. In second stage women are encouraged to long hard pushes. Midwives are 'helpful', 'kind', 'confidence-inspiring'. Are expert at avoiding episiotomy and need for stitches. Some midwives delivered babies over 9 lb without tear. Some writers had legs in stirrups for long time during suturing. One mentions a period of 1 hour, including 20–25 minutes during which she was waiting for the doctor to scrub up and repair.

Postnatal Very attractive wards. Sister welcomes each mother. Baby is by mother's bed all day although at night must go to nursery. But nursery staff go to great pains to discover what each mother wants for her baby and will wake her for night feeds. Mother has freedom to walk about or go to bed as she wishes and can feed and cuddle baby when she wants. Plenty of staff to give help if required. 'Contented, peaceful' atmosphere with busy hum of noise. Writers felt well cared for. Auxiliaries are 'attentive' and 'relaxed'. 'Everyone friendly', including tea-ladies. 'Nothing is too much trouble.' 'I was sorry I only had 48 hours.'

Food 'absolutely dreadful'. Choice in theory, 'but nothing ever arrives as ordered'. Menus sound imaginative on paper 'but all food reduced to same sawdust taste and texture'; 'particularly awful soup'. Writers suggest getting food parcels sent in.

Visiting 3–4 p.m. and up to 9 p.m. for partners; 'a scrum on Saturday but fun'.

Suggestions More sympathetic understanding of women's emotions by obstetricians. Woman who was admitted to antenatal ward said that she was subjected to emotional blackmail and told that it was her baby and if she wanted to risk losing it, it was up to her; she suggests that any statements about the need for different kinds of treatment or about development of baby should be carefully explained and fully substantiated.

Penrith New Hospital, Penrith, Cumbria   MO

Antenatal Not enough material about antenatal care to warrant including it, but antenatal classes described for couples together, at which such subjects as sex after childbirth are discussed; much appreciated.

Labour Shaving not compulsory. Midwives 'most helpful', 'very supportive', 'make the whole experience personal'. Some are sympathetic to NCT-style preparation. 'Midwife kept saying, "You are doing fine . . . good", etc.'; 'They were willing to let me do things the way I wanted.' Partner is present during prepping, though some writers said midwives objected initially; he is one of team and couple are kept fully informed. Some writers said epidurals were encouraged by obstetrician: 'But I wasn't told about the likelihood of forceps. Had I been, I would not have opted for one.' In second stage midwives seemed to urge mothers to push longer and harder, and keep pushing. 'She told me I wasn't trying hard enough.' Baby delivered on to your tummy if you wish.

Postnatal Again, not enough letters about postnatal care to include material here.

Peterborough Maternity Unit, Peterborough   MO

Antenatal Overcrowded clinic and 'time wasting' but staff 'very helpful and discuss difficulties'.

Labour Shave/enema. Some writers said they had to ask about what was going on and state of cervix, but were told readily when they did. One woman whose enema did not work when she was already 4 cm dilated said she was given another one while having 'contractions with a vengeance'. After prepping partner can be with woman throughout. Midwives try to avoid episiotomy. Baby is handed to mother immediately.

Postnatal 'All staff helpful'. 'Nursery nurses obviously love babies and give a lot of assistance with breast-feeding.' Baby is in nursery first 2 nights, but given only water if breast-fed. Forty-eight-hour discharge can be arranged.

Suggestions Partner should be able to spend more time with woman and baby.

Alexandra Maternity Home, Plymouth, S Devon   HO

GP unit. Home births can be arranged in this area. DNO writes, 'The Flying Squad can be rapidly assembled to answer obstetric distress calls, which are infrequent nowadays.' Domino system operates here.

Labour 9% of women have ARM in labour; 26% episiotomy rate.

Postnatal Over half of mothers breast-feed. Mothers are transferred here for postnatal care from Freedom Fields, Plymouth.

345

★ **Freedom Fields, Plymouth, S Devon**

DNO writes, commenting on first edition, 'Although your book is so pleasantly written, you have obtained your information from satisfied "customers" and it would have been quite possible to have had adverse comments. Consequently it was decided to send you some official information.' Large hospital, old buildings, but clean; antenatal clinic, labour, delivery and postnatal wards redecorated 1980. 'Quite easy to get lost on first visit.' Staff under terrific pressure, bed shortages at times. On the whole 'efficient', 'pleasant', and 'helpful'. 'We try to meet the mums' wishes all the way.'

Antenatal Very busy clinic, long waits. One visit can take 2½ hours. Same appointment time given to five or six women. Routine ultrasound. 'Things are rushed and there is no time to ask questions.' But one writer said she saw same consultant most times. Amniocentesis available on request after age 35 and suggested after 40. Normally consultant only seen on one visit and registrar or houseman at other times. Domino scheme in operation. Tour of unit offered; evening classes for couples.

Labour Pleasant first-stage room. Partner allowed and can stay for forceps delivery. Surgical induction 18%; ARM in labour 33%. Mothers encouraged to walk round in first stage. Midwives 'very considerate' to partners and 'very helpful' in encouraging woman to cope with contractions. 'I cannot fault the kindness and attention I had.' Women can labour without drugs for pain relief. Epidurals 13%. 'Very understanding' anaesthetist; 'he even held my hand when a contraction came'. Epidural is not topped up at end of first stage. Couple may be left together for periods alone. Electronic monitoring may be used; not enough machines for everyone. Woman has to be moved to another room for delivery. 'I was encouraged to push when I felt like it, not to worry how long I took, and to do things my way.' Women have given birth squatting on mattress on floor. Leboyer birth possible: low lights, delayed cutting of cord. Baby is placed on mother's abdomen and left there about 10 minutes. Then taken to be labelled next to delivery bed, wrapped and given back to mother for 15–30 minutes. Forceps 14%; Caesareans 9%. Father can hold baby while woman being stitched but is sometimes sent out. 'The sudden contrast from giving birth, holding my baby with my husband with me, to being alone with a doctor I had never seen at my feet, stitching away in silence. I felt bereft . . . cheated.' Then baby to nursery, women to ward; 'I wish I could have had him with me.' 1983: work starting on labour and delivery suites with curtains/wallpaper/camp beds for fathers.

Postnatal Nurses very helpful with breast-feeding, but sometimes 'run off their feet'. Good follow-up by obstetrician. Woman is meant to stay in bed for first 6 hours, but mothers arriving in ward in early morning find everyone up and about and cannot sleep. Baby is sometimes not brought to mother until several hours after birth. Woman is encouraged to cuddle baby and is 'always made to feel that she was mine and not the hospital's'. Baby is with mother all the time unless she wants baby in nursery. Mothers do things in their own way. Babies can be on and in the beds with mother for cuddle. No mother who wrote was ever told that she should put her baby down. Mothers have charts for feeds/bowel movements. Demand-feeding with no restrictions during meal or visiting times. One nurse sat with breast-feeding mother at every feed until she could cope. 'Always someone to help if there is a difficulty' and 'all nurses very friendly'. Test-weighing sometimes done. Women can have bath whenever they like. Fathers often stay after official visiting and writers' partners had not been told to leave. Both father and mother can handle baby as much as they like. Several writers stressed that there was plenty of time to rest and sleep, which is an unusual comment on postnatal wards. Relaxed and caring atmosphere. Food good. Excellent salads and wholemeal bread always available (1980) but not enough protein. Drinks trolley goes around several times a day and at meal times. Visiting afternoons and evenings only. Other children encouraged. Most women stay 48 hours.

Suggestions Better staff–patient ratio in antenatal clinic to prevent long queues. More staff on postnatal wards since existing staff are very over-worked. Bidets and salt for treatment of perineal pain. Paediatricians should have more contact with mothers. More food, especially for breast-feeding mothers.

★ Maternity Unit, Poole General, Longfleet Road, Poole, Dorset

There has been enormous progress in last five years in this hospital. Earlier reports said that relationships between staff and women were poor and writers said things like 'I felt just a number'. Very different now.

Antenatal Midwives 'friendly'. Writers say they were in and out of clinic in not more than 45 minutes. Shared care usual. Partners welcome to attend ante-natal classes.

Labour SNO says induction when 'medically indicated'. Monitoring appar-atus is used selectively. No shaving, no routine enema. Writers suggest that ARM is done automatically after examinations. Midwives 'friendly', approve of mobility in first stage, 'let me do my breathing and change positions', 'encourage natural birth', Pethidine and gas and oxgen offered but woman can refuse. 'No persuasion to have drugs.' Epidurals available. Midwives skilled at avoiding episiotomy and tears; 15% forceps deliveries; 6% Caesarean sec-tions. Father can be present for forceps delivery. Baby given to mother while placenta being delivered and then to father while mother cleaned up. Baby is bathed next to parents.

Postnatal SNO writes that there is rooming-in and a flexible approach to breast-feeding, with demand-feeding in many instances. Nurse helps with first breast-feed; no complementary feeds given usually, though dextrose if mother asks for it. Woman looks after her own baby. Baby is removed first night, but after that is next to mother day and night. 'Friendly staff' take time to talk with women. 'I don't see how I could have been better cared for.'

Shortage of bathrooms. Evening visiting for partners only, but on first evening other children can come too by arrangement with sister. Normally own children visit in afternoon. Food 'good' and 'hot'. Choice of menu for next day; also choice of portions, small/normal/big, which seems a good idea.

★ St Mary's, Portsmouth, Hampshire   MO

STOP PRESS. Dramatic changes. Waiting time in clinic much reduced. Exceptionally flexible. If you want something, ask beforehand. Staff try hard to meet individual woman's needs. No routine shave/enema. Will deliver in any position. Birth chair available.

Preston Hospital, Preston, Lancs   HO

Acting DNO writes, 'Two lady interpreters work full time in the antenatal clinics, postnatal wards and in the maternity and child-welfare clinics, to assist Asian patients and their families . . . Three courses per year, entitled "English for Pregnancy", are held to teach parentcraft and language skills mainly to pregnant Asian ladies . . . In-service training now includes seminars for midwifery staff and health visitors on Asian culture and communication problems, and teaches basic Asian language skills. Three evening sessions in parentcraft course, which partners are encouraged to attend.'

Labour She writes: 'Induction and acceleration of labour, episiotomy, forceps delivery, vacuum extraction, Caesarean section are only practised within this district when medically indicated.'

Postnatal Community special-care baby service for the mothers of babies who have been in SCBU, so that they can be transferred home sooner.

★ Royal Berkshire, London Road, Reading, Berks

Modern, clean, pleasant building. Staff busy but 'most agreeable'. 'Overall impression of professional competence'; 'staff encouraging and have enthusiasm for what they are doing'. Women having second babies here say hospital has improved greatly from several years ago.

Antenatal Morning visits seldom last less than 2 hours; 'depressing to walk in and see at least thirty worried-looking pregnant women waiting'. Afternoon visits quicker. Comfortable chairs/pleasant carpeting/large box of toys for children. But women say they rarely see same doctor or midwife: 'Only one doctor introduced himself'; 'he was not prepared to discuss pros and cons of induction'; 'gives no information, just directions to nurse'. On the other hand one writer said woman doctor said to her: 'You only want labour induced if baby at risk . . . I don't blame you.' Writers say that as woman arrives, file is put in tray, so one is seen in order of arrival and it is random which doctor one sees. They complain of conveyor-belt atmosphere and say: 'Only time you have any feeling of individual care is if you are interesting medically.' Some doctors 'reassuring', but younger ones 'do not like to commit themselves'. One writer says receptionist 'tells you off' if you forgot a specimen and this was hard on Asian women who did not speak English and could not understand what was required of them. Apparently receptionist 'takes a poor view of husbands and friends who accompany expectant mothers'. Midwives 'usually very pleasant' and 'have time to talk'; 'all questions answered'. But in general 'efficient', 'impersonal' care. 'I'd have so much liked a bit of continuity in care.' One problem with doctors, particularly consultants, is that they are 'very hurried' and have opinions which conflict. Some writers like doctors' attitudes. One said there was 'no waffle', others disliked 'offhand manners'; 'He came in and said "The terrible Mrs X!"' Writers advise asking questions for 'they usually assume that you have none'; 'you have to be completely firm'. Scans appear to be ordered frequently. A very pleasant ultrasound unit with caring staff. Good screening for abnormalities. Urinary oestriol tests also seem to be done frequently. Can be done at home. Writers found them a nuisance. Woman with breech said procedure for breech delivery was thoroughly explained. Antenatal classes 'useful'; can visit delivery rooms in advance. Women having shared care go to hospital clinic for booking at about 9 weeks and then not until 33 weeks. Writers suggested that induction rates seemed to be high. Several women admitted overnight for induction found that a rush of spontaneous births delayed induction: 'I had my tea and toast at 6 a.m. and waited . . . and waited . . . and waited.' Writers advise asking if there seem to be hold-ups. Information only given when you inquire. Woman is not given food, in case, but you can ask for another cup of tea.

Antenatal ward: staff 'friendly', 'relaxed'. Dietician 'charming'. Cleaners 'very efficient'. 'On admission I was asked to sign consent form agreeing to Caesarean section. As I was only 33 weeks, not in labour, I said I would rather not sign this until the occasion arose. Nurse reluctantly agreed. Not a very reassuring welcome.' TV lounge always smoke-filled.

Labour Partners sent out during prepping, but otherwise in all the time. Couple have time alone together in pleasant delivery room with crib in corner; 'very touching'. Dim lighting, complete privacy, comfortable bed. 'They did everything in their power to let me enjoy my birth.' Writers say atmosphere is 'calm', 'relaxed', 'reassuring', midwives 'gentle'. You can choose any position in which comfortable. No pressure to have pain-killers. Can ask for half-dose pethidine. Epidurals available. Midwives 'strictly respect' woman's wishes: 'I could do what I wanted . . . didn't feel I was being "bossed" at all'; 'midwife was quietly encouraging'; 'midwives were helpful in discussing way I wanted to do things'. Women say they are told about everything that is going to be done. If you don't want something, *say so*. Electronic monitoring often employed but woman can sit in chair. Amniotomy appears to be routinely done. Many writers also described oxytocin acceleration. One woman consented to doctor breaking waters but asked him to leave drip to see if it was really necessary. He agreed and labour proceeded normally. Some writers were very happy not to be 'plugged into' anything. Woman can be delivered on back or side, as she wishes. Partner and midwife hold one leg each if on back. Midwife may deliver baby up on to woman's abdomen. Far fewer episiotomies are being done. Baby given to mother to hold: 'I held her fingers before she was taken to be cleaned . . . fed her straight after her bath.' One writer who had forceps delivery said there was 'a sea of faces and a flurry of midwives, one holding my hand'. She was completely flat on her back and it was 'difficult to see what was going on below'. Her husband was outside, though the baby was taken to him after delivery. When in the recovery room her husband joined her. 'It was very peaceful' and parents had time alone with their baby and mother could breast-feed. Several writers comment on rush to get third stage completed, pulling on cord, which in one case snapped off. This woman had to have general anaesthesia for manual removal 1½ hours later. Meanwhile she could not be moved and baby was left in crib: 'It spoiled the post-birth experience.' Father present during stitching. Several women describe being sutured before anaesthetic had time to take effect. Once mother is on postnatal ward baby is brought to her immediately.

Labour: GP unit Antenatal care with own GP and midwife for woman not at risk, though it is possible to arrange delivery here for first babies and if you are over 30. Mini-shave/enema in labour. Single room with partner present all the time. He may be brought meals and 'is made to feel a member of the team'. Setting 'very intimate'. Many women have few or no drugs. Woman is asked if she wants drugs for pain relief and it is her choice. Can arrange Leboyer-style delivery with baby lifted on to mother's abdomen. Many women do not have episiotomies. Parents hold baby immediately. Can arrange for cord not to be cut until it stops pulsating. Mother encouraged to put baby to breast. Baby not taken away to be bathed, is left with parents all the time. Midwife brings trolley up to bed and baths baby beside it. Whole atmosphere 'gentle'.

Postnatal Attractive wards. Variable experiences and although some writers say 'everyone was pleasant', they also say things like: 'never saw same face twice', 'treated as though I were a mindless idiot' and said they needed more care than they received. Mothers who choose not to bottle-feed are not made to feel guilty. Modified demand-feeding is practised and women are told to feed not less than 5-hourly or more than 2-hourly. 'Unfortunately many nursery nurses seem to lack experience of breast-feeding.' Writers sometimes said that babies in nursery were fed bottles to allow mother to sleep. 'Height of hospital bed was ridiculous considering the need to be up and down looking after baby.' A writer who said postnatal care was 'a complete farce' described how she was taken up to single room and dumped, 'with no call button and baby out of reach'. Another said she was 'in tears of exhaustion by evening'. Writers complain of excessive heat. One writer said the radiator was 'jammed on and it needed muscle power to shut it off'. Bidets available. Food 'poorly presented' and some writers thought 'inedible'. Can arrange 8/24/36-hour stay.

Postnatal: GP unit 'Very friendly atmosphere.' Rooming-in and staff wake mother to feed if she chooses not to have baby beside her. Help with breast-feeding is 'relaxed' and 'progressive'. 'Sensible advice from midwives, most of whom were mothers'. 'Staff care for emotional as well as physical state of mother.' Here too, food is criticized as being 'awful', 'tinned stodge'. Writers advise taking in bran and wholemeal bread. Unrestricted visiting for fathers. It is extremely hot and one writer said she got 'appalling dry throat and cough'. Can arrange to be home again 24 hours after delivery.

Redhill General, Redhill, Surrey MO

Friendly, helpful staff. Though there are routines writers say they did not feel 'regimented'.

Antenatal Writers welcomed the chance to ask for what they wanted in childbirth and to have their requests noted down. 'SNO couldn't have been nicer or more helpful, wrote "no episiotomy unless medically required" on notes.'

Labour Midwives 'cheerful', 'friendly', 'take trouble to explain what is going on', 'make you feel at ease'. Electronic fetal monitoring seems to be used frequently and once electrode attached woman may spend much of the time alone with her partner, though staff come if called. If woman does not have electrodes attached may be allowed to be mobile, but this depends on staff on duty. Pethidine sometimes offered very late in first stage, but can be refused. Can use as many wedges as wished for pillows. Father allowed at forceps delivery. Couple have time alone together with baby after.

Postnatal 'Relaxed atmosphere' and writers say that nearly all mothers are breast-feeding. Nurses spend a lot of time helping mothers with difficulties, but conflicting advice is sometimes given. Some writers say baby was given sugar water at night till third day (1981). Demand-feeding encouraged and mother can make her wishes clear by putting note on cot; these wishes are respected. Some writers said there was an official maximum 20-minute sucking time, 'but no one stands over you with a stop-watch.' Baby in nursery at night and mother called for feedings. One woman said she was reprimanded for carrying her baby across the ward: 'We always wheel them.'

Suggestions Less routine monitoring. Some writers asked whether the rules on postnatal ward were really necessary.

Rochdale

Birch Hill, Littleborough, Rochdale, Greater Manchester   M O

'Unfailing kindness of everyone.'

Antenatal Shared care possible. Comprehensive conducted tour of unit with 'ample opportunity to discuss hospital routine . . . when I eventually arrived to have my baby, I felt as though I was going to a familiar place and knew what to expect'. Woman who had raised AFP count and amniocentesis said that this was 'handled with great tact and consideration' and consultant ensured that she had 'all information about what was happening and why'.

Labour Partner can be present at all times, including examinations. Pain-relieving drugs available when woman feels she needs them, but she is not 'pushed'. Is given choice as to whether fetal monitor should be set up. If drip is set up she is given full explanation. One writer describes ventouse (vacuum) extraction and forceps lift-out with husband present. 'Ironically I had requested a Leboyer delivery but the doctor and midwife did what they could, dimming lights.' Mother can hold her baby while being stitched and father is encouraged to cuddle baby too. Staff 'very friendly', 'supportive', 'informal'.

Postnatal Midwives involved in labour visit woman on postnatal ward. Meals kept warm for breast-feeding mothers (demand feeding is norm), but 'inadequate' for anyone breast-feeding; typical of large institution cuisine. Writers advise food being brought in by visitors. Babies wear their own clothes.

SCBU Very busy. Staff 'took time to teach me basics, like changing a nappy, and generally helped me to feel confident in handling baby'. Advice and help with breast-feeding. 'The sister stayed with me when I breast-fed and very gently assisted both of us, so successfully that on leaving SCBU she was on full-time breast-feeds immediately with no supplements.' Pump available. 'The night staff welcomed me whatever time I turned up.' Mothers have access at any time and fathers can take an active part in caring for their babies.

Suggestions Mothers who want to breast-feed at night should always be woken for feeds when babies are in nursery. Proper drying facilities on postnatal wards.

Harold Wood Hospital, Harold Wood, Romford, Essex

Consultant and ★ GP unit. 'Exceptionally clean'; shortage of staff seems to be a problem here.

Antenatal Head of midwifery services states that 'evening parentcraft sessions for mothers and fathers are well attended . . . A mothercraft/lactation sister sees all mothers when they book giving information on parentcraft classes and advice on infant feeding.'

Waits of up to 2 hours; 'never the same doctor'; 'I asked a doctor if he could note that I didn't want fetal heart monitor during labour. He glared at me and kept repeating, "Most extraordinary!" It was not noted down and made me feel antagonistic to the whole system.' Several writers say there is no opportunity for discussion: 'Doctors give impression that they have no time for conversation.'

Labour GP unit has been incorporated in hospital. If you opt for GP/midwife care you can be delivered by your own community midwife and get to know her during pregnancy. Baby's mucus not routinely suctioned. Syntometrine not always used before delivery of placenta. Baby handed to mother and cord not cut until it stops pulsating. Then to father before being put in cot or returned to mother and put to breast. Couple have about an hour together in delivery room with their baby. Then woman walks, if she wishes, to her bed in ward. 'Birth is something the woman does for herself, not something doctors do to her.'

Postnatal Head of midwifery services states that 'The number of agency nurses used has been greatly reduced, only used for emergencies . . . Babies delivered by forceps or Caesarean section are not taken to SCBU, but remain with their mothers if well . . . The mothercraft/lactation sister visits wards while the mothers are feeding and gives assistance and advice if the mother wishes. Normal deliveries and forceps deliveries are transferred home on sixth day to the care of the community midwife, Caesarean sections on tenth day . . . Providing it has been requested in the antenatal period and that the general practitioner and community midwife are willing to accept the care of the mother arrangements can be made to go home 6 hours after birth . . . Evening visiting time has been lengthened so that the first half-hour can be for husbands enabling them to see their wives alone and to cuddle their baby . . . A postnatal reunion club has been started where mothers and babies meet . . . A twin-club has just commenced.'

Baby is with mother day and night. Atmosphere 'homely', wards 'light'; 'everyone was friendly'; 'You felt you could talk about problems without a feeling of pressure'; 'fabulous'. Father and mother encouraged to caress, talk to, sing to, touch and cuddle their baby. Both parents helped to appreciate baby's psychological needs. Ward opens on to patio where mothers can sit in garden chairs in the sun for coffee and iced drinks. Mother need never lose sight of her baby. If she is sleepy, baby is washed and looked after for her; 'I was soothed and cossetted more than I have ever been in my life.' Staff give mothers their time, sit and talk informally about birth, 'become friends, not fleeting shadows'. Own GP visits. Mutual respect and understanding between GPs and midwives. No noise, women comment on tranquillity. Own children can hold baby when they visit and are encouraged to do so. No rigid rules. Flexible visiting hours. Anybody allowed to visit provided they don't all come at once. Each mother encouraged in any decision she chooses to make concerning her own baby. SNO says: 'It is your baby and your experience. We are privileged to be able to assist you.' Also: 'The staff . . . have job satisfaction and the pleasure of sharing in the uncomplicated "everyday miracle" of birth.' Can book in for 4 days or 1 week; encouraged to stay till you feel ready to leave: 'The best holiday I ever had.'

Suggestions Some writers would have preferred not to have enema. Father should not need to wear sterile garments, especially masks.

Rushgreen Maternity Unit, Rushgreen Road, Romford, Essex   MO

Fairly modern; writers say there is rapid turnover of staff.

Antenatal Long queues, 1–2 hours waiting.

Labour Staff 'friendly'. Routine episiotomies not done but several writers said that if they had been encouraged to relax more in second stage and take their time they think they might not have torn. There is lots of encouragement by midwives to push.

Postnatal Some women suggested that there needed to be more care and attention to individual needs, e.g. a woman whose baby had died was put in a room off corridor where mothers were with their new babies. Her husband was allowed in any time, 'but I was virtually left alone as everyone was too embarrassed to come in to see me'.

No SCBU, babies go to London Hospital if they need special care.

Postnatal check-up Antenatal and postnatal clinics seem to take place at same time in same place. Some writers felt lack of communication. The woman whose baby died was twice asked how many weeks pregnant she was, which she found 'very distressing'.

Suggestions A gentler approach to second stage with no commanded pushing. More understanding of grieving by postnatal staff.

Rugby Hospital, Rugby, Warwickshire   MO

Antenatal Conflicting advice given; 'depressing'; some writers remark on lack of coordination. One writer said she mentioned that if possible she would prefer to have baby without episiotomy, but 'my comments were disregarded' . . . 'I was more or less told that it would be out of my control and what was I doing bothering about things like that anyway?' One writer was induced without any apparent medical reason except that she was 30 and 3 days over her date; she suggests that hospital is 'induction-happy'.

Labour Some writers had been given pethidine without first being asked if they wanted it: 'I would have liked to have been far more aware of the birth of my baby and more in control.' Some women started pushing in good positions in which they were comfortable, e.g. on hands and knees. Commanded pushing seems to be general in the second stage: 'The midwife kept telling me I wasn't working hard enough.' Some writers thought episiotomies were done frequently. They are sometimes done without consulting mother: 'She did one before we realized what was going on and gave no reason.' 'The midwife had given me an episiotomy before my husband or I even realized what was going on and she gave no reason. The baby was coming so quickly and easily that we felt she did it more as a matter of course than as a necessity.' Some women said they were told that there was a limit of 1 hour on pushing. When mothers said they wanted their baby to be put straight on their bodies after birth it was not always done. One writer had waited 8 hours before she was stitched after birth: 'The doctor could not understand the midwife not calling him as he had been on call all night but she hadn't wakened him.'

Postnatal Women are urged to breast-feed but some thought that not enough help was given.

Suggestions Treat mothers as adults and involve them in all discussions and decision-making. Allow a more natural, unforced approach to second stage.

★ St Albans City Hospital, Normandy Road, St Albans, Herts   MO

Old, brick-built and 'unimpressive-looking unit'. But 'small and friendly place' and 'looks far worse from outside than it is inside'.

Antenatal 'Cheerful', 'helpful' staff. Waits not long; 'If it gets long, they apologize and explain.' Booking clinic takes about 1 hour. Subsequent visits quick, some writers were in and out within 15 minutes. Ultrasound has to be done when needed at Watford or Hemel Hempstead. Consultants 'discuss matters and explain things when asked'. Physiotherapy department runs course of eight relaxation classes with details of what to expect at each stage of labour and what you can do to help yourself. 'Very useful.' Partners invited and expected to attend last session where learn how to help. Also parenthood classes, two for women only, discussion with sister about health in pregnancy and feeding the baby. Two for fathers as well, one with birth film, other guided tour of progress rooms, labour rooms and postnatal ward.

Labour Enema usually waived. Mini-shave. Labour/postnatal staff rotate, 'careful and concerned', 'extremely friendly', treat women with 'kindness, sympathy and understanding'. Couple may be in room together for some time and told to call midwife when they need her, who comes immediately. Pethidine and gas and oxygen offered. Midwives *ask* before doing anything. One writer who asked to have pethidine without tranquillizer says she was told by midwife: 'It's you who's having it. You can have what you want.' No epidurals. No pressure to have any pain-relieving drugs. Fetal heart monitor may be used. Episiotomies seem to be done rather readily and it seems that some midwives feel it is disgraceful to have a tear. Baby can be put straight to breast before cord cut. Couple have a few minutes alone with baby. Partner may be asked to go outside while woman is washed and baby may be taken to nursery to be washed and weighed, but then can go with mother to postnatal ward.

Postnatal First 24 hours, meals in bed. Allowed out of bed 6 hours after birth. Unobtrusive help with breast-feeding. Policy of demand-feeding and no timed sucking. Baby can be with mother or in nursery as she wishes. Baby can be in nursery at night and brought to mother for feeds. Most women breast-feed. One writer who was ill with a bad reaction to an epidural had to lie flat for 3 days. She said a nursing auxiliary made toast 'to tempt my appetite' and ward housekeeper phoned kitchen for special sandwiches. Staff 'friendly', 'unofficious' and mother can choose how she wants to care for her baby. Help is there if she needs it; no interference. Paediatrician examines baby day of birth and day before allowed home. 'They made me feel I and my baby were special.'

'Menu has three to four options for each course, chosen day in advance, and with a bit of luck woman will get the meals she ordered.' 'About 2 hours after my baby was born I was required to choose all my meals for the next two days, when I really had not the appetite for anything.' Food is 'fairly good'.

Visiting 7.30–8.30 p.m., afternoon visiting Sunday and Thursday. If husband is shift-worker he can visit in mornings.

SCBU Baby goes to SCBU only if necessary, not routinely after forceps or Caesarean section.

Postnatal check-up Although examination was quick, one mother and baby had to wait nearly three hours before doctor saw baby: 'Everyone seemed to have been given an appointment at the same time . . . about half the waiting my baby was undressed waiting for examination, as requested. We were sitting in a corridor and it was late January.'

Suggestions Midwives should not have to feel it is disgraceful to have small tear. Postnatal check-ups should be done more speedily.

Buchanan, St Leonards-on-Sea, E Sussex   MO

Consultant and GP unit; old cottage hospital with modern additions. Small; friendly atmosphere; staff helpful.

Antenatal Booking interview friendly with chance to ask questions. Low induction rates among GP patients, who sometimes persuade women *not* to be induced. Some women went 3 weeks past their date. Consultant patients seem to be induced when about 10 days 'overdue', according to writers. Six antenatal classes plus two evening sessions for fathers are 'adequate', though one writer says women are treated 'like schoolgirls'. Fathers' participation encouraged.

Labour 'Gloomy' first-stage room. Partner can be with woman, including when she has bath. No enema if woman feels she does not need one; no shave. One woman who went in at night said she was given two Mogadon tablets and told to sleep. She was having strong contractions and felt she did not want them but took them 'in the end, not wanting to cause trouble'. After this her partner was told to go home. He stayed, but was sent to fathers' room in converted lift-shaft. Writers advise fathers to be well prepared with sandwiches. No pressure to have pethidine. Midwives 'attentive' and 'helpful'.

Small stool for partner to sit on may be uncomfortable. He must wear gown and mask. Delivery table high and hard and some writers who wanted to move around found it impossible to get off it. Partner can be present for forceps delivery sometimes. If you ask baby can be delivered on to abdomen before cord is cut. Midwife will help put baby to breast on delivery table. Some GPs do their own deliveries here.

Postnatal Ward 'old and dreary'. Annexe for GP patients 'bright', 'cheerful', 'modern'. Freedom to care for your baby in your own way. Mothers can feed their babies when they like and are left to 'do their own thing'. Ask if you need help. Can change and bath baby when you wish, but help available when required. Nurses 'friendly', 'helpful'. Baby is supposed to be in nursery first night, but if you want your baby to stay with you, say so. Women who asked to be woken during night to feed say that they have seen from chart that baby has been given glucose water during the first night. After this staff wake mother to feed. Generous, 'but exhausting' visiting times 3–5.30 p.m., 6.30–7 p.m., husbands 7–8 p.m., own children allowed and visitors can cuddle baby. Exercise classes taught by physiotherapist who also does antenatal relaxation 3 times a week and everyone 'rounded up' for them. Helpful, but some writers felt they were being 'talked down to'. Food 'good' and 'hot'. Choose from two to three dishes day before. Generous portions. Seven-day stay normal but GP patients may be able to go after 6 days.

Suggestions Brighten up delivery rooms; include pictures. Encourage rooming-in of mother and baby from start. More baths, lavatories and bidets.

Hope Hospital, Salford, Greater Manchester MO

Consultant and GP unit. Very modern, 'rather like a hotel'; writers indicate that there are severe staff shortages.

Antenatal Modern clinic, very busy, long waits of up to 4 hours on hard chairs and a 'feeling of anonymity'; seen 'for 20 seconds'; questions 'fobbed off', 'treated with suspicion' and 'as if stupid'. Woman rarely sees same doctor or midwife twice. Scan at 16 weeks is explained in detail by operator, 'marvellous!' Shared care possible.

★ *Labour: GP unit* Woman is in single room with partner; very friendly atmosphere. She can 'deal with contractions as she feels best'. If she does not wish to have pain-relieving drugs she will not be offered any, though gas and oxygen is in room. In long-drawn-out early labour woman is 'plied with cups of tea and toast' and both she and her partner are provided with meals. Midwives 'treat one as a person' and 'a friend, not a patient'. Transfers to consultant unit are 'handled with kindness'. Can arrange 24-hour discharge.

Labour: consultant unit Full shave is described by some women and enema. Partners welcomed: 'the midwife was very nice to my husband'. Some writers felt midwives were 'offhand . . . treated me like a child'; 'told me "pull yourself together, girl!'' when I cried out with pain'. Father can help with breathing, may be told by midwife to time contractions. He is also encouraged to massage and give the woman drinks. Lights in delivery room very bright; baby may be delivered up on to mother's abdomen. Father can help lift woman's shoulders to push. May be encouraged to be present during forceps delivery. One writer describes a 'very considerate' forceps delivery in which her head was lifted between contractions so she could see baby's head. Mother given baby immediately, can put baby to breast after cord cut and can hold baby during stitching. Couple have time alone with their baby. Then baby to nursery at night and mother to ward. One woman who delivered at 5 a.m. and was taken to a single room on postnatal ward with her husband, who was allowed to stay till 8 a.m., wondered why their baby could not have come too.

Postnatal Huge windows/sunny rooms/'pleasant even in bad, wintry weather'. Baby in nursery first night, but if mother insists she can have baby with her: 'Their attitude seemed to be that he would be my baby *after* I'd had my 6 hours rest, which annoyed me.' Women can demand-feed and are encouraged to feed as long as baby wants. 'Benign neglect' welcomed by experienced mothers, but hard on first-time mothers, some of whom needed more encouragement. 'Many mothers gave up breast-feeding about the fourth day and were given very little support over this difficult time.' Many writers comment that postnatal staff were not as helpful as they might have been and say that it was left to mothers to teach themselves. 'Different answers from different people when I asked for help; I became very confused.' But special praise for one older midwife who helps with breast-feeding, a motherly auxiliary nurse and a young doctor 'who was very kind when I had the weepies'. Writers say babies were offered glucose water after every feed. Women who were engorged found it difficult to get advice. 'Very noisy at night.' 'Nursery door left open with babies screaming and lights left on.' All doors left open and rooms 'very, very hot', 'too hot to sleep'. Food 'awful', 'completely tasteless' but numerous cups of tea very welcome. Far too few bathrooms. One writer said that officially only mother allowed to pick up baby, but this is not enforced. 'Rigid' visiting 3–4 p.m., 7.15–8.15 p.m. Some women said they went home after 5 days extremely tired.

Suggestions Greater alertness to help with breast-feeding problems. Have separate rooms for bottle-feeding and breast-feeding mothers. Turn down heat.

★ Odstock Hospital, Salisbury, Wilts

'Very friendly' atmosphere; DNO writes: 'Efforts are made to ensure that patients are treated with care and concern and that the atmosphere in the unit is happy and friendly.'

Antenatal Clinic; doctors 'kind', 'rushed' but 'will explain things if asked', though 'not much time to talk'. Midwives 'friendly and helpful'. DNO writes that: 'The volume of work . . . does sometimes mean that less time is spent on every individual patient than one would like . . . A senior nurse is specifically delegated to deal with the patients' problems and to listen to their anxieties.' Most women have shared care with own GP and go to hospital for only two visits. Long waits, but pleasant separate rooms and not cubicles; plenty of plants around; chairs haphazardly placed, giving general air of informality; toys for young children. Induction rate under 20% of which more than three quarters are performed by the use of prostaglandin pessaries. Woman who asked to be induced when 2 weeks past EDD was told by obstetrician, 'Oh, I believe in things happening naturally. Let's give it another week.' She said: 'I could have hugged him.'

Labour Writers describe shave/enema. If labour induced and has not started with prostaglandin gel woman may be offered breakfast before going to labour ward for amniotomy and oxytocin drip. One writer was not fed and since she had not eaten since previous day thought this was not good way to start hard work of labour. Yet another took in honey in early first stage and was told she could not eat it: 'The acid would upset your tummy, dear.' Woman can wear her own nightgown, 'so I felt more myself . . . not a product of an institution'. Midwives 'helpful', 'kind', 'superb', 'encouraging', 'understanding' and explained things to couple; 'will provide extra pillows if asked'. Pethidine offered but with discretion; some writers admitted in early labour at night were heavily sedated. Epidural rate 20%. Woman has to be moved to another room for delivery; partner wears gown, overshoes, but no mask; can be present at forceps delivery and suturing. Writers describe lying flat to push. Midwives skilful at not doing episiotomies and avoiding tears; will let cord stop pulsating before cutting if you ask. Father given baby to hold. Midwife will show placenta to parents and explain it. Midwife may do her own stitching. Mother encouraged to put baby to breast after third stage and midwife helps. Father can stay as long as he wishes and couple have long time alone together with their baby; he can go up to postnatal ward with mother.

Postnatal There were not enough descriptions of postnatal care to include this. But it should be mentioned that woman who had baby with multiple handicaps who lived only six days said that this traumatic experience was eased by 'the care and attention of the staff'. Very early discharge possible and a Domino scheme.

Suggestions Some writers felt that staff encouraged epidurals, and questioned the wisdom of this. Felt that sometimes drugs were used in place of emotional support. Women should not have to be moved to another room for deliveries.

Savernake – see Marlborough

Scarborough

Scarborough Hospital, Scarborough, N Yorks   MO

Staff 'super'.

Antenatal Not enough material from women to include this. Though woman to whom induction was proposed (for hypertension) asked to wait another week and said consultant was 'very reasonable about this' and gave her extra time.

Labour Partner sent out while woman has full shave/enema, according to writers. 'Long run from bed to loo.' Midwife runs bath for woman and provides 'pretty blue-and-white flowered gown'. Induction preceded by prostaglandin to soften cervix, ARM next day and syntocin drip. Breakfast provided before induction. Midwife happy to let mother and father listen to fetal heart. But woman who asked midwife what her blood pressure was could not get answer. Several writers said two midwives in attendance most of time and they were not left alone for more than a minute or two. Woman is able to choose her own position but is in bed. Can have as many pillows as she wants and is helped to move when she wishes. Partner may be sent out before amniotomy, electronic monitoring and epidural and only allowed in after. Epidurals are given expertly. Several writers said they felt midwives were 'on their side'. One said consultant remarked that she had been to 'those funny classes' and sister said: 'NCT? They're very good.' In second stage there is no 'shouting or cheer-leading'. Midwife and partner may take turns holding woman up to push. Space is at premium and instrument trolleys, boxes of stores in corridor; delivery room opens off main corridor, so all noise from outside comes in and all noise from inside out; 'visitors have good look in as they pass if door is ajar'. Door is opposite foot of delivery table. Baby handed to mother after delivery but already wrapped: 'A towel with a face inside it was dumped in my arms.' Father can hold baby too. Mother can put baby to breast helped by sister who 'came in at a gallop, hopped up on to the delivery bed and off we went'.

Postnatal Antenatal and postnatal patients in same ward. One writer commented on 'many teenage girls'. Staff keen on breast-feeding and 'very helpful', but 'easy-going'. Water may be given to baby after feeds. Help available with feeding whenever mother wishes. No rules about 2 minutes each side. First 2 days baby is with mother till 10 p.m., except that on main ward babies go to nursery after lunch, but in private room can stay with mother during rest time. First 2 nights mothers given 2 sleeping pills and babies go to nursery. Paediatrician checks baby over at side of mother's bed. Food 'good' with choice, but have to order one day in advance, so first day's food ordered by someone else. On one occasion night nurse went round taking orders for curry and chips at 11.30 p.m. Women may have to queue for bath. Visiting twice a day and children can come at father's visiting time. When full women may be discharged after 48 hours or moved to St Mary's. Forty-eight-hour discharge can be arranged.

SCBU If baby goes to SCBU father can go with baby.

Suggestions Some writers thought that electronic fetal monitoring was used too frequently and would have preferred more choice. More privacy needed. More bathrooms/showers/bidets and lavatories.

Jessop Hospital for Women, Leavygreave Road, Sheffield   M O

Antiquated building with extra bits added, but antenatal clinic more modern and fairly pleasant building. In middle of city. High proportion women doctors. 'Warm, friendly atmosphere.' Large proportion high-risk cases.

Antenatal Staff 'competent, pleasant and efficient' but 'too busy to answer questions'; 1½-hour maximum length of visit reported. Women describe seeing two or three doctors through pregnancy. 'Inconsistent advice' given and 'emotional needs not considered', but 'a caring atmosphere on the whole'. In fact, writers seem best pleased with care when students present because this 'encourages explanations' and under these circumstances writers were more likely to say doctors were 'attentive' and 'willing to explain things in detail'. Shared care possible. Good psychoprophylaxis classes but 'rudimentary' parentcraft classes. Fathers can attend both. Visit to unit and seeing a 'real baby' being bathed.

Labour One couple, arriving at 2.15 a.m., could find no one in reception and waited for 15 minutes before encountering human beings. Flexible approach to what were previously prescribed routines, though partners asked to wait outside for lengthy period in some cases. Electronic monitoring usual. Woman put in side room until she feels ready to go through to delivery suite. Writers say there is lack of continuity in side ward and delivery room, e.g. woman who found her midwife 'courteous' and happy to accept that she wanted to have her baby naturally 'didn't realize that going through [to delivery room] would mean an immediate active management of labour, waters broken, fetal monitor put on my baby's head.' Though individuals are described as 'kindly', 'helpful', 'reassuring', 'extremely helpful in encouraging breathing patterns', and 'lovely midwives explain everything' and treat couple as 'intelligent adults', no single member of staff is likely to stay with woman throughout labour, and writers keenly felt lack of continuity in care, especially those who said partner was allowed in but was kept 'in a corner'. Or where member of staff was 'brusque' and 'offhand' with an anxious husband and 'didn't explain to him what was going on or put him at ease'. This, however, was the exception, and most writers said that 'staff make a great effort at all times to help you understand what is being done and why, and take your views into account'; 'We were kept well informed by the doctor and midwife'; 'Throughout my husband was made to feel that he had a vital part to play.' Some writers comment that since the Jessop is a teaching hospital it attracts keen staff who are likely to be 'pleasant' and 'supportive' and give mothers a feeling of confidence. One writer, who felt she had 'superb midwifery care', said that, 'I was able to make the decisions . . . there was a minimum of interference in the first stage . . . no drugs were offered . . . I was allowed to be in any position I wanted, and didn't feel under any pressure. The midwife shared my delight in being able to cope.' But some midwives were overruled by senior members of staff and mothers then felt 'at sea'. One woman heard a doctor mention 'forceps', who then went out of room. She was 'completely in the dark about what was happening', asked and was told 'fetal distress'. Another said 'no one explained why I needed forceps at the time or later'. Some writers say that only pain relief offered was epidurals. 'We were told that it could not affect contractions when we asked. "Don't be silly!" But they stopped.' (This woman had forceps delivery.) Epidural Caesareans done. Woman is expected to lie down in labour: 'another position would have been more comfortable'. Several writers said that no one explained about artificial rupture of membranes, 'staff were confident in their routines and approachable when I asked questions, but did not give explanations or options unprompted.' In second stage woman may push with legs on partner's and midwife's hips. Other writers said they were 'encouraged to sit up and push the way I had been taught'. And that staff was 'fully cooperative when I said that I was doing NCT breathing'. But here, too, midwives may be overruled by senior members of staff. Eight writers who sent reports said there was time limit of half an hour on pushing. 'Sister kept coming in, telling the midwife my time was up.' 'Doctor has to be called to check everything OK after ½ hour and there is possibility of forceps delivery.' Some writers had been told by staff that 80% of women have episiotomies. Several wondered if their episiotomies were really necessary, though some were told by midwives that they were not done as a matter of course. Baby can be delivered on to mother's abdomen and into her arms. Paediatrician checks baby in front of parents. Then baby put in crib. 'But it would have been nice for my husband to have held her longer. He seemed pinned in at my bed-head.' Writers say partner cannot be present at Caesarean birth: 'A big disappointment'; 'Yet students can crowd in. Why is one father extra so undesirable?' Sister takes baby to father as soon as possible.

Postnatal Good support for breast-feeding, though some writers say nursery nurses are 'didactic' and 'professionally rigid' about baby care. Rooming-in, so writers think it may be best to carry on and do it *your* way, not asking for advice. Then 'you feel it's your baby and you are in charge of it'. Doctors 'very ready to explain things', again especially when students present. Nurses 'patient' and 'kindly' on the whole. Writers criticize 'crazy' routines. Mothers are woken to have temperature taken at 6 a.m. and tea. 'Then nothing happens till breakfast at 8 a.m.' Lot of noise at night. No blinds on windows. 'Constant stream' of doctors, orderlies and cleaners in day, 'making it impossible to catch up on sleep missed at night. Even in mandatory, post-lunch rest hour, and with "Do not disturb" notices on door people come in to empty waste baskets.' Mothers say they got very tired: 'above all I needed sleep and couldn't get it'. 'There were constant interruptions.' 'First someone would come to put the bed rest up, then someone to take the litter bin away.' Writers advise making sure bladder is catheterized after epidural; one had 'hours of pain' before anyone realized what was the matter and had a litre of urine drawn off. Some writers suggested there was 'considerable staff turnover', which in addition to shift changes, some found disorienting. Antenatal teachers come to postnatal wards to get 'consumer reactions' in order to improve their classes.

Food 'quite good for institutional catering'. Order choice day ahead; meal kept warm if you are feeding baby.

Suggestions Some writers felt that position in which midwife and partner were supporting woman's legs was neither comfortable nor most effective for pushing. Suggested exploring different upright postures. Couples should be able to be together for epidural Caesarean. On postnatal ward more explanations needed. Though writers said it was lovely to have baby beside them, some became distressed by noise and bustle, and they felt they needed more time to be quietly alone with their babies.

★ **Netheredge, Osborne Road, Sheffield**   MO

Very modern, 'airy', 'pleasant', 'bright', 'efficient'. Writers say they were treated with 'courtesy and sympathy', though some feel that staff are 'obsessed with routine'. Contrast here between doctor-managed and midwife-managed births. Radical midwives have strong effect on style of midwifery in this hospital.

Antenatal 'Fantastic', 'open and honest'. Those who have had babies there before say whole atmosphere of clinic has changed. Doctors mostly 'kind', 'patient', 'sit down when they talk' though a few are 'abrupt' and seem short of time. Some writers found it difficult to have any discussion about birth but most said there was plenty of chance to ask questions and they were 'treated as adults' and full explanations were given. Waiting not more than about 10 minutes to 1 hour on rush day, though occasionally woman reports much longer wait. Classes, 'both midwife and physio tried to be encouraging', but one writer says 'midwife read from notes and seemed completely out of touch with women, often using difficult medical terms'. Some writers said there was not enough detail in relaxation classes and no help as to 'when' to use 'the breathing'. Emphasis on how doctor always knows best and how wonderful epidurals are. 'They make a big thing about how they have six televisions for watching in labour when they have epidural.' Antenatal ward 'very boring', 'depressing', but staff 'understanding' and 'provided us with much-needed laughs'. Some writers were made anxious for baby by 'sleeping pills and pain-killers offered round' but said that you don't have to accept them. One asks, 'Is there any proof that bed rest reduces high blood pressure? It would appear not, if the women in our ward were anything to go by.' Gentle induction is done by prostaglandin pessaries. One woman who was told she was having a trial of labour did not have the term explained. 'I would have been happier if I'd known exactly what was going on.'

Labour No routine shave, enema or rupture of membranes. Midwives 'cheerful', 'emotionally supportive', extremely kind, 'sensitive' and some 'so good it seems almost a betrayal to criticize the hospital in any way'. Though most women said things like, 'she was keen to help me manage the labour *my* way', there were a few who said midwives seemed to be more interested in the monitor 'than in the lump of meat having a baby. She only came near me to take my blood pressure.' Pleasant first-stage rooms, but not sound proofed; 'I could hear absolutely terrifying screams . . . very frightening for a first-time mum.' Partner encouraged to be present and some husbands were there all the time, but others told to leave when doctor comes in, felt forgotten and had to ask when they can come in. Some writers found this very upsetting. Several writers said they were asked their feelings about fetal monitors and were consulted at every phase of labour. On the other hand, others said that when fetal monitor was free it was used; 'They gave the impression they felt I was being given the best treatment possible by the use of them.' One writer said her husband, a doctor, was not allowed in until she was 'strapped up'; he was also 'kicked out' before epidural set up. Writers tell of being urged to have epidural, and no other pain relief being offered. One woman who did not have epidural was not offered TV, but asked for it anyway and it was brought for her. Some women said they had good, constant support and were not left alone for more than a few minutes. Others were not so fortunate. One woman said she was alone for about an hour with monitor and TV for company. Monitor worked 'erratically'. Another said she was told by obstetrician she would have ARM only to see if labour started, but also was given oxytocin drip without being informed what was in drip and without her consent; 'they just went ahead without asking or even telling me'. Epidurals available 24 hours; 'I wanted to know the facts before making a decision, but too many different doctors were involved. I felt very helpless.' On the other hand, several writers said that no one mentioned drugs at any time. Recent writers say that midwives help with relaxation. Doctors 'pleasant', 'friendly', 'very, very gentle'. No cheer-leading in second stage. Some women have delivered squatting on mattress on floor. Cord is left to stop pulsating before being clamped. Theatre is cream and green, 'clinical, windowless, airless'. Mother can usually hold baby for a while, even if baby goes to SCBU later. After delivery couple have time to be alone together. Several writers said doctor did not speak to them when suturing; 'while sewing me up the doctor chewed gum noisily'.

Postnatal Feeding on demand encouraged and flexible regime. Some writers felt they had inadequate help with breast-feeding. Baby is with mother but is taken to nursery first 3 nights if she asks. There is a valuable discussion session on feeding, encouraging women to share experiences. Midwife who does delivery may visit on postnatal ward and some midwives came several times. Nurses seem to vary; some 'helpful', others 'give no emotional support at all' and woman is left 'to get on with it'. One first-time mother said she felt 'frightened and insecure' because she could not get help. 'Quite honestly, the worst week of my thirty years.' Another writer said, 'a feeling of insecurity and fear was brought about by the uncaring approach of the night staff towards breast-feeding. Most who were trying to instruct me were unmarried women with no sensitivity. A lot of women are put off breast-feeding in the first few days because of these hospital staff.' Very difficult to get sleep on wards. 'I emerged a nervous wreck . . . I wish to wipe this week from my memory.' Women with stitches said beds are too high while lavatories too low; 'we all wondered if a man had designed the maternity ward'. Savlon baths advised and Panadol 'handed out like sweets'. Food 'diabolical'; writers advise getting food sent in. Visiting ½ hour in afternoon, ¾ hour in evening for fathers only.

SCBU Staff 'marvellous'; everything is explained. Women write about 'atmosphere of love'. A mother of handicapped baby who lived 27 hours writes movingly of exceptional emotional support and loving care she and her husband had, 'but they never overwhelmed me with sympathy . . . we were asked our wishes about seeing and holding Elizabeth before she was born. They shared our grief, and wept with us . . . flowers were placed by her cot.' After her death 'we were given a lock of her hair and her arm band. There was good, thorough, down-to-earth follow-up too.'

Suggestions Thought should be given as to how to make labour less mechanized and adjust care to individual needs. More positive understanding of mothers' emotional needs after birth; 'they should remember that hospitals exist for patients, not the other way round'. More pleasant auxiliaries. More extended visiting.

★ Northern General, Sheffield

Antenatal Women's impressions of care vary widely. A few wrote that it was 'dreadful' because they saw different people on different visits and felt there was no continuity. Most of those who wrote, though, said it was 'friendly', 'caring', 'humane' and some said it was 'fantastic'. There is time to talk. Children's play area. Obstetricians reluctant to induce, though some women put pressure on them to do so: 'It was the doctors who hesitated or refused.' Induction rate less than 20%. Good course in psychoprophylactic preparation for childbirth.

Labour SNO writes that there is 'minimal perineal shaving'. No rigid routines. Can wear own nightdress. Partners encouraged. May be sent out during VEs. 'Staff encourage you to play as big a part as possible.' One writer said that she wished more attenton had been paid to her husband's comfort; 'Labour was long but he was not provided with food and there was no possibility of a bed for him.' Midwives 'calm', 'friendly', 'gentle', 'sympathetic' and most go to courses in psychoprophylaxis themselves, so can give good support in labour. Some midwives encourage women to squat in second stage. But some writers criticized 'hearty' approach. Said they were told that second stage was not supposed to go on longer than 1 hour, when forceps would be applied. 'I was disappointed that at no point was I told *not* to push. I was pushing with all my might when the head was born, and therefore tore.' Partner can be present for forceps delivery. Episiotomies not performed routinely. Modified Leboyer birth, but midwife may insist on cutting cord immediately. Lights dimmed. Mother can put baby to breast immediately.

Postnatal Friendly atmosphere. Nurses 'very helpful' with breast-feeding and give good, consistent advice. Babies fed on demand. Baby often in nursery 1–2 nights, but if you want your baby with you, say so. Wards uncomfortably hot in warm weather, but mothers have access to hospital grounds and in heatwave deckchairs provided. One writer said routine enemas were given for constipation. Food 'appalling', 'processed'. Visiting 1 hour in afternoon and 2 hours for fathers only in evenings.

Suggestions Better food; bran cereals for breakfast. Writers who were on ward where bright lights from corridor shine through glass cubicle so that they cannot sleep suggest thick curtains.

★ Shepton Mallet, Somerset   MO

Cottage hospital. GP unit. One writer describes it as 'perfection'.

Antenatal With own GP. Couple invited to hospital together for booking visit, meeting with sister and have guided tour lasting 30 minutes or more.

Labour 'A woman retains her own identity as a person.' Baby delivered up on to mother's abdomen. 'I shall always remember kissing her on the top of her head as soon as she was born . . . we established communication even before the cord was cut.'

Postnatal Staff look after the mother and let her care for the baby as she wishes. Few rules and what there are adapted for each woman. 'I was always asked how I wanted the baby treated.' Visiting at any time: 'I never felt shut away and still felt part of the community.'

★★ Southlands, Upper Shoreham Road, Shoreham-by-Sea, Sussex

Busy general hospital; cramped, but 'relaxed atmosphere'. Modernized 1979. Staff 'friendly', 'sympathetic'.

Antenatal Overcrowded clinic. Different doctor or midwife each time; sometimes difficult to get clear information. Long waits frequent, including trek over to pathology lab for blood tests. Shared care possible. Antenatal classes available include relaxation/breathing/talk on labour/tour round maternity unit, but are 'not as comprehensive as NCT classes'.

Labour Several writers said they had shave and suppositories. Others did not. So if you do not want either or both of these it is worth asking. Woman stays in same room through labour and delivery. 'A relaxed atmosphere is offered.' When labour is induced prostaglandin gel is used. Some writers described this with electronic fetal monitoring. Woman can wear her own nightdress. Staff are 'concerned to make birth a positive experience'. Midwives happy for women to use techniques learned in antenatal classes outside hospital, but need more help to learn how to support them. Pethidine offered (sometimes late in first stage) can be declined. Partner can be present throughout, does not have to wear gown or other special garments. Writers describe delivery as 'informal' and 'cheerful'. Visitors no longer have to pass labour beds on way to and from ward. Midwives skilled at avoiding episiotomies and stitches. Leboyer-style deliveries are now done on request. Baby can be put to breast soon after delivery and woman can walk back from delivery room if she likes.

Postnatal Help given with breast-feeding and nurses are especially good at getting baby 'fixed'. Almost every woman breast-feeds. Writers appreciated being left to do things in their own way, and being able to make their own decisions about feeding. Policy of demand-feeding. Baby is by bed 6 a.m.–10 p.m. Mother keeps record of feeding times. Hospital leaflet states: 'Remember that you and your baby are individuals' and goes on to give guide-lines, not rules. Urges 'leave baby to decide how long to feed'. Guide-lines for nurses state that mothers should be able to breast-feed in delivery room as soon as possible, that mother and baby must not be separated and that both parents should be encouraged to caress the baby. The baby should be unwrapped while feeding and given as long as s/he wishes to suck. 'Once the midwife is satisfied that a mother is managing to breast-feed well, nothing is gained by hovering near her.' Additional bottle-feeds may be suggested if a baby cries a lot, according to writers. Leave a note on cot if you want to be woken at night to breast-feed. Smoking is forbidden on wards; separate room for addicts. Visiting 2.30–3.30 p.m. when own children can come; husband or one special person 6.30–8.30 p.m. Arrangements for visiting at other times can be made with sister. In fact, writers say that fathers come and go at any time and that visiting times are 'relaxed'. Washing and toilet facilities 'not very good'. But DNO writes that now 'there is an adequate supply of hot water for showers, baths and bidets as the system has been overhauled and updated'. Food 'poor'.

SCBU Expressed breast-milk is tube-fed if baby cannot suck. Breast-feeding is encouraged – also frequent visiting by parents.

Suggestions Some writers felt that 'doctors could explain procedures more'. They felt they did not do so because they might have been afraid that to do this would increase anxiety; not so – women want truthful information.

★ **Copthorne, Royal Shrewsbury Hospital,**
Mytton Oak Road, Shrewsbury, Salop

Consultant and GP unit, 'lovely hospital'. SNO writes, 'Shropshire has an integrated midwifery service where midwives work both in the hospital and in the community.'

Sidcup

Antenatal Very busy. Writers describe waiting plus appointment takes 3 hours or more. See different doctors each time. Staff 'polite', 'helpful' . . . 'if you can manage to actually stop one of them'. They are 'piled high with paper work from cleaner to consultant'. All antenatal care shared between consultant and GP for women booked for consultant units. Ultrasound scan. Creche in clinic. Midwives visit patients at least three times during pregnancy. Relaxation and parentcraft classes 'helpful'. Are for couples or women alone. Include prospective adoptive parents. Antenatal ward: 'unstinted devotion to care.'

Labour SNO writes, 'Induction of labour has been reduced considerably . . . with approximately 25% of consultant and less than 20% of total deliveries requiring this.' 'Pleasant', 'friendly' atmosphere. Staff 'kind', 'calm', 'sympathetic', though one writer said she felt that she was expected to 'sit and obey'. Two writers comment on welcome from night porter. Iced water provided. Epidurals available. SNO says that 'less sedation is required' than several years ago. She says, 'Fetal monitoring is undertaken when indicated and when possible this is intermittent rather than continuous . . . the majority of husbands sit with their wife during labour and many stay for delivery, including some instrumental deliveries.' Forceps 11%; vacuum extractions 1%; Caesareans 9%. SNO writes, 'Episiotomy is not a routine procedure and is performed for approximately a third of patients.' Midwives can do their suturing. 'The majority of patients are delivered in a quiet environment . . . babies are put to the breast after delivery whenever possible and may be bathed in the delivery room.' Writers describe babies being delivered on to mother's abdomen.

Postnatal Mother and baby can be transferred following delivery to a GP unit near home. 'Like an excellent hotel'; women say they are given 'encouraging, supportive care', that there is 'friendly efficiency' and that staff show 'kindness and love'. Woman whose baby was of very low birth weight says that nurses and doctors gave her comfort and encouragement and she was grateful for 'loving and thoughtful care'. Both breast- and bottle-feeding on demand with, says SNO, 'flexibility over duration of feeding'. Writers say there is a 'relaxed attitude'. Breast-milk bank and SNO writes, 'We have the invaluable support of the local branch of the National Childbirth Trust in maintaining a good supply . . . Both parents are encouraged to learn to care for their baby either on the ward or in the special care baby unit.' A writer who wanted to keep her twins with her all the time says nurses gave her help and support to do this. Open visiting. SNO writes, 'There are no rigid policies.'

SCBU Members of family may visit baby. Flat attached for use of mother. Midwives visit postnatally up to 28 days after delivery with minimum of three visits between 10 and 28 days.

Queen Mary's, Frognal Avenue, Sidcup, Kent

Very modern; pleasant surroundings; 'general air of friendly efficiency'. Hospital purpose built and senior midwifery officer writes: 'Efforts are made

368

to make it less clinical.' She says that community and hospital services are well integrated.

Antenatal Efficient booking system. At least 50% of mothers have shared care. At hospital clinics 50% are seen by midwives at midwives' clinics, where 'plenty of time for questions'. Parentcraft classes include partners at three evening sessions in early, mid and late pregnancy. Writers say these are useful mainly for 'those with little knowledge of birth process or babies', and that exercises taught are 'inadequate'. Couples encouraged to tour hospital and see a film. One writer commented on 'amateurish presentation' of couples classes. 20% induction rate, for medical reasons or 10 days past EDD. One writer said Saturday is popular day for induction done with Prostin gel.

Labour Women wear their own night clothes. Partner, relative or friend may stay throughout labour. Pethidine may be encouraged, sometimes late in first stage, 'because you still have a long way to go'; epidurals on demand but rate only 6%. Woman may spend much of first stage alone with partner, with midwife popping in occasionally, which some writers liked very much. Midwives 'friendly' and 'talkative'. Writers felt free of pressure or control from midwives, except that some felt they were urged to push too soon and too hard. 34% episiotomies; 18% forceps; 7% Caesareans. 71% are normal deliveries conducted by midwives. Baby put on mother's body immediately and can be put to breast. 'They are trying to make labour a pleasant experience, but are some way behind Leboyer!' says one mother. Mother can cuddle baby while waiting to be stitched; midwife baths baby in front of mother. Senior midwifery officer states, 'siblings are encouraged to visit immediately after delivery'.

Postnatal Between 80% and 90% of all mothers breast-feed; policy of demand-feeding. Staff 'very positive' and 'helpful'. Mothers left to breast-feed in their own way, but 'very helpful' breast feeding counsellor available. Complements given only if weight loss on fourth day is great. But some writers found postnatal care generally 'inflexible': 'Some nurses are schoolmarmy, others very friendly.' Great insistence by day staff on changing baby before feeding. Why? Night staff allow reverse procedure. Baby must be in nursery for afternoon visiting. This meant that one woman's mother who had travelled 250 miles could not see baby close. One writer said there was 'great emphasis on opening bowels. Sennacot is thrust at you if you haven't performed after 2 days.' Auxiliaries 'often give more practical advice than nurses, though all are keen'. 'They are trying to be up to date but have far to go', but there is in general 'pleasant atmosphere'. Senior midwifery officer writes, 'There is always a midwife on duty on each ward 24 hours a day. Patients may sit in the grounds, weather permitting. Tea can be obtained throughout the night from well-sited tea-urns, alleviating the need for early morning wakening by staff. Some visiting time is reserved for father of baby only, for him to handle his child, or one visitor only.' First-time mothers stay 7–10 days; after second and subsequent babies 2–6 days.

SCBU Two-bedded flat attached to unit includes sitting-room/bathroom/kitchen for parents. Babies needing phototherapy are nursed with their mothers on the wards. And 'every effort is made not to separate mother and baby'.

Suggestions Women should not be urged to push baby out as quickly as possible; allow more time in second stage and gentler approach. On postnatal wards all nurses should give encouragement to mothers to work out their own ways instead of following rigid rules. Let babies be with mothers all day, including afternoon visiting. Women who said their babies were given dextrose at nights would have preferred this not to be done. Facilities for washing underclothes.

Solihull Maternity Hospital, Solihull, West Midlands   MO

'Very busy', but 'friendly/helpful'. Consultant unit and GP unit. In latter 6-hour stay is possible.

Antenatal Very long waits, especially for booking appointment and scans. 'After my scan I had to wait for 3 hours before seeing the obstetrician, by which time my blood pressure was soaring.' In this hospital various writers stress it is important to make sure you are not 'overlooked, to speak up, ask questions and not mind about being a "nuisance"'. Inductions appear to be frequent and every writer had her labour accelerated.

Labour Mini-shave and enema. Partner is made to feel welcome. Can stay during stitching. Epidurals on request; are not topped up at end of first stage if possible. Some writers said that labour was accelerated with little explanation: 'Rigged up with contraction and fetal heart monitors it was very uncomfortable. I was unable to change position and the thick rubber belt made me sweat.' Women report malfunctioning monitors and say that staff seemed to rely more on monitor's record of contractions than on what women in labour are experiencing. Midwives skilled at avoiding episiotomy. But some writers say doctors did episiotomies and forceps deliveries without their consent. Some writers described delivering their babies themselves up on to their bodies. One writer says: 'I immediately fed him but had a bit of a tussle with the staff who wanted to cut the cord first.' One writer who was lying flat being stitched wanted to put her baby to the breast, but was given no help and could not manage. Mother has extended time with baby in delivery room and can feed as she wishes. Then is taken to ward with baby.

Postnatal Very busy. A mother sleeping for a few minutes after delivery said she was woken to answer questions about the method of feeding. Writers say not much help is given with breast-feeding. One member of night staff 'forced bottles on breast-feeding mothers the second their baby cried'; if the baby was fed recently said, 'ten sips won't put him off the breast'; one mother, not able to get her baby to latch on for a night feed, told staff nurse of her difficulty; she 'thrust a bottle into my hand and left me to get on with it'. Electric pump available. Rooming-in but baby usually in nursery first night. If you want to keep your baby with you that night, say so; 'You might have to fight for this "privilege".' Topping and tailing demonstration compulsory, which one mother of two small children thought odd; says she was firmly told 'things have changed you know' . . . in 16 months? Some writers say that if you are worried about baby you should know that you can ask to see paediatrician. Apparently you may have to be firm about this. Own children can visit in afternoon only. Writers find this restrictive as husbands at work then. Hospital can arrange 2–3 day discharge, which writers advise.

SCBU Baby who goes to SCBU can be visited by father immediately. Mother can go as often as she wishes.

Suggestions Improve antenatal clinic system. More pillows on labour beds. Staff should have more knowledge and understanding of breast-feeding. Fewer rules and treating mothers as adults would make postnatal stay less 'irksome'. More staff needed.

The Fenwick Hospital, Southampton, Hants   MO

Cottage hospital GP unit. Staffed by many part-timers. Lack of continuity in care.

Antenatal See same midwife throughout pregnancy. Writers appreciated being able to discuss with her how they wanted to have baby.

Labour 'Old-fashioned' care. Woman offered pethidine and gas and oxygen, but encouraged to cope wthout it if she does not want it. Midwives helpful and cooperate in giving the type of birth women want. 'The midwife talked things over with me.' 'She adopted a policy of non-interference.' Women can choose to have no shaving and no artificial rupturing of the membranes. Atmosphere is 'calm', 'quiet': 'I felt like a person whose feelings were taken into account.' Writers speak highly of midwives here and say that they know each woman's wishes and try to meet them in labour: 'She was an experienced, competent midwife, well-versed in the traditional arts.' Woman can choose her own comfortable position.

Postnatal Writers advise being very definite about what you want. Staff/patient ratio good, and there is time to help and advise. Some writers say they were woken on 'rigid four-hourly schedule to feed' though they said they were demand-feeding: 'I don't believe that all the babies in the nursery woke at 2 a.m. and 6 a.m. and not in between.' Two women in a shared bedroom said that they both wanted their babies with them all the time, but they were 'whisked away at night regardless'. Food varies 'medium to good, depending on cook of day'. Get milk and other protein foods brought in if breast-feeding. Writers advise early discharge; though they were warned that they would regret it, they didn't. Six-hour discharge can be arranged.

Southampton

Princess Anne, Southampton MO

Opened October 1981. Large, 'characterless' teaching hospital, 'well organized despite its enormity' and 'pleasant enough'; very busy.

Antenatal Shared care can be arranged, but even so women have to go to hospital clinic six times: 'appalling'. New clinic is on outskirts of town. Old clinic was central, close to where members of immigrant community live. Some concern that those most at risk in pregnancy may not attend new one. Reception and nursing staff 'friendly and thoughtful'. Booking visit involves lengthy wait – up to 3 hours. Waiting area hot/crowded. But care is 'efficient' and 'clinical atmosphere is reduced to minimum'. Writers say they were seen by different doctor at almost every visit: 'May see same doctor twice if lucky – disconcerting.' Many writers said they were told at clinic that most people had episiotomies, 'I mentioned that I did not want an episiotomy. They would not write my request on my notes.' 'During pre-labour visit to maternity unit I asked the sister who was showing us round what the hospital policy on episiotomies was. She made it clear that they were performed routinely. I put to her that I did not want to have one unless absolutely necessary, to which she patronizingly replied, "Well you can always ask, dear. It will depend who is in charge."' Several women said that doctors were approachable: 'A sympathetic doctor answered all my questions.' One writer who said she had a lot of questions said all were answered and staff were 'kind, helpful and informative'. Several women whose labours were induced for post-maturity said they were told afterwards: 'We needn't have induced you.' One writer went 3 weeks past EDD and cervix was then 'swept' by consultant. Antenatal classes 'worth attending'. Fathers' night. One father said 'training with gas and air machine beforehand would be beneficial', and recommends that anyone offered a 'go' should accept opportunity.

Labour No enema or suppositories but mini-shave. Partner there throughout. One writer, whose waters went before she was admitted, says she was 'told to walk about hospital in hope that labour would start'. Medical students may be present, with couple's consent: 'Two medical students actively *helped*.' Writers who did not have students with them sometimes felt that shortage of staff led to 'lack of attention'. 'Left alone without any further examination for about 5 hours.' (This writer was the one whose membranes had ruptured and was in early labour.) But 'once the midwife took over I felt I was in capable hands . . . care was good and sensitive'. 'Midwife was encouraging and took time to explain to me what was happening.' Writers praise 'relaxed attitude'. Some felt they could have done with more help with breathing: 'They seemed more concerned with delivery of baby than with my well-being.' One woman who felt she had been left too long without guidance said she panicked and there was no reassurance. Pain-relieving drugs offered 'but not forced'; epidurals available. One husband said, 'I found it worth while watching the gauge on the gas bottle as nobody else was and once they had taken it away for replacement I had to ask the porter to bring another bottle in immediately, otherwise he had been planning to collect all the empties before he replaced ours, and I am sure M. would have been left without any pain relief for a considerable time at the worst part of her labour.' Some writers said they were never shown how to use mask correctly. No drinks allowed during labour, which distressed some women. It seems that midwives were not always aware of progress of labour. Several writers were told they 'had a long way to go', when they were on the point of delivering.

Second stage: delivery rooms austere; 'I had an excellent midwife who encouraged and urged me and guided me throughout. I was told to push with contractions as long as contractions lasted.' A few writers say they were coaxed to push hard. Others said they were allowed to go at their own pace and do 'their own thing'. Some wished they had not been urged to push so hard, often up to delivery, as they had tears which they think could have been avoided, sometimes extending episiotomies already made: 'It would have been better if she had eased the head out more slowly.' Most writers had episiotomies. 'I was not consulted. Midwife assumed I would need one and had anaesthetic ready.' Writers describe pushing on side, semi-sitting, holding on to thighs and with feet on hips of midwives on either side. 'During second stage the doctor suddenly asked me how tall I was and on hearing 5 ft 2 immediately reached for the cutting implement.' Woman who had a breech baby said: 'There were too many people around. I began to feel confused. Too many chefs.' Some writers described how they were told to put their hands down before delivery and feel the baby's head being born. One writer who asked to have Leboyer-style delivery was told she could have it but didn't. Baby's mucus was sucked out before being handed to her husband. Another was told baby would be too cold if not wrapped immediately and must be checked over before being handed to her. But baby is given to mother and can suckle on delivery table; midwife may help but is sometimes 'too busy'. 'My baby was born crying and cried for 35 minutes before anyone thought of putting it to the breast. Mothers should proceed with feeding and not rely on the hospital staff.'

Postnatal 'I kept pestering the staff to let me have the baby for her to try sucking, but I was not allowed to hold her (other than for 5 minutes or so initially) until she was given to me to feed after about 2½ hours.' Policy of breast-feeding on demand. Conflicting advice given. Student midwives particularly helpful with breast-feeding. Writers said they had to ask for help they needed or they did not get it. 'Women are left very much to their own devices.' Others appreciated 'unfailing kindness and understanding of all staff'. Baby is allowed to suck as long as s/he wants. Postnatal wards 'short staffed and busy'. And among things writers did not like were: 'Being told something would take place and then it never did'; 'Asking for assistance or a question, being told someone would be back in a minute and they never came'; 'Being treated as a "body" rather than a person'; 'Being told nothing whatsoever and offered no assistance unless particularly requested'; 'The general feeling that everyone was too busy to really bother and consequently one felt a terrible nuisance whenever one asked for anything.' Rooming-in, which many writers liked but others said that this made sleep impossible: 'It was noisy at night, it was difficult even to doze.' One writer, giving overview on care, said it was 'bewildering and Kafkaesque'. 'There always seemed to be plenty of nurses around, but they were involved with *all* the patients with the result that none of them knew anyone well, or the results of tests, or when they could be discharged.' Wonderful bidets. Rubber rings and lots of pillows provided for women with stitches.

Food 'very good with range of choices' ordered in advance, so you start off with whatever person in bed before you has ordered. Writers advise having prunes and bran brought in.

Can be transferred to local GP unit on third day. Arrangements can also be made for early discharge home. But there are sometimes long waits for ambulances. One woman who had a 2-hour labour, then 'waited 2 hours to be stitched', was taken at last to a ward and given permission to leave that morning but 'had to wait till evening for an ambulance to take me home'.

Suggestions More continuity of care between antenatal clinic and delivery suite. Some doctors should be more ready to share information with mothers. A father who says he was 'disconcerted soon after our arrival to hear the midwife ask how she could be expected to cope with so much all on her own' suggests that more trained midwives are needed. Some writers who said they were given conflicting information and advice by different members of staff suggest that better communication and coordination between staff is needed. One suggests that an attempt could be made in interior decoration to counter immediate impressions of 'endless corridors'. Replacement gas and oxygen should be immediately available when one has run out. Two writers describe problems with thermostat on air-conditioner/heater in delivery room – it was either 'cold' or 'tiny, hot and stuffy . . . couldn't breathe'. (Presumably this has been remedied by now.) Skin contact between mother and baby immediately after delivery and woman should be able to plan ahead with her midwife so that she knows this will be done.

Airedale Hospital, Steeton, Nr Keighley, W Yorks   MO

'Modern, bright, cheerful.'

Antenatal Clinic arranged so that one midwife does weighing and urine tests and women get to know her. Appointment system seems to work. No long waits. 'Longest was about 15 minutes.' One writer says, 'There seems to be no provision for ambulances to take pregnant women to the clinic . . . I had to take two buses or go by taxi . . . the hospital is in a rural area and people travel long distances to get to it.' (This woman had very high blood pressure.) Though questions are not encouraged in clinic, they are answered. Women are encouraged to breast-feed. Those having shared care visit hospital only about five times. Relaxation classes include partners at one class only, but are 'helpful'.

Labour Writers say preparation includes full shave/enema, 'but midwife good at stopping during contractions to let me breathe'. Some women queried full shave and were told it was hospital routine. It is taken for granted that partner is there and he is not asked to leave at all. Pethidine and Entonox available but not 'pushed'. 'The doctor suggested a drip to speed things up but didn't object when we said we would wait a bit and see how things went.' (This doctor made this suggestion after only two hours of labour.) One writer said doctor wanted to use vacuum extractor at second stage, though everything was going well: 'Even with my lack of experience I felt this wasn't necessary.' Baby was born 5 minutes later. Some writers heard discussion about episiotomy, doctor wanting to do one, but midwives 'much more relaxed' about it. Baby may be put in cot on other side of room and not given to mother. Writers describe their husbands holding the baby while they were being stitched. Mother and baby moved to ward together.

Postnatal Staff 'very kind' but 'different opinions on almost everything, how much water, dextrose, artificial milk baby should have until established on breast'. Most writers stayed 6 days.

Suggestions Lavatory for partners near labour ward. More consistency in advice about breast-feeding.

★★ Steppinghill, Stockport, Cheshire   MO

Consultant unit and GP unit. Modern, well-decorated building, wards bright and cheerful. 'Feels small, friendly and informal', 'fresh and cosy'. Cleanly designed, well run, 'emphasis on retaining mother's individuality and self-esteem'.

Antenatal Well staffed. 'Most caring'; 'efficient', 'friendly'; 'staff remember your name from previous visits'. But 'booby prizes to unpleasant receptionist and nurse with a voice like a BR announcer who reads out names on the run'. Midwives' clinic has no long waits. Longest reported was 20 minutes!' Antenatal care couldn't be better.' Staff are 'friendly and helpful'/'considerate'; 'nothing was too much trouble for anyone'. Women say they have plenty of opportunity to ask questions. Nurses 'eager to mind tots while mums see doctor'. Room with lots of toys for small children adjoining waiting-room: 'nothing is hurried' and midwives 'reassuring'; 'very keen to preserve modesty'. 'Good atmosphere among staff promotes confidence.' Doctors' clinic 'slightly more formal'; in fact, one writer speaks of it as 'conveyor belt'. It may take 1–1¾ hours to get through. Cubicle bench is 'designed for person with 6-inch-long bone in thigh and 2 ft-long bones in lower leg'. 'Doctors should talk *to* mums directly, rather than about them and baby to nurses.' There are three consultants here and women may see as many as five different doctors throughout antenatal period. One writer felt that some doctors had 'ignored' her as a person. Private tour of the hospital wards can be arranged; ask parentcraft sister.

375

Labour Warm welcome given. Routine shave/enema according to writers. Partner welcome and can stay whole time. Is given plenty of tea. Is not asked to leave when drugs given or for examination. Continuity of care and same midwife stays with woman as long as possible. Midwives are 'helpful', 'considerate', 'reassuring' and 'nothing seemed too much bother'; 'I got the feeling that many midwives were mothers themselves.' Pethidine offered, but not in high enough dose to knock woman out; also gas and oxygen. Drugs 'not pushed', but available if wanted. Electronic fetal monitoring may be used. Many writers described acceleration of labour, but in each case it seemed to be carefully controlled. No epidurals given. Bright, individual first-stage room with own lavatory. Writers said they were offered tea or soup if labour was not advanced. Woman is moved to different room for delivery apparently. In delivery she can choose between lying down or being propped up. Some women would have liked more choice of position, but 'I was made as comfortable as possible'. Partner wears gown and overshoes. Second stage is 'calm' and 'unhurried'. Woman who had elective Caesarean said she wished she had chance the night before operation to talk to someone who had had one. Everyone in theatre and anaesthetist were 'reassuring' and 'charming'. After delivery midwife helps woman put baby to breast. Ask for this to be put in your notes if you want to be sure it is done. Stitching is 'very gentle' and while woman is stitched baby may be wrapped and handed to father. 'Nothing is rushed.' Both parents have time alone together with baby. One father said doctor first congratulated him and then carefully explained episiotomy. Baby is by mother's side from delivery till she arrives on ward.

Postnatal 'Fantastic'; light airy rooms, but tend to be too hot. Woman who had emergency section with general anaesthesia wrote, 'Nurse from special care came up to see me when I was coming round properly to tell me all about baby and brought me a photograph.' Policy of demand-feeding and staff very keen on breast-feeding. 'They spent ages getting breast-feeding established with those mothers who were keen.' Though there may be some conflict between midwives and nursery nurses 'who like to give the baby a bottle'. Women stay in bed 6–12 hours after delivery. Baby normally in nursery first night and then with mother at night. Tea is served: she gets up to wash and baby is brought to her. 'Plenty of help always available through day' from 'warm', 'supportive', 'encouraging', 'friendly' staff. Wonderful 'friendliness and informality'; 'more like hotel than hospital'. Writers say also that cleaners and auxiliaries 'could not do enough for you': cleaning could be more thorough: 'shower room filthy, all slimy and bloody'. Six a.m. start each morning which some writers found tiring after noisy nights. Paediatricians 'a bit grunty' and 'not forthcoming'.

Food 'adequate', but 'often cold' and 'people come to collect tray' before mothers have had time to eat: 'If you are wise have salad and icecream'. Tea served in plastic mugs. Choice of 3–4 main courses.

Visiting very informal and flexible: 'Don't need to watch clock.' Writers say postnatal wards are too hot.

SCBU Staff 'exceptional'. 'They were unbelievable.' Lots of help and advice. Breast-feeding greatly encouraged and help given when asked, though some writers said advice was conflicting. Mother can visit SCBU whenever she likes: 'I used to just sit there by him for hours.'

Suggestions Paperback library for antenatal ward. Women are extremely bored there.

★ Mary Stevens Maternity Home,
Oldswinford, Stourbridge, West Midlands   MO

Small, relaxed GP unit in quiet grounds. Interior 'bright and warm'. All facilities for mothers on ground level. Wards open on to gardens with benches to sit on in warm weather. Threatened with closure.

Antenatal Care with own GP except for two visits, one booking clinic at about 3 months and again at 32 weeks. Chance to talk to midwives, who are 'friendly and willing to answer questions'. No long queues and appointment times kept. Can have tour of Home. In good weather women sit outside in lovely grounds, 'I can't think of a more pleasant and relaxing place.'

Labour Mini-shave rather than full shave/enema if woman asks for it. Midwives 'relaxed', 'pleasant', 'gentle', 'helpful', and understand breathing techniques learnt in classes. Partner welcome and is fully involved. Woman can wear own nightdress. Amniotomy may be done. Pethidine and gas and oxygen offered, 'but neither is pressed on you'. Midwives interrupt examination while woman is having contractions. Must be moved to another room for delivery, but this room has 'a relaxed feel'. No arbitrary time limit on pushing. Midwives often 'encouraging' and supportive, let woman take things at her own pace, though some are criticized for being 'abrupt and offhand'. Baby handed to mother immediately and she can put it to breast if she wishes. 'No rush to get father out of way', but when mother goes to ward baby may go to nursery and some writers lay awake all night longing for their babies.

Postnatal 'Pleasant', 'relaxed', 'homely'. Good breast-feeding support from midwives and determined mothers can now demand-feed 'within reason' (?) but not at meal and visiting times. Baby with mother 10 a.m. to 10 p.m. except when ward cleaned and during mother's rest time. If mother wants to feed baby during night she can be fetched to nursery if she makes it *very* clear that this is what she wants, but expressed breast milk collected during the day is sometimes fed to baby at night if mother does not want to wake. Baby is weighed on fifth day, but mothers do not feel under pressure about weight gains. They say they get 'sympathetic care', 'friendly guidance' and that nurses are 'helpful', 'kind', 'efficient' and on hand at feed times to answer questions and give advice. 'The Ovaltine, which arrives just when it is needed, is out of this world!' Breakfast and lunch of high standard and plenty of food, except tea-time, when some writers said they could have eaten more.

Stroud

Suggestions At the moment nurses have to do ward clerk work and act as telephonists and receptionists as well as looking after mother and baby. Writer suggests clerical staff should be hired to take over this work. Baby should be able to stay with mother inside ward first night.

Stroud Hospital, Stroud, Glos   HO

GP unit. Nursing officer writes, 'The patients are very susceptible to the atmosphere created by staff, and much appreciate the happy relationships staff have with one another.'

Antenatal First-time mothers between 17 and 30, those having their second, third or fourth babies under 35 and women who have had previous low forceps are booked here. Surgical inductions (i.e. without syntocinon infusion) 15%.

Labour Nursing officer writes, 'Minimal shaving is now done, or not at all if the patient so requests. Partner welcome. 60% of women receive pethidine; 5% forceps deliveries; 55% episiotomies. Epidurals not done here. Baby is delivered into mother's arms and mother herself is allowed to discover the sex. 'Putting baby to suckle is now routine procedure.' Baby transported to ward in mother's arms.

Postnatal Mother gets up after 6 hours. Rooming-in of babies practised. Demand-feeding; nursing officer says, 'the mother is called to feed baby if necessary during the night'. 72% of babies are breast-fed on discharge. Mothers not wakened till 6 a.m. (antenatal rest patients not till 7 a.m.) Mothers have a choice, with their doctor's and midwife's approval, of 24 hours'/48 hours'/5 days' or 10 days' stay. Choice of food and menus filled in daily.

Good Hope Hospital, Sutton Coldfield, W Midlands   MO

Antenatal classes geared to couples.

Labour Women say care is good and there is a full explanation of what is happening. Partner can be present and is 'made to feel very welcome'. Some writers said they found it offputting to hear other women screaming down corridor.

Postnatal Not enough information from mothers to warrant including it.

SCBU One woman wrote, 'I had no opportunity to breast-feed or to put her to the breast until the third day. I felt the early stages of mother–baby relationship very strained as there was constantly someone else in the room. I felt my baby had already been labelled HOSPITAL PROPERTY. One nurse went to put her back in the incubator but before she did held her face close to mine and said "Give mummy a kiss before she goes." It sounds soft and sentimental but those few kind words brightened up a very weepy day!'

378

Suggestions Mothers-to-be should be treated like capable human beings. Labour rooms should be soundproofed.

Princess Margaret, Okus Road, Swindon, Wilts

Consultant unit which takes medical students seconded from St Mary's Hospital, London, and University Hospital, Southampton. DNO writes, 'Aim of all staff is to fulfil the expectations of the patients.'

Antenatal Induction rate now less than 20% and aim is to reduce it to 10–14%.

Labour DNO writes, 'The husband or another person of the patient's choice is encouraged to stay with her during labour and delivery. It is our intention that patients are not left unaccompanied during labour, but in times of busyness this may happen . . . Shaving is not routine. Patients are not given pethidine or any other analgesia against their wishes. 11% epidurals. She says, 'Ward is attractive and women can walk about and are encouraged to be as active as they wish.' Have to be transferred to another room for delivery. Artificial rupture of membranes may be done. 40% of all women have electronic monitoring. 'Continuous fetal monitoring applies only to high-risk patients. Patient's wishes are taken into consideration as far as possible and the aim is that all deliveries are conducted in a relaxed atmosphere.' Midwives keen for women to deliver in alternative positions.

Postnatal Policy of rooming-in. If you wish to have your baby at bedside and feed at night discuss this with staff. DNO writes that 'feeding is on demand', and 'whenever possible complementary feeds are from the human milk bank.' 'Friendly' wards.

Visiting 3–5.15 p.m. and 6.15–8 p.m. and at other times by arrangement with ward sister. 7.15–8 p.m. is for fathers or next of kin. Own children can visit every day.

SCBU DNO writes that 'Parents are encouraged to visit frequently and help with care of their baby.'

Musgrove Park, Taunton, Somerset

Large proportion of high-risk patients. Though old army camp, warm and welcoming.

Antenatal Friendly care. 'Midwifery tutor chatted to us, noted our interest in NCT, Leboyer, etc. Scans done. 16% inductions. Antenatal ward – women in for long periods can go home for weekends or for special evenings.

Labour Some writers described enema. Most couples were able to be together all the time. Most midwives 'helpful', 'encouraging', though one writer found her midwife 'lacking in sympathy' and another, whose baby was posterior, said midwives 'evasive' and refused to give her accurate information about her baby's position. Other writers said they were able to obtain detailed information. One who was having her baby 5 weeks early wrote 'everything was explained all the way'. Women who are having a possibly complicated labour or with a baby at risk felt very well cared for. 'During the 2 nights and days that my husband was at the hospital he was given a bed and meals and always allowed to be present. Doctors discussed my condition with him and encouraged me to have a natural birth rather than a Caesarean.' 'My GP popped in frequently through labour and the next couple of days, which I found helpful.' (Such cooperation between GPs and hospital obstetricians is unusual.) Women are asked if they will agree to continuous electronic monitoring. Many had intravenous drip and said it was difficult to change position though in early part of first stage they were encouraged to walk around in day room. They seemed to be allowed no food, even in early phases. SNO writes that 'patients wear their own night clothes, husbands stay, and are very welcome, wearing their own clothes and staying for most procedures including forceps and vaginal examination but not for Caesarean sections.' Epidurals are 'available for selected cases, mainly for medical reasons', and that 'mothers are not given sedation unless requested'. Some writers said there were not enough pillows for backs, though SNO says that 'there are foam wedges if required'. Some writers felt very uncomfortable pushing with legs raised in stirrups; 'I wondered if severe muscle strain in my thighs when pushing might have been less severe without stirrups'. Room is not sound-proofed. Women were expected to push lying flat on their backs and found this difficult. Mothers said they were very uncomfortable with their legs raised on two people's hips even though this position was 'insisted on'. A writer who had a planned Caesarean section under general anaesthetic with a breech baby wished that her husband, rather than the nursing staff, could have told her that their baby had been born; would have liked epidural and her husband present to share at the moment of birth. Writers who were delivered by midwives usually said they did not feel under any pressure to 'perform' and could go at their own pace in their own way; 'they let me do as I liked and just encouraged me'; 'I could relax as I felt right, and could see the baby being born.' 'Midwives were familiar with NCT methods and sympathetic and helpful.' 'Tried to let you do it how you wanted and the midwife told me to put my hands down and deliver his head myself, and she helped him up on to my tummy still all wet and warm and they cleaned his nose while he laid there. He opened his eyes and looked straight at me without crying.' But some women said they were told there was a time limit of 1 hour on pushing. Some said episiotomy was done without asking them or telling them it was about to be performed. Most, however, said they had an opportunity to discuss it and were given a choice as to whether or not to have one. This was much appreciated. One woman wrote, 'I am still unsure whether the fact that the night shift was over in 8 minutes had anything to do with my having an episiotomy.' One woman who had a Syntocinon drip said that midwife tried to get her to push before she was sufficiently dilated and then 'because of the drip I couldn't stop pushing as the baby was born' so that this put a lot of strain on the perineum. SNO says that episiotomy 'is never done as a routine, only at a midwife's discretion'. Forceps deliveries 10%; vacuum extractions occasionally done; Caesarean sections 15%. SNO writes 'Babies delivered normally and by forceps are delivered on to the abdomen and the baby is put to the breast as soon as practical in the delivery room.'

Postnatal Breast-feeding on demand encouraged. SNO says that hospital 'is now more understanding towards the different views of the individual'.

Suggestions More midwifery staff. Some writers suggested that doctors should listen more to way midwives wanted to do things. Food needs improving.

Tavistock Maternity Home, Tavistock, S Devon   HO

GP unit about 15 miles north of Plymouth. DNO writes, 'The national policy is to encourage all expectant mothers to come into hospital to have their babies delivered under the care of a consultant.' She adds 'The Flying Squad can be rapidly assembled to answer obstetric distress calls, which are infrequent nowadays.'

Labour Midwives do all deliveries here. No inductions, no ARMs in labour and no forceps deliveries.

Postnatal Mothers are transferred here from Freedom Fields, Plymouth, for postnatal care.

Wrekin, Wellington, Telford, Salop   MO

Small GP cottage hospital; 'relaxed feel about it'.

Antenatal Woman attends her own GP for antenatal care and has one check-up at hospital. Relaxation and parentcraft classes available.

Labour Admission procedures 'relaxed and informal'; partial shave/suppository. Staff 'cheerful', 'lovely'. 'Explain everything' and 'all my questions were answered'. One writer says her midwife was 'smashing' and student midwife 'delightful'. Labour room small but not austere and woman may be delivered there rather than being moved to delivery room with hard, high bed. Partner can stay throughout and is encouraged to participate. Drugs 'not pushed'. Baby put immediately on mother's body and staff 'tactfully leave' so that father, mother and baby can have time together, before taking baby away to be cleaned up.

Postnatal Generally pleasant atmosphere. Plenty of help with feeding when wanted, but 'independence encouraged'. Unfortunately much conflicting advice about how to do things, 'which eventually forces you to go your own way'. Some mothers have been able to breast-feed at night if they were keen to do so, but some members of staff 'disapprove strongly'. Father welcome and can help bath baby. GP visits regularly.

Suggestions More lavatories needed and showers which don't break down so often.

Mayday, Mayday Road, Thornton Heath, Surrey   MO

Staff 'charming', 'very helpful', 'approachable consultants'.

Antenatal Waits may be 2 hours or more. Staff 'very cheerful', 'friendly', 'helpful', 'pleasant'. Questions answered 'in straightforward way'. Scan 'clearly explained'. Some writers thought they had 'perfunctory examination'. Writers said they were seen by different doctors each time. Antenatal classes: emphasis is 'on explaining hospital routine'. Some writers thought that atmosphere 'not very friendly'. 'Staff apologetic that Mayday has only three fetal monitors and not everyone can have an epidural.' Mothers encouraged to visit labour and postnatal wards before admission. Useful tour. 'Midwife who showed us round was prepared to answer a lot of questions.' Large number of writers had been induced. One woman's consultant proposed induction when she was 1 day overdue and with no other indications.

Labour Partner made welcome but may be asked to leave during admission procedures. Some writers said they had full shave, some with blunt razor. Staff are 'uninformative when asked about induction procedures' after admission. Epidurals available and most women requesting one get it. Woman with planned Caesarean would have preferred epidural but did not have option. Electronic monitoring used; one writer says it was put on but staff did not switch machine on for 1½ hours (1979). Amniotomy seemed to be frequent. Pethidine offered. 'Midwives seemed to find the idea of natural childbirth hilarious . . . persisted in talking to me through contractions.' One writer who said she did not want electronic fetal monitoring was told she must have it because midwife was distracted by another patient's alarm clock when trying to listen to baby's heartbeats. Writers seemed much less happy with care in labour than in antenatal clinic, which is unusual. Some said midwives were 'very pleasant' but others that they had 'offhand' midwives. One writer said that her midwife was 'obviously terrified' of senior midwife who was 'bossy, uncommunicative and short-tempered to the point of rudeness'. A father says midwife would not answer his questions and that 'no one smiled or looked at me during entire labour and delivery'. Delivery table is in middle of room with no back rest. A mother who wanted to squat was told she could not and others who asked to be propped up said they were told this was not possible. One writer said she enjoyed pushing and was shouting to her husband, but was told 'sharply' to stop. When she touched her baby's head 'I got the worst ticking off of all'. Most writers had had episiotomies. Very helpful woman doctor is praised. Baby may be laid on mother's abdomen. Can be put to breast soon after birth, but one writer said, 'I was allowed to suckle her, but this request was granted as if it were an enormous favour. One minute each side, no more.' Others said 'I had my baby, put him on to the breast and almost immediately he was taken away.' Yet another: 'when I tried a surreptitious suckle later on in delivery room baby was snatched away from me and put in a cot on the other side of the room'. Couple may have a chance for extended time alone together afterwards; '2 blissful hours', but if somebody else has to be moved into room this may be much curtailed. Some fathers helped wash their babies after delivery. Some husbands went to ward with mother and baby. After Caesarean, baby is taken to ward with mother if all is well. Birth chair available.

Postnatal Nurses 'kind and helpful with babies'. Baby goes to nursery first night and is with mother as soon as she feels she can cope after that. Stays with mother throughout the day. 'Relaxed atmosphere.' Some writers said staff took some convincing that they really wanted babies with them non-stop. Demand-feeding encouraged and 'usually someone to help'. Some writers found it difficult to make sure that their babies were not given artificial milk or water. Baby waking on first night is brought to mother as soon as wakes; 'Baby was brought to me at 3.30 a.m. and I asked if she could be left beside me after I had fed her, as I thought I would sleep better with her there.' This was allowed. Women said they found it very difficult to sleep in hospital because of general disturbance, noise and lights and 'ridiculous early waking system'. 'I had about 7 hours sleep in 6 days, in all.' One woman said she had fed baby and had 1½ hours sleep, and was then woken to have temperature taken at 6 a.m. Complaints of not being given enough to drink; given 'tiny glass of orange squash after I had been stitched. I needed at least a litre of water when I was eventually moved to ward 3 hours later.' Nurses are 'friendly' and 'unobtrusive'.

Food 'not too good'; 'had worse'. But one woman thought it was 'appalling'; 'my first meal was baked beans, tinned tomatoes, boiled potatoes and jelly and ice cream' (vegetarian). One woman said she was not given anything to eat until 7 hours after her baby was born and became 'quite desperately hungry'. Another who said she thought the food was 'dreadful', said it was diet of 'fried potatoes, greasy meat, soggy vegetables, stodgy puddings' which was unsuitable for nursing mothers. Frequently entire meals were sent away by mothers who said they were 'hungry'. This, writer suggests, is 'appalling waste'. Writers suggest taking in bran, 'all need laxatives every day'.

Suggestions Writer who says she was shaved when fully dilated 'when only half on bed in first-stage room' suggests that shaving is unnecessary. Writer who says midwife 'kept shouting at me as if I were dead or drugged "PUSH! PUSH!"' suggests that whole approach to second stage should be 'gentler and less rushed'. Mothers should always be examined before being encouraged to push. Writer who said she felt she was treated 'like half-wit' suggests that staff should treat patients as adults. Improve food. Offer something to eat after delivery if mother wants it.

Torbay, Torquay, Devon MO

Writers say they are usually treated as 'an intelligent human being'.

Antenatal Writers say no long waits. See same midwife each week. Prostaglandin gel used for induction, and if nothing has happened waters broken following morning. Partner can come in after that and drip then inserted. Writers say inductions take place on antenatal ward with delivery rooms on either side of corridor off main ward; 'I became anxious and upset listening to the shouts and moans of pain . . . I kept thinking "I have to go through with it the following day."'

Labour No enema or shave. Lots of encouragement given by midwives. Partners can stay throughout examinations and for forceps delivery. Some women said they have been given pethidine without being examined beforehand, and as a result have received it late in labour. One writer being electronically monitored says she was not checked by human being for 2 hours, and only then by auxiliary nurse who made sure that drip and monitor were working correctly. Most writers were not asked to push in second stage any more than they felt they wanted to, but a few said that they were commanded to push and midwife 'tried to make me push harder and longer than I sometimes wanted to'. Generally midwife tells mother to work with contractions. Baby can be put to breast immediately after birth. Baby washed in front of parents.

Postnatal Very busy postnatal wards; 'it was more like an army camp than a mother and baby unit'. Some writers would have appreciated more help. On day of birth one woman says nurse put baby to breast and told her to feed for 5 minutes, and went off and returned after 15 minutes, 'presuming everything was alright', and then took baby away again for night. Some writers had little help with sore nipples. For first 3 days baby is with mother during day, but taken away at night. Auxiliary nurses are 'kind'. Some writers said it was difficult to get information or guidance. Some staff were 'domineering', 'reduce inexperienced mums to tears'. Father and grandparents can hold baby.

Suggestions Some staff on postnatal wards should have more understanding of new mother's emotions. More flexible visiting for partners.

Trowbridge and District, Seymour Road, Trowbridge, Wilts MO

Clean, well kept. Small ward was built to accommodate extra mothers when Bradford-on-Avon hospital closed. Building adjoining the large waiting room, comfortable chairs, carpets.

Antenatal Woman has shared care with GP and sees GP, except for booking visit at about 14 weeks, seeing consultant at 36 weeks and final visit before EDD. Some writers did not feel sufficiently at ease in this clinic to ask questions. One woman said consultant 'was man of few words' and she 'submitted' to him. One woman went to clinic at EDD plus 2 days. After examination was asked, 'how about stirring things up then?'; she declined, and was told she was overdue. She said she would prefer to wait 10 days; and was told 'no'. Asked if she could wait till weekend; told 'no'. Then doctor looked at her notes and told her that she gained no weight in last few weeks and was putting baby at risk. She asked if it could wait until after she had seen her GP, told no; 'I had no time to get accustomed to the awful thought I was not going to be allowed to give birth to my baby naturally . . . felt too afraid of his authority to argue. He said, "you're coming in tomorrow, alright?"' Labour was induced following day.

Labour Women report shave/enema. Partner can be present throughout. Electronic fetal monitoring may be used: 'I had nothing to fix my mind on except the flashing red fetal heart lights. It goes off now and again, and we gasped.' External monitor may be used; 'tight, elasticated belt'. Several women said they were not allowed to lie on their sides because it interfered with readings on print-out. Woman who refused drip was told that she could not have waters broken without drip and that doctor would not do anything that she was not happy about. She was summoned to office of senior member of staff and 'treated like naughty child'; told 'you are 4 days late and it is doctor's policy to start women off if they are 3 days late'. Large doses of pethidine seem to be given sometimes, because women report feeling 'disoriented' and they 'cannot control thoughts'. 'Staff wander in now and again, turn drips speeds up.' Some women said they were told they were allowed 1 hour in second stage and then intervention would take place. Episiotomy is not done routinely. Mother can hold baby on delivery table, then baby is taken to nursery and mother to ward.

Postnatal Several writers said there were many rules and that they felt 'intimidated' by system. 'Kind' nurses help establish breast-feeding but writers felt 'they treated the babies as if they were theirs', and some felt estranged from their babies 'because there was so little contact'. 'It was like being in prison'; 'I was told the baby book I was reading was rubbish.' 'Staff should be aware of how emotionally sensitive mothers are.' At time of writing women said that there were no night feeds during first 3 days and women could not go to nursery to get baby out. One woman 'sneaked' her husband into nursery to hold baby, but he was seen and 'thrown out'.

Food 'good'.

Suggestions The whole of postnatal care should be looked at so that it is not 'an emotional and physical endurance test'. There should be complete rooming-in of mother and baby.

Wakefield

Manygates, Barnsley Road, Wakefield, Yorks

Small, older type of hospital; most staff 'very pleasant' but short staffed. Head of midwifery services writes, 'as far as the midwives are concerned every effort is made to meet the individual patient's expectations of the birth process'. Home births can be arranged.

Antenatal Shared care with GP. Hospital clinic often entails 2-hour wait and clinic is crowded. 'Personal identity gets lost', 'difficult to discuss anything worrying', 'emotional needs not met', but writers say they are told how they are progressing. Writers said they were given no advice or encouragement on breast-feeding. Some writers were seen by as many as nine members of staff on first visit. But care is 'thorough' and 'conscientious'. Some writers commented on inadequate cooperation' between consultant and GP; 'my GP was not informed of the results of either the scan or oestriol except by me. The hospital had not even noted them on my cooperation card.' Relaxation and parentcraft classes available.

Labour Head of midwifery writes, 'husbands are encouraged to stay with their wives during labour and delivery and if the husband is not available another person may stay . . . the first stage of labour is conducted in single/double rooms where the husband and wife may watch television together. The patient is moved to the labour room for delivery . . . pubic shave is not done routinely . . . acceleration and induction of labour is undertaken in selected cases for medical indications only. Fetal monitoring is undertaken.' Writers say they had shave/enema and partner was sent out during this. But when couples were together again they were left in pleasant room with 'midwife popping in and out'. 'The midwife was super . . . made the delivery informal and relaxed.' Woman is free to decline pain-relieving drugs. Head of midwifery says, 'episiotomy is done as necessary but not routinely'. Forceps 8%; Caesareans 7%. Woman can breast-feed on delivery table and father is handed baby to cuddle too; some women who were stitched say that lithotomy stirrups were very uncomfortable.

Postnatal Very relaxed atmosphere. Mother has baby with her, but baby taken away for checks, sometimes for as long as 1½ hours (why not in front of mother?), for rest periods, when paediatrician comes and when going for baths. Policy of rooming-in and demand-feeding. Mother can care for her baby her own way, can get up in night to breast-feed and need give no complementary feeds. Writers advise, 'have the courage to ask for what you want'. 'They had a fetish about complementary water after the breast-feed "until your milk comes in."' One woman, whose baby did not want water, says she was told by two members of staff that she 'must try and get it down her'. One writer says that life is rather hectic on the ward with activity going on from 6 a.m. till midnight. Food 'awful'. Visiting 3–3.30 p.m. and children can come then too. 7.30–8.30 p.m. husbands only; as head of midwifery writes, 'we believe that it is in family interest that husband and wife have the opportunity to be together alone for some period of each day. If husband is unable to visit another visitor may do so.' It visiting times are not suitable 'no reasonable request is refused'.

SCBU Head of midwifery says, 'parents are encouraged to visit frequently, handle their babies as soon after birth as possible and participate throughout in the care of their own baby'. Brothers and sisters can visit with their parents. Postnatal stay of 48 hours to 7 days.

★ Wallingford Hospital, Wallingford, Oxfordshire   MO

Small, 'happy', 'relaxed' GP unit, with excellent safety record, where women can 'do their own thing'; 'lovely family atmosphere'; natural birth encouraged. Was threatened with closure but now redeemed. Caring midwives with flexible attitudes. Antenatal care with own GP. Based on adjoining GP surgery, with one of community midwives attending most clinics. Genuine continuity of care throughout pregnancy, labour and postnatal period.

Labour Midwives 'very supportive' and 'friendly'. 'She let me know all along what was happening – seemed to know by feeling my tummy rather than by internal examinations and use of machines.' Father welcome throughout labour. Woman encouraged to move around during first stage; breathing and relaxation encouraged. Pethidine offered in 50 mg doses, gas and oxygen available. Sonicaid (ultrasound) may be used. NCT mothers welcomed. Can wear own nightdress but pleasant shoulder-opening nightdresses available. Woman walks to another room for delivery or may be delivered in progress room. Delivery by own midwife and GP. Midwives are patient in second stage and 'willing to wait'. Plenty of pillows. Episiotomy not done routinely; one midwife has not needed to do one since her training over twenty years ago! Woman can help lift baby out on to her abdomen and father can cut cord. Encouraged to put baby to breast after delivery and couple have an hour or more together with baby. Writers say this is 'as near as possible to home birth' in 'an enlightened atmosphere, flexible to adapt to each individual's wishes and needs'.

Postnatal Everyone who wrote commented on personal care. Policy of demand-feeding and general help with it. Baby is with mother by day, in nursery at night and can be woken to feed baby. If you want your baby to stay close beside you all the time, say so. Electric breast pump available. Mother looks after her own baby with midwife's help. Midwives give a great deal of time and offer good emotional support. Women can transfer from hospitals in Reading and Oxford for postnatal care here. Some writers appreciated bidet. Generous visiting may mean that mother finds it hard to rest. Visiting hours are flexible: 10.30–11.30 a.m. and 2.30–4 p.m.; 7–8 p.m. for fathers only. Children are welcome and 'made to feel at home'. Ancillary staff 'friendly', 'helpful'. The great thing about this hospital is that all writers say that midwives are 'friendly' and have time to give to each mother and baby. Separate day room no longer available but it is needed, as children can be noisy and disturb other mothers.

Watford

Schrodell's Peace Memorial, Watford, Herts

'Efficient', 'spacious', 'pleasant' high tech hospital with 'active management of labour' and geared to the abnormal, in which obstetric staff are very conscious of public relations, but many writers say that they feel care is 'impersonal'. Hospital looks 'clean', 'jolly and modern on first sight, but fraying curtains and dirty walls on closer inspection'. Signs of greater awareness of women's needs.

Antenatal Long waits to see doctor 'about 2 hours and sometimes 3'; then seen 'very quickly' and by different doctor on each visit (1979). Hospital staff are themselves concerned about this and are trying to arrange continuity of care; things have much improved in the last few years according to writers. Everyone is 'friendly', 'helpful', and 'willing to discuss labour', says NCT teacher, who saw that consultant had written on her notes, 'treat this lady with kid gloves. She's an NCT lecturer [sic].' Some writers thought they were 'treated like an idiot' by most doctors, but some women who had babies there before say there is increased openness and flexibility now.

Ultrasound used frequently. May be asked views on epidurals at first visit. There are a few soft toys for toddlers, but otherwise no facilities for children. High induction rates in this hospital. Good antenatal classes, with excellent talk on baby bonding.

Labour Birth room available. Writers who had labour induced not always well informed; 'my baby was induced because I was 1 week late. No one explained what they were doing. I did not seem to have a choice about being induced' (failed induction; Caesarean section). Epidural offered with induction. One writer who missed antenatal class about epidural says she received no facts on which to make an informed decision, 'no warning about side-effects such as slowing of labour'. Another says she didn't realize forceps delivery would be highly likely. Some writers said they were not given information about other forms of pain relief. Epidural rate is 75%. 'The hospital made it very easy to say yes to an epidural.' Epidural Caesarean can be arranged. Partner can often be present all the time, including, sometimes, for suturing, if he has seen film at fathers' evening. One writer had her husband and her sister (midwife) except for catheterization and suturing. Writers describe partial shave/suppositories unless nearing second stage when they went in. (Why can't you insert suppositories yourself?) Amniotomy seems to be done routinely. Midwives 'very kind', 'easy-going', 'most caring'. 'Whatever I wanted was OK with them'; 'the midwife was very helpful and included me in all discussions with pupil midwife concerning my progress in labour'. On the other hand one writer, having her third baby after two previous, happy births, wrote, 'it was a fight to get my wishes respected concerning the presence of my husband right through, not breaking the waters, and him being present while I was stitched.' Several writers asked for half dose of pethidine and got it, though some said midwives insisted on 100 mg. Electronic monitoring no longer routine. There were some problems with epidurals; one writer would have preferred to go to lavatory when epidural wore off, rather than having catheter passed twice, but no one told her. Some writers said epidural was timed well so that they could push; others would have liked epidural to be allowed to wear off, but it was not well timed. Writers sometimes said they were ignored by consultant with his retinue and advise asking doctor's name. Everyone agrees that hospital is 'very good at coping with the abnormal'. But those having straightforward labours often felt under threat of intervention; 'drugs were constantly being offered when my husband left the room . . . I was hooked up to the fetal heart monitor which I did not want . . . and I did not appreciate arguing with staff while having contractions.' Woman has to be moved to another room for delivery, but is wheeled on same bed and then changes to delivery table. A few writers said they could get in whatever position suited them, but most said they had to push lying on their backs: 'I couldn't push properly, being nearly flat and lop-sided. As I had only two or three pillows I couldn't sit up properly.' A woman who said the intravenous drip in her arm made getting into a comfortable position difficult added that the unit 'had a policy of semi-lying-down rather than more upright position'. Some writers said midwife told them to push non-stop and some said 'never told to stop pushing at delivery'. Many found second stage stressful; 'midwife kept accusing me of not trying hard enough'. Mothers generally felt that birth in this hospital was something doctors did to them, rather than something they were supported to do for themselves; 'the obstetrician was taking bets with his entourage on the size of baby before delivery, and generally doing a Morecombe and Wise act with the registrar and sister. I felt left out.' Episiotomy sometimes done without local anaesthetic (is this because they are so used to having women with epidurals?) Rate is 43% in primigravidae and 22% in multigravidae. Some writers said, 'the midwife and I agreed not to have an episiotomy unless absolutely necessary'. Writers said they were told they were not allowed to be in second stage longer than 1 hour. One writer who had removal of placenta under general anaesthetic 'as it broke up as they tried pulling it out' wrote, 'I objected to the insinuation that it was my fault that I had to have the placenta removed under general anaesthetic because I did not have an epidural.' 'The midwife stalked out in a huff when we wanted to hold our baby while waiting for a theatre to be free.' Some women had to wait a long time to be stitched. One said birth took place 'at 19.27 and I was finally taken down to the ward after stitching at 23.30'. Occasionally woman was put in stirrups ready for doctor well in advance of his arrival: 'having to wait 20 minutes with my legs in stirrups in a bare delivery room all on my own was very uncomfortable'. After stitching couple can have about ½ hour alone together with their baby; 'a relaxed and happy atmosphere'.

Postnatal Wards 'spacious and airy' but amenity beds recommended for those who want privacy and freedom. Short staffed. Writers say one whole wing is closed (GP wing) and GP patients mixed with consultant patients. Atmosphere 'very relaxed', staff 'helpful'; 'mothers come first and are encouraged to do what they think best' and relationships 'happy' on the whole. Policy of demand-feeding, but some writers said they were readily advised to 'top up at the slightest hint of trouble'. 'Staff prefer it if baby demands every 4 hours and mothers need to be very firm.' Writers also say that dextrose is *'de rigueur'*; several wrote that though told to give glucose water 'until the milk comes in' you do not *have* to do this. Some mothers felt hurried, some that they needed more mothering themselves in first day. Though impression from recent writers is that care has much improved recently. Bonding with baby is encouraged, but occasionally a writer says she was 'told off' for picking up her baby too often. Staff assume second-time mothers can cope unless they ask for help. Fathers can bath their babies. Baby can stay by mother's side, including during visiting, and first night too, if you *ask*. Breast-fed babies often test-weighed apparently. First-time mothers said they got conflicting advice.

One mother's day;

6 a.m.	Woken, temperature taken, tea, feed baby.
8 a.m.	Breakfast, tea, bread and butter, cereal, boiled egg.
8.30–9.30 a.m.	Ward cleaned, baby goes to nursery, where bathed and/or topped and tailed.
9.30 a.m.	Tea.
Midmorning.	Feed baby.
Noon.	Lunch, fish and chips, icecream.
Afternoon.	Feed baby, discharge/stitches examined, tummy felt, 'bowels opened?'
3.30–4.30 p.m.	Visiting, cup of tea, feed.
6 p.m.	Supper, e.g. soup and round of egg sandwiches, coffee/cold milk.
7.30–9.30 p.m.	Visiting, night feed.
10 p.m.	Milky drink, pill.

Writers say that two distalgesic or Panadol tablets were given every 4 hours for perineal pain and pain-killers at night. Food is 'unappetizing', 'nutritionally unbalanced' (e.g. potato pie with mashed potato and chips) and often cold; 'icecream melted'. Choice of about three items and order night before; one writer who ordered cheese was sent pork (she is Jewish). Writers say you need to supplement food with fruit, salad vegetables, but wholemeal bread available. Writers often missed meals when breast-feeding. A woman who had Caesarean section said she would like to have known in advance some after-effects of operation and what she could expect. She was very much at sea. Sisters, nurses and auxiliaries 'all delightful' and 'charming to talk to'. One writer said that when she told sister she was 'disappointed with the birth, she said that childbirth was overrated, like sex'. Bidets in all lavatories and bathrooms; showers very hot, be warned.

SCBU One writer who was expressing breast milk for her baby was disappointed to learn that it was never given to baby.

Suggestions Greater flexibility generally. Women should have choice whether to have electronic monitoring in labour or not. Writer who said a student 'stitched me up very painstakingly but on completion was not satisfied with it', and that 'the registrar decided to take out the stitches and do them again' suggests that medical students should only suture under careful supervision.

More open visiting for partners. Restriction of number of visitors at any one time in first 2–3 days. Woman with baby in SCBU, who says she 'got depressed looking at blank wall' in her private room suggests that those in single rooms should be able to bring pictures from home and hooks should be provided (or pin-board, so they can put up cards, etc., too?)

Wellington Maternity Home, Wellington, Somerset

Small GP unit which had two stars in the first edition of the *Good Birth Guide*.

Antenatal Staff are 'positive' and 'encouraging', but one senior member is criticized as 'severe, brusque and controlling'. 'Reading books – biggest crime you can commit.'

Labour Staff 'kind', 'reassuring', 'interested' and 'concerned', but 'general atmosphere unrelaxed', and writer says staff are 'noisy', 'rushing about and crashing and banging'. 'I was staggered at the insensitivity'; however 'I always knew what was going on and what was going to happen.'

Postnatal Difficult for mother to arrange to have baby with her at night unless she is in room on her own, and then not until after the first 3 nights. Some mothers said that nobody fetched them when the babies woke. 'They told me that babies at Wellington just don't wake at night after the first couple of times when they get a nappy change and then if they fail to settle, a bottle of water'; 'I was assured that by the time I went home after 10 days I would have a baby that slept through the night'; 'I was told that babies didn't need to feed at night.' Some writers thought that there was too much reliance on the clock and breast-feeding regime too rigorous.

Queen Elizabeth II, Welwyn Garden City, Herts

Modern general hospital; large, pleasant. Rebuilding completed and another layer added on top for SCBU. Ante- and post-natal wards 'with superb views'. Admission, progress and delivery rooms 'very clinical'.

Antenatal Efficient but 'Awful'. Writers often found it difficult to get what they wanted, though 'questions answered willingly. Reception staff helpful; auxiliary staff pleasant. Wait of 30 minutes–1 hour, but longer to see consultant. Large parentcraft classes, mainly in evening. Tour of department included.

Labour Suppositories. Partner often sent out when doctor examines. Writers said that partner was out of the room a long time on these occasions, 45 minutes plus. Some were upset. 'I would have been more relaxed if my husband had been with me all the time.' But once in again husband is welcome and encouraged to help. May be allowed to stay for forceps delivery. Some doctors 'extremely gentle' and 'understanding'. Though one writer, her husband sent out of the room, being sutured after episiotomy, said it was terribly uncomfortable as she was in stirrups and 'kept getting cramps in my leg' . . . 'the doctor completely ignored my comments, not at all tolerant of the extreme discomfort'. Woman cared for by midwives only is likely to have birth with maximum technology. Midwives 'emotionally supportive' and when they are in charge are very positive about couple being together'. Explain what they are doing and why. Some writers described being wired up to various types of equipment linked to intravenous drips. This they found restrictive; 'I had a syntocinon intravenous drip which was faulty. Every time I moved my arm it stopped.' Some writers found second stage hectic: 'It was disturbing when the midwife was shouting during the pushing.' But midwives are expert at avoiding episiotomy and stitches: 'She was very firm about getting me to pant, not push.' Writers said they were able to have baby tucked up in bed with them in delivery room and had a long time with their partner to get to know their baby. Baby is cleaned up and weighed only after this.

Postnatal Very attractive wards. SNO says there is 'flexible feeding regime', but some writers say not all staff are happy with this and top-up bottles may be offered freely. Night nursery regime still exists. 65% leave hospital fully breast-feeding. Waking time now 6 a.m., not 5 a.m.: but 'killing routine' till 11 p.m. when babies taken to nursery. One writer says: 'Staff are thin on the ground . . . Auxiliaries give most help with breast-feeding.' Staff will keep meals hot if you are breast-feeding. 'Help is there when you want it' but otherwise 'left to own devices'. Food 'abysmal'. 'Desperate need' for more bathrooms: 'long queues every morning'.

SCBU Some writers said policy was to give artificial milk after every breast-feed.

Suggestions Some continuity of care between antenatal, labour and postnatal wards. More rest on postnatal wards.

Roy Hartley Maternity Unit, Billinge Hospital, Nr Wigan, Greater Manchester

'Modern, impersonal' and 'fond of gadgets'. Some writers said that they waited nearly 3 hours in booking clinic and at least 1 hour for subsequent appointments; 'a bore', 'a worry if there are other children to collect from school'. See different doctor each time; in five visits did not see same doctor twice'. Women who asked questions, however, said everything was ex-plained.

Labour Partner allowed to stay throughout. Usually perineal shave only and enema for all. Women may be able to walk around in first stage. Wears own nightdress. Pethidine may be encouraged, but second-time mothers say drugs are no longer pushed as previously. Continuous fetal monitoring often used. Most women have partners with them but some without partners said they were left alone with monitor for prolonged period; 'I was left plugged into monitor for 5 hours, in which time not a single person came in to check the print-out.' Area administrator says it is 'most unusual for patients in labour not to have a partner with them. Difficult to accept that they were left alone for prolonged period because of the necessary examinations which have to be carried out frequently and recorded in the case notes. When patients in labour have been given sedatives and analgesics the time factor can be very confusing for them as they are drifting in and out of sleep. Five minutes can seem like an hour or vice versa.' Delivery room 'white-tiled', 'massive' and 'like mortuary'. Day staff treat women with 'great kindness and consideration', but some night staff have been criticized for being 'impatient', 'lacking in sympathy' and even 'rude'. They prefer machines to keep check, rather than an occasional friendly face to see if everything is OK.' Writers stress that it is 'vital to have a partner with you'. Pushing is encouraged enthusiastically. Some women said they had to wait for a long time after delivery before going to ward, their baby separated from them. Area administrator says 'Once the patients have held their infants on delivery, the infants are then returned to them after bathing for them to hold and the infants are then transferred to a warm nursery on the postnatal wards or the special care baby unit.'

Postnatal Modern, pleasant ward. Some writers say there is poor communication; 'she never answered a direct question. It was always "we'll see" or "perhaps" as if speaking to a child'; 'it is always the member of staff who has just gone off who knows the answer'. 'No one explained anything about my baby to me . . . they just brought her to me and that was it.' Some writers said it was difficult to get questions answered, obtain results of tests on baby or even sometimes to find out weight on discharge. Area administrator writes, 'Totally untrue. A full examination is carried out by the midwife in charge very morning and at any time during the day the midwives are available to answer questions . . . results of tests are given to the mother as soon as they are received from the laboratory. It is totally untrue that it is difficult to find out the birth-weight of the infant.' Some writers said it was far too hot and that their babies developed heat rashes. The area administrator agrees, but says, 'the mothers are averse to having open windows. When opened by staff, often closed by patients.' Writers describe temperatures of 78°, say water is warm to drink. Night staff tend to be noisy. Area administrator comments, 'this has not been the subject of formal complaints but is now being investigated'. Some first-time mothers felt they were treated like children. Area administrator's comment on this is 'In some cases this may have been necessary because of the attitude of the mother.' Food is good, ordered 2 days in advance, so first 2 days you eat something ordered by someone else. A husband who made a complaint about his wife's traumatic Caesarean section had to wait 'many weeks and several phone calls' for an answer and even then was not offered an opportunity for discussion with consultant.

Forty-eight-hour stay possible.

Suggestions Brighten up delivery rooms. Women should be 'treated like mothers, not children with new toys'. Hospital staff should 'realize that the baby is not theirs, but the mother's'. Mother should be allowed to put her baby on her bed.

★ **Royal Hampshire, Winchester, Hants** MO

Consultant and GP unit. Information on antenatal care was too sparse to include.

Labour Partner can be present, including for forceps delivery or vacuum extraction. His assistance is encouraged. 'They were much more enlightened than last time, my husband was not sent out at any point.' When labour is induced prostaglandin gel only may be used; 'I was pacing around until an hour before the birth.' Midwives and doctors 'very helpful', 'encouraging', 'reassuring', 'create, happy relaxed atmosphere', though occasionally women said they were treated as 'patients', that there was no discussion and that it was difficult for them to get information on management of pain. One writer who asked for pethidine said she was given 125 mg and *then* examined. She was 10 cm dilated and ready to push. This knocked her sideways and she had no energy to push, result was a forceps delivery. Writer who had GP delivery said, 'They all knew my feelings about drugs, low lights, Leboyer and relaxation, as I had good opportunity during the latter half of my pregnancy to discuss them.' She said there was good communication with midwives 'which made all the difference. I knew that they would not press me to accept drugs or interfere with the labour unless absolutely necessary.' Several writers describe moving around in labour and being encouraged by midwives at all times. One woman who lost control in transition says midwife reminded her of breathing learned in NCT classes. Another praises midwives because 'no one was making me lose concentration by asking daft questions'.

Second stage: some women longed to sit up more, but said wedges were too low. Position in which mother pushes with her feet against midwives' hips is disliked by many women. Most writers said they had to lie down on their backs to push or sat up leaning forward, and were enthusiastically encouraged to put everything they could into each effort. 'I did as I was told and pushed till I thought my head would blow off, but I did think the baby was making good progress by herself and wondered what all the worry was for. The midwife took over control of events in her own brusque, nonchalant way. There wasn't much time for communication. Urgent exhortation from the midwife. The midwife reinforced all my old habits of tensing up to cope with an extreme situation. Attendants gave the impression that they had more important matters to attend to . . . I wish now the whole thing had been done a little slower and that the staff had been more patient.' But other writers said that they were allowed to do second stage at their own pace. Some writers said they were told that episiotomy rate was 60%, that women having first babies had a rate of over 80% and that a woman who has had one is 'almost bound to need another'. Women also said position of stirrups for suturing was uncomfortable and they got cramp in thighs; 'when I told the doctor he wouldn't believe that I was in pain'. Some criticism of suturing; 'doctor who did the stitching seemed to do a good job kindly if a bit nervously'; 'I was the first patient the student doctor had ever sewn up. I resented this. As my doctor later told me, the student had not done a very good job.' Mother can hold and feed baby after delivery. Father is given baby to hold while she is being stitched; 'he could hold her as long as he wanted'.

Postnatal Nurses 'superb' at helping to breast-feed. Some mothers advise amenity room if you can get one; 'left on my own I *had* to cope with my baby and I feel this was important for our fast bonding'. Bidets available.

Suggestions Women should not be urged to push harder or longer than they find is helpful for them. Drugs for pain relief should only be given *after* a vaginal examination.

Bowthorpe, Tavistock Road, Wisbech, Norfolk HO

Small consultant unit.

Antenatal Clinic bright and airy, with homely atmosphere. Children welcome and toy-box provided. Most women have shared care. Local GPs hold antenatal clinics in hospital.

Labour SNO says that induction is performed 'for medical reasons only. Husband or other person is encouraged to stay throughout labour and they may stay during examination, or an abnormal delivery, at the discretion of the midwife or obstetrician. Patients may choose whether or not they have drugs for pain relief. An epidural service is available. Some Caesareans are performed under epidural. Husbands may be present . . . babies are put to the breast immediately after delivery.'

Postnatal Policy of feeding on demand. Baby is dressed in own clothes and is roomed in with mother at all times. Mothers are encouraged to get dressed while on postnatal ward. Visiting: 1 hour in afternoon, when own children may visit; evening visiting for husbands only. Babies who are ill are transferred to SCBU at Queen Elizabeth Hospital, King's Lynn. The mother goes too.

New Cross, Wolverhampton, West Midlands MO

Modern, very big, extremely busy high tech hospital; 'not very friendly, apart from the cleaners, who are a mine of information'.

Antenatal Crowded clinics, 'like a cattle market'; 2-hour wait usual; very hot in waiting area. Writers say they usually see different doctor each time, some of whom 'brusque', some who 'explain things'. 'The thought of New Cross antenatal clinic acts as a good contraceptive.' 'Appalling lack of communication' between doctors and mothers and lack of courtesy remarked on. Shared care possible.

Labour: GP unit GP unit especially praised; 'super' staff and 'relaxed atmosphere'. Midwives 'lovely', 'encouraging', 'motherly'.

Labour: consultant unit Part shave/enema; 'I asked if it was really necessary and told it was'. Some women who went into hospital at night were given sleeping pills. Partner allowed, but not when epidural given, for breech birth ('too messy') or if woman is in very early labour. One writer said she asked for her husband when induction was about to be done but was told that he had been instructed to return after 2 hours. Feeling trapped, she started to cry. Senior member of staff told her to read her book and left. Couple may be left alone together with midwife 'popping in'. Electronic fetal monitoring may be used and epidurals are available. One writer in labour with a syntocin induction drip, sphygmomanometer, a fetal scalp electrode, and epidural syringe and a contraction monitor felt alone and frightened. Her epidural had not taken effect and she says the fetal monitor was registering the baby's heart at irregular intervals. She could not find a bell and shouted, 'excuse me' when she heard footsteps. Usually a senior member of staff came and asked furiously, 'Why don't you ring the bell instead of shouting like that?', handed her the bell, which had been out of reach, adjusted the monitor, told her that the machine was always going wrong and walked out. Writer who had breech baby would have liked more explanation. Baby delivered 'gently' and laid immediately on mother's body on its back. (Mucus drains naturally if baby is on *front*.) Woman usually encouraged to suckle baby after delivery, but some had to ask. Partner allowed in after stitching, and mother, father and baby had time alone together.

Postnatal Pleasant room. Demand-feeding, including during visiting time if mother wishes. One woman said she was warned that she would get sore nipples if she breast-fed so often. One writer took artificial feeds and threw them down the sink when staff had left the room. Mother is not allowed to walk around with baby in her arms but can cuddle baby in bed. Writers appreciated midwifery staff who were on duty during labour coming to chat with them afterwards.

Food 'dreadful'; some writers thought there was not enough. 'You can smoke if you want to', one writer says.

Children can now visit their mother every afternoon instead of only Saturdays as previously.

Suggestions Re-organize antenatal clinic. Obstetricians should never criticize junior staff in front of other staff and patients. Staff should 'listen to mothers more' on the consultant wards and one writer suggests that they need to learn how to relax themselves. Postnatal staff need to learn more about basics of breast-feeding and understand bonding. One writer says rubber of only breast pump available was perished and suggests that more should be available and in good condition. Improve food.

Ronkswood, Worcester   MO

Buildings 'dull and antiquated', but most staff 'cheerful', 'informal'. Some writers, however, speak of 'petty authority' and feeling bullied'.

Antenatal Modern clinic, production-line procedures; 'cattle market'. 'At least 3 hours for routine urine, blood pressure, prod session.' One writer said she lay on a couch 'sans knickers while all and sundry wandered by and got black mark for not knowing dates of last period. When I lightheartedly said that the babe would arrive when ready was told by humourless doctor that he would not then be able to induce me accurately . . . at each subsequent visit induction was mentioned except when I saw consultant, only doctor to introduce himself.' Writers say that doctors seem 'at pains to discover something wrong' and do not realize that women can have babies without doctors. One woman, asked which classes she was attending, said 'NCT' and says consultant's comment was 'Those are the ones who read books and think they know it all.' All those writing about this hospital mentioned induction; some said they thought it was 'induction-happy', and that labour was induced more often than necessary. Some writers had been induced when 7 days overdue, no other reason being given, and some when 2 days past EDD. 'Pupil midwives explained how much easier labour would be if induced and how much more painful if baby grew any bigger.' One writer, discussing attitudes among staff, comments, 'Their problem seems to be in coping with normality when their expertise and power base is with the abnormal.' She felt that staff used 'moral blackmail', suggesting that she was damaging the unborn infant and 'asking her if she could forgive herself if anything went wrong'. One woman whose cervix was not ripe, told how it took 3 days of pills, drips and having the waters broken to get me into labour. Three days in a labour ward, being allowed only that disgusting milkshake, surrounded by wailing women, does no one's morale any good.'

Labour Staff 'considerate' on the whole and 'helpful reassurance' from mid-wives and consultants. Some writers felt regimented. But on the whole women had very good relations with their midwives: 'I was lucky that I had a midwife who believed in allowing things to progress naturally. She didn't try to rush me at all'; 'I cannot stress enough how kind the staff were and how much trouble they took to explain everything (they were all women)'; 'they tried to adapt to patient's wishes'. Partner can be present, may be sent out before prepping and not be called in for long time. One writer counsels 'courage' in asking for him to come in again. One women without a partner said she laboured alone for much of the time. There are shared labour rooms and two women may labour together. Several writers described enema: 'Large, hot enema *de rigueur*.' One writer said she would have much preferred not to have had full shave. Into 'morgue-type gown . . . when I worked in psychiatric hospital we used them for laying-out!' Several writers wondered whether lying in bed in early labour is good idea: 'put to bed, told to lie down. Surely it would be better on the move?' 'Threatened with drip if won't drink nauseating fluid called Build-Up.' Some writers report labouring without having pain-relieving drugs. Others seem to have had large doses of pethidine, as after having them their minds were 'a blank' or were 'frustrated by being unable to make my body obey my head'. Epidurals available and anaesthetist very helpful and pleasant, describes what he is doing. Several women told how epidural was allowed to wear off for second stage so they could push. It may be chance, but sixteen out of twenty women described a good deal of obstetric intervention.

Second stage: some writers felt they were not upright enough and would have liked to be more propped up. Others said they were allowed to adopt position they found most comfortable. One writer said 'officious SEN used force in making me lie flat on my back'. When she tried to explain dangers of supine position, she says she criticized her for 'reading books'. One writer said she had to answer questions during contractions. Another said, 'When I wanted to push we rang the bell, 35 minutes later someone appeared.' This seems to be the exception, for most mothers found a vigorous approach to second stage. 'I was hectored by jolly midwife who seemed to have done her training on the lacrosse fields of some girls' public school.' Another woman who said her husband was trying to help her, wrote that 'nurse told him to shut up'. Vacuum extraction may be used instead of forceps and 'everything was explained'. One writer says she was told that 'all fair-haired women with first babies have episiotomies'. Mother has immediate contact with baby, usually even if baby has to go to SCBU after. Couple have time alone together with their baby. 'Tea, but no toast,' comments one woman, 'after a whole day's starvation.' Some writers waited inordinately long time to be stitched, e.g. one said she had to wait 2½ hours and then, 'A lad who looked as if he'd been out on the trawlers gutting herrings, besmirched in someone else's blood, arrived and sewed me up without washing first.'

Postnatal Atmosphere 'pleasant'. Baby must sleep in nursery first night, even if mother in single room. One writer who asked to be woken to feed said she was not. One woman had to ask 'constantly' for her baby before she appeared following delivery. Morning after birth one writer says she was rebuked for changing her baby's nappy without supervision. Modified demand-feeding practised: 'I was told "We do believe in demand-feeding, but only every 4 hours."' One writer said she tried to breast-feed while nurses 'stood about discussing the small size of my breasts, insisting I would never do it . . . a public trial', and that she had to cope with 'constantly proffered bottles.' (1979) Staff referred to one mother in front of her as 'the woman who reads books'.

SCBU Woman with baby in SCBU can have room across corridor from unit. Parents can visit any time. Regular staff always helpful, though busy: 'They make you feel it is your own baby.' Sister 'superb'.

Suggestions Induction policy should be reviewed – one woman suggested it produces problems for staff and puts them under pressure, since on the day she had her baby three induced women and one not induced entered second stage all at the same time. Food and drinks should be provided for women in early labour and for partner during a long labour. Women should be able to drink plain water during labour. One writer, who said she could only hold baby 'for all of 5 minutes' suggests longer time for getting to know baby. Baby should either not be taken away from mother at all, or should be brought when she asks after delivery.

Yeovil Maternity Hospital, Yeovil, Somerset MO

Modern, 'very pleasant'.

Antenatal Staff 'friendly and caring', 'efficient'; 'At first I got the impression of just being a number, but when my blood pressure rose slightly they seemed to take more notice'. Writers said they felt 'free to ask questions, and never felt rushed'. Receptionist 'really pleasant', 'helpful', 'acts as if she knows you'. Mothers advise making appointment first thing in morning if you do not want to 'wait for ages'. They say staff are 'very apologetic' about long waits. Hospital has good car service, boon to mothers in rural area who do not have a car. Women having shared care see own GP but also have about six visits to hospital. Women for whom induction has been suggested say they have had 'ample opportunity to discuss' this and decline offer if they wish. One writer who discussed episiotomy with sister says she was told: 'As with all hospital procedures, you do not have to accept it.' No facilities for children: 'You spend the time trying to amuse them and keep them from annoying other people.'

Antenatal ward: 'I thoroughly enjoyed my stay.' One writer who started labour on antenatal ward appreciated being given hot drink before being taken up to labour floor.

Labour 'Pleasant' environment. Partial shave. Woman has bath and can spend long time in it if she wishes. Partner can stay throughout, including for VEs, amniotomy, forceps delivery. 'Calm, quiet atmosphere.' 'Everything was explained.' Yet this seems to rather depend on the midwife, since there were some writers who advised 'making a stand' and who said they felt 'swept along by the tide'; 'If you want anything done your way you have to dig your heels in.' One woman wrote that once the midwife heard she attended NCT classes and she asked questions she was treated as 'awkward'. Pethidine given 'if you ask for it'. Sometimes given much too late at onset second stage. Minimal intervention: 'I was able to cope with my labour in my own way' and though some labours are accelerated, this is done 'reluctantly'. Woman is moved to different room for delivery: 'very clinical', but everyone 'quiet' and 'relaxed'. Wedges and pillows available so woman can sit up for birth, but some women wanted more than were provided. Midwife may suggest that woman puts her feet on her and her husband's hips; 'At times just one foot was given support and midwife wandered off somewhere, so I was uncomfortable.' One writer said, 'The midwife seemed as enthusiastic about birth as we were ourselves.' Baby is put on mother's body while cord cut; can be put to breast; then in 'plastic box' while mother is stitched. If you want to pick your baby up, do so, as 'no one will object'. One couple said they were so tired and 'intimidated by the system', though, that they did not think of holding their baby during suturing. Woman who had Caesarean with general anaesthesia was delighted to wake up to find her baby was with her.

Postnatal Hospital has become much more relaxed (1981). Staff generally 'very helpful' and 'understanding'. Baby is with mother during day, in nursery at night. Policy of demand-feeding. Mothers can be woken during night to feed, but 'only ever once a night': 'It was a big shock to get home and discover that babies actually wake up rather more than once a night!' Mother is given hot drink when she feeds baby at night. Staff has stopped telling mothers to clean their nipples before feedings. Cleaners asked to leave ward so that a baby can be fed and mothers' meals are kept back if they are feeding. One woman whose baby had to go to another hospital for special care said she thought she might not be able to breast-feed, but was given 'bags of help and managed easily'. Women who have had Caesarean sections are helped to breast-feed and given much encouragement. But writers say there is 'a lot of conflicting advice': 'You can't pick him up every time he cries, you'd spoil him' on the one hand and 'Babies need to be cuddled' on the other. 'One soon learned who to avoid.' Most staff are aware of feelings of new mothers: 'After the first few days I became more confident and started to treat the baby as if she were mine and not theirs.' One mother, with her second child, says she was severely 'ticked off' for daring to change nappy before she had been shown how. Staff do everything for baby first 3 days; and then mother takes over. Everybody has to be in bed when consultants come round. Staff are praised for friendliness, particularly auxiliary nurses. Staff 'seem to change daily'; some women found it difficult to cope with 'lots of different faces'. But on the whole 'very happy atmosphere'. A night nurse did not wake ward till 7 a.m. Babies had woken 4–4.30 a.m. and were sleeping so she ignored normal getting-up time of 6 a.m. and left women to sleep. This staff nurse had a baby 5 months old herself and mothers very much appreciated her understanding. Bidet, 'great relief' and 'sheer bliss' for sore perineums.

Wales

Bronglais, Aberystwyth, Dyfed
MO

'A gentle wind of change in the air, perhaps more of a breeze.' Little birth technology and doctors only at birth if problems arise. Clean and bare; 'terrible taste in curtains and paint'.

Antenatal Very long waits; short examinations. One writer says she was told that it was up to midwife on duty whether father allowed in. In fact, fathers present for normal labours, but staff may not commit themselves beforehand. Women can have tour of unit. One woman's husband came too but staff tried to turn him away. He stood his ground and they relented. Induction 13–20%.

Labour Partner cannot be present during prepping. One woman described dry shave with blunt razor. But mini-shave only, suppositories, occasionally small enema. 'Midwife did not stop during contractions.' Some couples felt 'anxious' or 'alienated' because sheet of orders for fathers handed out which instructs them not to interfere in any way during birth, to carry out midwives' orders, e.g. to leave the room at once without discussion if asked. Woman can deliver without drugs for pain relief if she wishes. Those who have asked for pethidine at end of first stage have been advised not to have it because there is not time. Epidurals not available apparently. Those who wrote mentioned noticeable absence of drips to induce or accelerate and electronic monitoring. Staff 'pleasant', 'kind' but some a bit 'brusque'. SNO particularly mentioned as being 'understanding'. But some staff 'made it clear that the conduct of birth was their concern, not ours'; 'Most delicately worded questions were interpreted as sinister threats'; 'They fiercely defended their professionalism.' Some women disliked position they were asked to adopt for second stage, flat on their backs, holding their legs in the air, arms under their knees and found it uncomfortable. 'Kitzinger cushion available if woman wants to sit upright, but may be used only at mother's request.' Some writers had episiotomy without being asked and wondered if it was necessary. If mother asks baby is put on abdomen, cord still intact. One writer who asked if she could put baby to breast after delivery says midwife helped her to do this, but 'I wasn't allowed to hold her. Midwife held her wrong way up with feet by my ear.' Partner sent out for stitching up. Baby may then be taken to nursery for several hours. One woman who asked for her baby says she was told senior midwife had gone to lunch and those remaining had no authority to fetch baby. Remarks on 'rigid hierarchy, those at the bottom, the cleaning staff, being the most friendly'.

Postnatal 'Very kind and pleasant.' Staff 'tactful' and supportive about breast-feeding. Meal kept hot for feeding mothers. But 'each midwife has her own opinions, always given as fact, though varying from one to another and

401

sometimes contradictory'. Some writers were confused and worried about this; those who already had their own ideas could cope. Each mother can breast-feed in her own way. Water brought with each feed. Some writers say that first night baby was given bottle (soy milk). It may be offered second night too, but at least one mother 'firmly refused it'. Some writers advised asking for amenity room if available. Baby is with mother during day and may be at night if midwife on duty agrees. One woman said she was told baby was cold and nursery warmer. 'I should have thought she would have been warmer snuggled in with me.' Food 'awful; but lovely to have it brought on tray'. 'Why can't hospitals apply simple rules of good nutrition?' Visiting 1 hour evenings only, but those in amenity rooms can 'stretch this a bit'. Some writers were concerned that their husbands only saw mother and baby with other visitors present. 'I would have liked more time alone with my husband.' Other children in family can visit weekend afternoons and at other times on request.

Suggestions Greater flexibility generally. A woman who does not want to be separated from her baby should not have baby taken away at all. Free visiting for fathers.

Brecon Hospital, Brecon, Powys HO

GP unit which functions as mini-district-general hospital and deals with its own abnormal cases. Inductions with ARM 3%; with syntocinon 9%; with prostaglandins 11%. Forceps deliveries 7%; ventouse (vacuum extraction) 8%; Caesarean sections: elective 4% and emergency 9%. SNO writes: 'We still aim to offer a home-from-home atmosphere and try to accommodate all the mothers' requests and wishes. Fathers stay in for forceps deliveries if they wish.'

West Wales Hospital, Glangwili, Carmarthen, Dyfed MO

New building, staff 'friendly'. Good layout, with delivery rooms at end of long corridor away from wards.

Antenatal Waits of 1–2 hours; can discuss problems with midwife. Some doctors described as 'impersonal', 'bossy', 'tend to shout questions at you as you lie undressed on the other side of a screen', 'clearly disliked giving explanations'. Domino scheme functions here. Writers think there is a good deal of induction for mild hypertension.

Labour Labour and delivery take place in 'one bare room with greyed-out windows'. Midwives 'friendly'. In consultant unit 'it is taken for granted that woman will need drugs for pain relief'. One woman says she was asked: 'Have you had your injection yet?', was offered pethidine and when she was firm that she did not want it, it was not insisted on. Partner welcome and can be present except for prepping and ARM. Mother given baby to hold immediately and can suckle on delivery table.

Domino delivery: partial shave. No drugs if woman does not want them. But writers say they had to accept continuous fetal monitoring. Domino mothers feel they are 'very special as compared with routine interventions for other women', but even so, insist that 'you have to be firm about what you want'. No episiotomy unless necessary. Woman stays in hospital overnight and then goes home.

Postnatal Light, airy wards. Breast-feeding, according to some writers, 'is not fully understood by some members of staff'. A woman who asked if she might have her baby with her a couple of hours after delivery said she was told: 'Alright, but it's your responsibility if it chokes and dies.' One writer who was breast-feeding in bed, said senior member of staff came and 'snatched the baby off my breast with no warning'. No babies are allowed in bed. Baby is with mother in day, in nursery at night. One woman writing in 1978 says baby is brought 3-hourly for feeds and taken away at visiting times. 'Not much understanding of bonding and how to encourage a mother's relationship with her baby.' Food 'mediocre' but there is menu and choice.

Suggestions Antenatal clinic waiting room, row of chairs along corridor, could be replaced by room where there is somewhere for children to play. Rooming-in choice for those women who want it, with women who decide on this sharing ward together.

Griffithstown County, Griffithstown, Gwent — MO

Aged, prefabricated buildings, but light and airy inside. Antenatal and postnatal wards split into three sections separated by board and glass partitions. 'Not intimidating.'

Antenatal Visits 'a pleasant experience'! Same staff each week, who work 'quickly and efficiently'. 'Their close working relationship involved witty repartee . . . I spent a large amount of time grinning and joking.' Visits usually not more than 30–45 minutes and 'sister in charge apologized for delay'. But women rarely encounter same doctor twice.

Labour Women describe enema/shave. Immobilized position 'in labour and compulsory electronic fetal monitoring. Monitor with wide strap round abdomen may be used: 'very uncomfortable'. And this may be further tightened as labour proceeds. Women tell of being given pethidine automatically 'to relax you'. Large doses seem to be given and writers describe being in 'semi-stupor'; or 'unconscious'. Some said they were left alone for long periods. Labour may be accelerated with oxytocin intravenous drip. Mother can sit up and watch birth, sometimes even with forceps delivery. Can then hold baby.

Postnatal 'Everyone very enthusiastic about breast-feeding, but every shift has own ideas of right approach', and women describe conflicting advice. 'No adverse comments made to women choosing bottle-feeding.' Some nurses 'kindly', some 'authoritarian': 'as if afraid we'd get out of control'; 'one or two didn't seem to like babies'. Mothers have to adjust instantly to different personalities and different sets of unwritten rules. Rapid turnover of nurses on different shifts produces 'oppressive atmosphere'. Women describe cramped space: 'Climbing over stools and squeezing past people is no fun with stitches, worse for those who had had Caesareans.' Seats padded but 'uncomfortable'. But 'not enough personal care'. One woman said no one offered to wake her to feed her baby in middle of night. She was too timid to ask, so another mother got up and woke her. A doctor came to discuss implications of baby's weight loss with one mother and handled baby 'with loving care'. Ice-cold milk or Guinness for breast-feeding mothers mid-morning delivered by lady 'always courteous and kind'.

SCBU 'Inauspicious start to breast-feeding. Comments on my nipples: "The right one is very poor",' wrote one woman. One mother whose baby had died was asked by staff nurse when her baby was coming out of SCBU. Another mother whose baby went to SCBU with jaundice said she could not get information and her husband's inquiry 'was rudely repulsed'.

Suggestions Staff should 'sit down and thrash out common policy about breast-feeding'. Modify shift system 'so that mothers can relax and enjoy their babies'.

★ Llandrindod Wells Hospital, Llandrindod Wells, Powys

SNO writes, 'We aim to offer a home-from-home atmosphere . . . and try to accommodate all the mothers' requests and wishes.' Inductions with Syntocinon 8%; ARM 15%. No use of prostaglandins is reported here. Forceps deliveries 5%. SNO writes that partner can be present for forceps delivery.

Postnatal Writers say there is a high standard of care. Women are transferred here from large hospital for postnatal care. Some writers say care is 'fantastic'. One midwife, on call for emergencies only, offered to get up in night to give baby bottle of expressed milk for mother who felt ill.

Suggestions Put more money into this hospital and upgrade it.

Glyn Garfield, Neath General, Neath, W Glamorgan   HO

Antenatal Shared care. SNO writes, 'A great deal of emphasis is placed on health education.' Midwife available at every antenatal clinic 'to give advice and deal with any queries'. Induction 17%.

Labour Hospital policy encourages presence of husband, friend or relative during labour and delivery, provided delivery normal. SNO states, 'The general policy regarding the active management of labour is still one of non-intervention unless . . . there is a clear indication that mother and/or fetus may be at risk. Routine procedures such as the use of suppositories are still used, but enemas are now performed only on medical request. Pubic and perineal shaves are no longer performed. Continuous fetal monitoring is used for selected patients whenever there is an indication of fetal distress . . . The consent of the patient is always obtained beforehand. Mother is transferred on bed from first-stage room to delivery room.' SNO writes, 'We have no experience of Leboyer-style delivery.'

Postnatal SNO says that 'Rooming-in is practised and mothers are encouraged to spend as much time as possible with their newborn infant and to do as much as they can for their babies themselves. We are very much aware of the importance of "bonding".' If mother intends to breast-feed, baby is put to breast very soon after birth in delivery room. 'Our interpretation of "demand-feeding" is that of a minimum period of 3 and a maximum period of 5 hours between feeds. This gives a period of 2 hours during which baby should be fed. However, each baby is also treated individually and fed as is deemed necessary.' Artificial feeds given to babies only at mother's request. Paediatric examination nearly always takes place in presence of mothers.

Visiting 3.30–4.30 p.m. and 7.00–8.00 p.m. daily, 'but visiting arrangements for husbands and close relative are flexible. Other children of family may visit in visiting room adjacent to ward. Fathers are allowed to hold their babies.

SCBU Accommodation for mothers.

Royal Gwent, Cardiff Road, Newport, Gwent   MO

Modern unit, 'clean and bright', 'cheerful atmosphere'.

Antenatal Writers seemed to wait about 2 hours. Most staff 'friendly' but in 'slightly impersonal way'. 'Cattle-market atmosphere.' 'Reasonably efficient.' Scan likely to be done. One mother told scan showed her baby would be small: 'He was a nine-pounder!' Women say they are shifted from room to room, see different doctor each time. Some writers mentioned difficulty of communicating with non-English-speaking doctors: 'This did not inspire confidence'; 'I found the lack of someone to talk to the most distressing aspect.' One woman said, 'I felt like a lamb going to the slaughter.' Can have shared care with GP, hospital appointments only about three times at end of pregnancy. Couple can see round labour wards if they ask. Those attending relaxation and parentcraft classes see round anyway. They appear to be well organized.

Labour Shave; one woman described 'horrific, 2-pint, soapy-water enema'. Staff 'quite caring'. Some midwives encourage women to walk around in early labour. One woman was taken to day room but found it 'embarrassing' to breathe her way through contractions among a number of pregnant women sitting watching her. Her husband asked if there was an empty single room; this was provided. Partner can be there throughout except for VEs. Writers advise having partner who understands exactly what you want and can speak for you. Pethidine and Valium offered to many writers. Women who accepted

Newport

it say labour was 'just a haze' after that and some kept on falling asleep. Women who asked not to have drugs believed they were considered odd – 'that natural childbirth lady' – and may be warned: 'you will never do it without drugs'; 'you are underestimating the amount of pain you will have'. Woman who asked for epidural says she was not able to have one because nobody could be found to give it. A writer who asked not to be attached to a monitoring machine said her wishes were respected. 'The staff were generally very kind, but impatient about waiting till the end of a contraction to examine me . . . they seemed not to understand the effort involved in changing position to be examined in labour.' Many women seemed to have had episiotomies, though one writer said the midwife waited as long as she could before doing one. One woman said that after birth they were not offered a cup of tea and 'it was just as if they were all glad the work was over'. One woman said how nice it was when a pupil midwife who had been with her in labour came in to see her next day.

Postnatal Writers say they have to stay in bed 12 hours after delivery. Baby roomed in with mother but removed to nursery if cries. If you want your breast-fed baby brought back for feed, make this clear. 'Staff pay lip-service to breast-feeding, yet give conflicting advice and no one has time to sit with you in the early days to help.' Wards have mixture of breast- and bottle-feeding mothers and one breast-feeding mother said it was bad for morale to see how easily bottle-feeders managed while she was 'struggling madly'. One senior member of staff 'told her off' for being over-eager to breast-feed and 'having read too much': 'You're a teacher, aren't you?' she asked. 'Nurses and teachers always make the worst mothers.' One woman booked for 48-hour stay discharged herself against advice. She said sister said she was not coping with feeding and 'did everything in her power' to keep her in but as soon as she got home everything was all right. Day starts at 5 a.m.: 'not at all restful'. Room 'very hot'; babies are 'soaked with sweat'. One mother said her baby was having convulsions and asked to see doctor. When he came baby was taken straight to special care suffering from dehydration. Mother said she was told she could go to SCBU to feed baby if he was well enough and waited 10 hours without news: 'We were sure by then that he was dead' (he was fine). One woman said care was 'a farce', and added: 'I would have had better care if I had been booked into a cheap boarding house.' Visiting 3.30–5 p.m. and 7–8 p.m. husbands only.

SCBU 'Staff marvellous . . . like being in different hospital.'

Suggestions More understanding of natural childbirth; some writers suggest more contact with NCT. Provide epidurals for those who want them. Turn down heat on postnatal wards. Breast-feeding mothers should be in their own wards; more personal help given with breast-feeding. One hour each evening is not long enough for fathers visiting – make it more flexible; some writers suggested open visiting for partners.

St Asaph Hospital, St Asaph, Clwyd   MO

Writers say this hospital is very short-staffed.

Antenatal Busy clinic; pleasant staff, but care 'impersonal'. Only curtains separate couches. One woman said 'no help was given in getting down from high couch'. One woman says she was asked by obstetrician, as she lay on the couch, who was 'putting ideas into her head' and says she was treated as if 'complete idiot'. As day of expected birth passed some women say they were warned of increased perinatal mortality when baby overdue and made to feel 'guilty', 'naïve', and 'irresponsible' if they did not want to be induced for post-maturity at that stage. One woman went with her husband to see nursing officer with lists of the routines they did not want 'imposed' and said they were told she saw no reason why they should not have what they wanted provided there were no clinical indications to the contrary.

Labour Shave/enema. Partner can stay whole time including during VEs and for stitching, but if you want this you will have to be quite clear and firm: 'My husband was told to wait outside . . . then without explanation the doctor put a glucose drip into my arm and then broke my waters and placed a monitor on to my baby's head. My husband was then allowed in.' Usually one midwife with each woman. She 'consulted us over every issue'. Midwives concerned to meet mothers' wishes. Writers say that those who do not want unnecessary intervention must be definite with doctors. Midwives ask mothers beforehand if they may perform episiotomies. Mother can ask for cord to be left until it has stopped pulsating; 'The midwife asked if she could use the suction tube to clear some mucus from her mouth.' Baby can be put to breast immediately, but some mothers found senior members of staff reluctant. Couple have time alone together with their baby in delivery room: 'It was just wonderful.' Women advise others having babies here to go ahead and do what they want and get the midwives' support, many of whom are 'marvellous'. Women wanting Leboyer-style birth will be helped to have it if they consult the nursing officer beforehand, writers say.

Postnatal One writer felt that it was a pity that she should have to go on to a busy postpartum ward just after delivering. Cleaners were in and very noisy: 'I couldn't keep my eyes open, yet was unable to sleep.' Writers describe glucose water given to babies after breast-feed. Staff are very good 'hunting for you if baby is in need of a feed'. One woman whose baby was crying said nurse tried to persuade her to give complementary feed 'as if it were the answer to everything'. Some staff are reluctant to wake mother at night to feed. Nursery is long way from wards.

Suggestions A writer who asked for pethidine late in first stage, was advised against it and told that 'it would not be long now' – she appreciated this and suggests that women should never be 'persuaded' to have pethidine against their better judgement and when they do not think they need it, which is what happened to other women in the hospital. After delivery a woman should be able to go into a single room with her baby and to sleep or lie cuddling the baby, as she wishes.

Morriston Hospital, Swansea, W Glamorgan   MO

Antenatal Women 'turn up in groups every 15 minutes'. Routine scans at 15–16 weeks. One woman said her partner was refused entry but another that radiographer developed negatives for her husband to see. Women say they had long wait to see consultant.

Labour Writers describe enema/shave and partner asked to leave for this and for internal examinations. Electronic fetal monitoring may be used. Women seemed to be expected to go to bed after being admitted. Some writers who wanted to sit up to push said they were not allowed to do so, though their partners could raise head and shoulders. 'In between contractions staff rushed to table on other side of room to write notes. Very distracting.' Episiotomies not done routinely. Baby can be put to breast on delivery bed.

Postnatal Baby goes to ward with mother, but may be then taken to nursery to be cleaned up. After return, is in cot by mother's bed throughout stay, unless she wishes baby to go to nursery at night. Mother looks after her baby after 6 hours. Staff are very busy and some writers said there was little or no help with breast-feeding. Night staff prefer babies to go to nursery rather than remain with mothers. Beds high and difficult to get on and off. Forty-eight-hour discharge can be arranged and writers strongly recommend this.

Suggestions A lactation sister.

Mount Pleasant, Swansea, W Glamorgan   MO

Main part of hospital converted Victorian workhouse, almost on top of steep hill. Very busy. No SCBU. If baby needs special care has to be moved to Morriston Hospital.

Antenatal 'Very pleasant' clinic building but according to some writers, 'inflexible attitudes' and 'fragmented' care. Little continuity. Some sad breakdowns in communication. Large proportion of doctors from overseas according to some writers. For scan, woman has to go to one of two other hospitals and this is 'inconvenient'. AFP tests not done routinely, despite high incidence of spina bifida in south Wales. Many women attending clinic come with toddlers; creche facilities. One writer said she felt she had to 'fight and argue and struggle every step of the way' not to be 'completely taken over'.

Labour Some writers had to wait a long time in waiting room when they were admitted in labour. One, who waited more than an hour, was then found to be 6 cm dilated. Enema given sometimes even in latter half of first stage. Pethidine seems to be given more or less routinely and in large doses. Some writers complained of 'medical hustling' and that labour was often accelerated with syntocin: 'My poor husband was so appalled by the sight of me covered in tubes and blood (heavy-handed injections and one nurse forgot about the drips and wrenched them out) . . . that he virtually passed out and couldn't stay for the delivery, which disappointed me very much.' Episiotomies not done routinely. Baby given to mother to suckle within 2–3 minutes of delivery.

Postnatal Writers deplore 'authoritarian' attitudes of some members of staff. Food 'awful'. Forty-eight-hour discharge can be arranged, but some writers said it was not easy to get discharge.

Suggestions Improve communication between women and doctors. Give more information, with greater accuracy and care, to women. Separate day rooms for smokers and non-smokers. Provide bidets and more bathrooms.

Scotland

Aberdeen Maternity Hospital, Forester Hill, Aberdeen MO

'Scrupulous attention to every aspect of birth.' Great interest in research and women as 'objects of research', with some notably caring people too.

Antenatal Waiting time nearly 1½ hours. Good playroom with supervisor where mothers can leave children. Usually see different doctor each time; all staff 'pleasant', but 'treat everyone as of little intelligence'; 'Male doctors do not understand that woman knows anything at all about her own body or whether labour is imminent.' Some women said there was not much opportunity to ask questions and discuss worries. Scans done. Several writers said they saw social worker on first visit. Shared care possible till late pregnancy and only visit hospital at that stage. Summerfield, auxiliary hospital, used for antenatal care; 'absolutely perfect'; 'marvellous nurses'. Antenatal ward in main hospital; many student midwives but some of them 'impersonal'. Obstetricians appear to have different and sometimes conflicting views on induction according to women. There seems to be a high induction rate and women indicate that it is done routinely for certain categories of women. 'Anyone due for induction was pumped full of Valium.' One woman said she was sent for induction three times, each time given enema and taken to delivery room, only to be told there was no room for her and she had to be returned to antenatal ward. She found this distressing.

Labour Husband can stay throughout. Student midwife sits with woman throughout if she wishes. Electronic fetal monitor seems to be used in most labours. One woman who objected to this because her labour was normal told doctor that she herself was born at home and says she was told 'You were lucky not to be brain-damaged.' Pethidine available, but if it is nearing end of first stage woman may be told not to have it. Other writers had it far too late and could not cooperate at the second stage. Midwives sometimes 'have all the knowledge but none of the experience, talk to each other and ignore woman in labour' according to one woman, herself a senior nurse. She says they 'do not tell mother of progress or encourage her'. It seems that ¾ hour is considered a normal limit of second stage and that woman is then given 'choice of forceps' if she has not delivered. Baby can be breast-fed in delivery room and sucking time not limited. Some women say they have been stitched with inadequate anaesthesia.

Postnatal care: Summerfield 'Impeccable care.' Daily visits from paediatrician.

Postnatal care: Aberdeen Breast-feeding 'approved of but not actively encouraged'. Some mothers felt they did not have enough time with their babies. Some writers found it difficult to get permission to contact by telephone relatives who lived far away. One woman from Shetland, who had her baby at

9 a.m., says she was not allowed to use phone to tell her husband till 7.30 p.m. But wards are 'friendly' and staff usually 'understanding' and 'flexible'. An unmarried woman was distressed at being asked if she wanted the baby adopted in middle of ward and about details of her relationship with father of child at dining-table; midwife and nurse 'most sympathetic' and 'calmed me down'. But some members of staff find it difficult to cope with experiences of loss and handicap; one woman, some of whose baby's organs were outside the body, was told of this by midwife who simply said, 'Your baby is deformed.' Lavatory and bathroom facilities 'not too new and not too clean'. Some breast-feeding mothers thought food was 'poor'.

Suggestions Reduce waiting time in antenatal clinic. Doctors should spend more time discussing birth. Make wards much more comfortable, with private rooms for those women who prefer them. Hospital staff should realize that baby is not their property – it belongs to mother and father. Women should be given longer notice of discharge; sometimes it is only about 2 hours.

Vale of Leven, Alexandria, Dumbartonshire   MO

Bright, modern, 'luxurious' with 'friendly attitudes'. 'Beginning to recognize that women have their own ideas . . .'

Antenatal Women coming from islands are booked in two days before EDD. Writers say practice is to induce 7 days after EDD, but in practice, if a mother came from far afield . . . she would be induced a day or two after arrival at the hospital. 'Most mothers accepted this rather than wait a week in hospital away from home and possibly other children.'

Labour Woman in one room throughout. Apparently routine mini-shave and suppository. Electronic fetal monitoring frequently used: 'Bandage holding on contraction transducer was painfully tight.' Partner can stay throughout. 'A doctor was automatically going to accelerate me (after 4 hours in labour) but made no objection when I said I would prefer not to be.' Student midwife may be with woman all the time. One woman who asked for pain relief said she had to wait 2 hours before she was examined 'because they were so busy'. She was then given 150 mg pethidine and was knocked out. Epidural Caesareans are done. Episiotomies seemed to be frequent. Baby is wrapped/face washed before being handed to mother or father. Mother can put baby to breast. Staff 'all friendly' and 'chatty'.

Postnatal Babies fed at 4-hourly intervals. 'I had written to the hospital in advance about rooming-in, complementary feeds and demand-feeding, and was told I could do it my way subject to medical considerations. I was the only mother who wanted her baby with her at night and I was told I would have to take it to the ward nursery . . . if he disturbed the other mothers.' Rule that babies are not allowed to feed in bed, but 'night staff turn blind eye to this'. Nurses very helpful in getting baby fixed on breast. Woman said that although she had been told that her baby would be brought to her for a feed at 6 a.m., 'they told me at 6 a.m. that he had already been fed . . . to check for abnormalities in his digestive system'. Normal practice to offer complementary feed but nurses supportive of women who want to do it their way: 'She said, "What do you think this place is, a concentration camp? He's your baby and you look after him the way you want to!"' Breast-feeding counsellor turns up occasionally, but not often enough to help mothers starting on breast-feeding. Staff 'generally friendly'. Hospital warm and food good. Views of Loch Lomond and Ben Lomond in the distance from some wards and labour suites. Common-room with television is full of smoke. Milk machine with as much milk as you want. At lunch and dinner three or four main course choices, always a salad, but little cooked green vegetables. Endless hot water and bidet with warm spray: mothers can pick up their babies whenever they want but are not supposed to carry them around or sit on the beds with them. 'A determined mother wanting to demand-feed could have done so if she quickly got the hang of the ward routines, meals, when the baths were likely to be free, staff nurses' rounds, doctors' rounds and found when her presence was needed.' Food kept hot for mothers who were late. Visiting every evening and some afternoons; children allowed two afternoons. Husbands from a distance can see their wives at any time and sit outside ward. Visitors not supposed to pick up babies, but some fathers do, 'and no one said anything'. Feeding not allowed during visiting hours, but a mother can always feed her baby in ward nursery.

SCBU Unrestricted visiting by parents.

Suggestions Breast-feeding mothers should be visited by breast-feeding counsellor within first 2 days of delivery. Breast-feeding mothers should be encouraged to suckle more frequently.

Ninewells Hospital, Menzies Hill, Dundee

Very modern; 'friendly atmosphere'; 'a go-ahead hospital'. Takes problem cases from wide area.

Antenatal Waiting area always full, but there is one clinic in suburbs visited by hospital doctors. Antenatal ward 'very relaxed', 'friendly nurses'; 'no do's and don'ts'. Food 'very good'. Heating sometimes turned up too high. Women say induction is done for specific medical reasons, but is sometimes done when mothers ask for it.

Labour No shaving. Staff 'very helpful throughout'. Epidurals available and Caesareans can be done with epidural and partner present. Electronic monitoring may be used. Single labour/delivery rooms and woman does not have to be moved. Partner can stay for forceps delivery. Midwives skilled at avoiding episiotomy and need for stitches.

Postnatal True demand-feeding, and no time limits. Mothers encouraged to breast-feed whenever necessary at night. Baby only moved from bedside at mother's request. Visiting flexible if mother has single room. Some women deliver here and move to local GP unit for later postnatal care (following day if all well).

SCBU Nurses 'understanding'. Unrestricted visiting by mother. 'My baby was in SCBU and I just had to lie there looking at the other mothers with their babies, which was very upsetting.' Some nurses on ward did not realize that baby was not with her and handed her bottles. 'I felt more or less ignored by the nurses who were busy with the mothers with their babies.'

Suggestions Community midwives should deliver in hospital and take women home after a few hours.

Eastern General, Seafield Street, Edinburgh

'Friendly little hospital'; 'not glamorous'. Because most women come from a wide geographical area, most antenatal care shared with GPs. Consultant clinics also at Haddington, Kelso and Galashiels. Most women have scan at first visit. All offered screening for spina bifida.

Antenatal Visits involved long waits, but staff, from receptionist up, 'helpful and friendly'. Some writers saw same doctor on almost every occasion. Questions answered fully and explanations given: 'I was in a position to make informed decisions about my own labour.' Women say they were fully consulted about proposal to induce; induction appears to be done for 'older primigravidas' 1 week after EDD. Younger mothers may get '2 weeks' grace'. Induction rate 22%. Six antenatal classes, 'excellent course' run by antenatal sister, with physiotherapists and consultants. Parentcraft taught by paediatrician stresses value of breast-feeding.

Labour DNO writes, 'Care during labour is as individualized as possible. All procedures are explained beforehand . . . No one is pressurized to take drugs if they don't want to.' Suppositories/half shave. Fetal scalp monitor may be put on. One woman with unripe cervix and very long induced labour says prostaglandin gel to soften cervix overnight was not used. Woman has single room through labour and delivery. Partner can be with her throughout, but is asked to go out when she is cleaned up afterwards. Teamaking facilities for husbands. Epidurals available. Women can ask for them, but anaesthetist not always available. One writer with epidural wrote, 'I was like something out of science fiction with oxytocin and glucose drip, intrauterine catheter, bladder catheter and fetal monitor.' 15% of women have epidurals. Pethidine or diamorphine also offered. Woman may push with partner holding one leg against his hip and midwife holding other; 'lots of encouragement and cheers'. Baby delivered on to mother's abdomen. Father can cuddle baby. Several women described baby going to nursery shortly after.

Postnatal Breast-feeding and bottle-feeding on demand. 'Complementary feeding discouraged', DNO says, 'No test-weighing unless there is a positive indication.' Baby stays in nursery for few hours, then 6 a.m. to 10 p.m. with mother and to nursery for night. DNO writes that 'night staff ascertain mothers' wishes regarding night feeds'. Some women said babies were given bottles in nursery; but you can ask to be wakened for night feeds. DNO says that 'if a mother is very keen to have her baby with her throughout the 24 hours, she will be put in a single or two-bedded room'. One mother said senior registrar brought baby to her after difficult labour and sister made toast and tea when she woke. Staff 'helpful', 'kind', 'nothing too much trouble'. Give physical and emotional nursing when necessary. 'We were not treated as ill.' DNO writes that 'husbands are encouraged to handle baby at all times'. Food 'institutional but acceptable'. Women seem usually to have 5–6 days' stay. Husbands may visit any time. Other visiting 3–4 p.m. and 7–8.30 p.m. Own children welcome.

Suggestions Mothers would have liked much more upright position for second stage.

★★ Simpson Memorial Maternity Pavilion, Lauriston Place, Edinburgh MO

Large unit in 'oldish' building, but clean and bright. 'Once you get used to it, a very friendly place'; several writers were very surprised at the atmosphere, including one who admitted she was 'very nervous of hospitals'. Staff 'efficient' and 'skilled'.

Antenatal 'Very helpful' staff, 'always willing to explain procedures'. AFP testing done and ultrasound used frequently. See one of two doctors, so good continuity; 'treated in human and understanding way'. 'Doctors seem interested in you, even though your pregnancy is normal.' In early pregnancy woman may be asked if she wants to book epidural, but it is 'not pressed'. Waiting ¾ hour·plus. Waiting-room is corridor with chairs facing changing cubicle. New patients have to sit in their gowns, which are very short, among other clothed patients. Nurses stay and chat rather than leave a mother alone in cubicle. Some 2-hour waits to see consultant. Induction seems to be fairly frequent. Prostaglandin pessaries are used to ripen cervix overnight if necessary, but some women describe painful amniotomy with unripe cervix. And some describe a very high dosage of oxytocin. Helpful evening classes; fathers encouraged.

Labour If woman is induced overnight, midwife 'pops in with cup of tea' if mother awake and makes her more comfortable. Inductions take place in small side ward, two or three women together. In morning membranes ruptured in labour ward. Staff ask woman when she wants her husband phoned. After some hours oxytocin drip. Highly competent midwives reassure, encourage, praise if woman wants to manage without pain-relieving drugs; never left without midwife for more than 5 minutes. When teaching of midwives takes place in labour, couple are involved in it. Partner never sent out. 'A great deal of support from every member of staff.' Drugs not 'pushed', but woman is asked if she would like epidural. Apparently diamorphine is used for pain relief. Woman is offered extra pillows. 'Every technical aid was available, but you can decline electronic monitoring.' Even after waters have broken some women are encouraged to walk about to get labour going well. Writers ate honey during labour. One woman, with backache labour, said nursing officer experimented with pillows to get her comfortable and turned her on her side with pillow for her 'drip hand' – 'sheer bliss!' – and stayed to chat. Woman is in same room for labour and delivery. Pushing encouraged and woman is given 'running commentary'. Iced water to sip with bendy straw between contractions, and cold flannel on face. Given baby to hold immediately after birth. Baby who needs resuscitation is taken away, but brought back by paediatrician who explains what has been done and reassures parents. 'Senior registrar popped in to say "Well done and see you on the ward."' Great care in making woman comfortable to be stitched. Couple have time alone together. Midwife who did delivery takes woman to postnatal ward, where she is welcomed by sister. Partner can go too to help her into bed and unpack. Baby brought and can be put to breast.

Postnatal All staff 'kind' and 'reassuring'. Baby may be kept in nursery first two nights, roomed in during day. Breast-feeding on demand encouraged, but bottle-feeders were given good help. Breast-feeders and bottle-feeders not separated. Dextrose may be offered, but is not 'pushed'. Most people felt they had plenty of help with breast-feeding but some first-time mothers said help was not always available when they needed it. Atmosphere 'cheerful', 'free and easy', 'casual'. A genuine feeling of concern and helpfulness from all staff. 'Never felt just another patient'; 'felt individual'. Nurses talked to babies while handling them and called them by name. Staff busy, but 'will always stop to answer questions'. Nurses check on babies beside mothers' beds during breakfast, so there is chance to talk and ask questions then. Mother can care for baby in her own way. No set lights-out: 'You could stay up all night if you wanted.' Baby can be put in nursery overnight if mother wishes; nurse will fetch her when baby wakes for feed. 'They offer to take baby into nursery the night before you go home so that you can get good sleep.' TV room 'very smokey'. Some women say there are poor toilet facilities. Occasionally, when wards are full, writers say there is no salt for baths, no early tea or late-night drinks. Food 'sometimes fairly good, sometimes disgusting'; plenty of choice; always salad and two other dishes. Food kept hot if feeding. Good physiotherapy and 'very nice physiotherapists'. Visiting at 2 p.m. and 8 p.m. A father travelling a long distance is allowed in at other times too. Women sometimes found it exhausting when a visitor came. Nurses 'very perceptive in removing a visitor who has stayed too long'; chat with husbands and grannies. Some writers said exit from hospital was rushed and this made them anxious: 'I was not told when I would go home until the actual moment, which made it rather a hectic exit.'

Suggestions More showers and bidets needed.

Western General, Crewe Road, Edinburgh   HO

Antenatal Most women have scans. Amniocentesis offered to all women over 35. Induction rate 22%. DNO writes: 'Open forum evening sessions, conducted by consultant obstetrician, consultant paediatrician and nursing officer, for expectant parents, continue to be very popular.' Antenatal ward also used for postnatal patients.

Labour DNO writes that 'individual care is given as far as possible. Minimal perineal shaving, omitted . . . if any objection is raised. Routine enema is not' given. Husbands are welcomed and facilities are offered to them to make tea or coffee in the sitting-room. Pethidine or diamorphine offered to patients but can be refused. Not sufficient anaesthetist cover for "on demand" service for epidurals.' Epidural rate 8%; forceps 14%; Caesarean 13%.

Postnatal DNO says that 'staff are enthusiastic about breast-feeding and there is policy of demand-feeding. Husbands are welcome into nurseries. But ward areas are not large enough to allow sufficient space to room in babies with their mothers. Husbands may visit at any time; other visiting is 3–4 p.m. and 7.15–8.30 p.m. Own children may come at visiting hours or at other times by arrangement with the ward sister.'

Glasgow Royal, Rottenrow, Glasgow

DNO writes, 'In the edition of 1979 the write-up for the hospital is unfavourable and, while I may admit that this may have been true at that time, the circumstances have dramatically changed to meet the 1980s.' Old building.

Antenatal DNO writes that 'aim is to cut the waiting time and to deliver a more personalized type of care and so midwives' clinics are in operation. Discussion . . . between patient and midwife regarding their participation in labour and their choice of type of milk feeds for baby takes place.' Hospital-based midwives work in community and so meet women antenatally. Doctors give time for discussion and note down women's personal birth plans. 'Day area, where patients come for continuous assessment and monitoring on a daily basis and return to their home in the evening if they are satisfactory.' Programme of talks and evening films for couples. Cassettes shown in pre-natal classes and on antenatal wards. On ward handicraft teacher also employed.

Labour Induction rate 35–38%; augmentation (oxytocin) 14%. DNO writes that 'patient participation welcome during labour and husbands involved and present throughout. Good nurse/patient contact and bonding of family unit is in focus.' Woman in single room and not moved during labour. Woman is *asked* whether she wants waters broken. Epidurals available on request. 'Forceps rate 25%; Caesareans 15%. DNO says, 'modified Leboyer-type of delivery available if requested'. Episiotomy figures not available. Birth chair available.

Postnatal DNO writes, 'Emphasis . . . is on a relaxed, friendly atmosphere for mother and baby, where bonding is incurred. Feeding with breast and bottle is on demand . . . on-going programme of mothercraft education . . . visiting times are very fluid and families are allowed to cuddle and fondle their baby.'

SCBU 'The aim here is to open the area for parents and relatives.' And mothers are encouraged to be fully involved with their babies.

The Queen Mother's Hospital, York Hill, Glasgow   MO

Antenatal 'Long waits most days' and clinic tends to be very hot. No gowns provided unless going for ultrasound: 'It would have been nice if we'd been asked to bring a cotton nightie to wear in cubicle while waiting.' Can ask questions 'if you are determined and insistent on not being rushed'. No facilities for children. On first visit sister explains everything in privacy of her office. Classes 'very good', 'informative'.

Labour Mini-prep; enema not used routinely. Partner can be present throughout and writers say their questions are answered readily. Never left alone. Everyone 'chatty', 'friendly'. Tea/coffee provided for partner. Women may be held up in admission and this seems to be badly organized sometimes: 'I was on hard, narrow couch in admissions for 2 hours waiting for doctor to come to admit me officially . . . very uncomfortable.' Pethidine offered and midwife says, 'I used to feel staff bullied women into having it'; epidurals available, midwife can top up. Writers describe intravenous infusions. Midwives do not always anticipate needs, so *ask* for ice or whatever you want. Some fathers are asked to go outside for forceps delivery, but can come back in as soon as head delivered. Can be there while placenta delivered and stitching done. Father can then go with midwife to see baby checked over and weighed.

Postnatal Well organized, and plenty of help with breast-feeding. Mother looks after baby herself. Baby is 'never carted off to nursery'. One midwife from hospital feels that some mothers are left to get on with it when they could do with more practical help. Looking back on her experience she says advice given was 'all text-book stuff . . . when I think of what I used to say!'; but writers say 'married staff with families gave great support and loads of useful tips' and are 'helpful', 'friendly'. Relaxed atmosphere. Busy nights. Writers consider physiotherapy exercises very good. Food 'deplorable'; 'lots of wee cups of tea and cocoa' between meals.

Suggestions Creche in antenatal clinic. Reduce long waits. Turn down heating. Install wider couches in admission suite. More baths needed on postnatal wards.

St Francis Maternity Home, Merryland Street, Govan, Glasgow   MO

Private maternity home. Old-fashioned building next to church, but care by sister and other staff 'makes up for surroundings'.

Antenatal Clinics 1.30–3.30 p.m. No appointment necessary: 'You just turn up and join the queue'. Long waits, but 'relaxed, friendly atmosphere'. Doctors are GPs. Will answer questions and 'there's no stripping off'.

Labour Appreciate sisters already knowing who they are when they go in in labour. Can wear own nightdress. Pethidine may be advised for relaxation. 'A holy medal was placed on my neck.' Husband encouraged to do back-rubbing and couples like 'being left to get on with it ourselves'. Woman who had elective Caesarean said she had no enema and only very small shave; pre-med. in her own room, then to labour ward, her husband sitting with her all the time; then to theatre where she could hold her own oxygen mask and anaesthetist explained everything. In second stage woman may be asked to push with her legs supported by sisters and her husband gives her gas and oxygen. Sisters expert at avoiding episiotomy. Woman who had section had her husband sitting beside her when she came round from general anaesthetic and he told her about baby. At normal delivery baby may be left between mother's legs for a few minutes and then taken to be wrapped up and back for cuddle.

Postnatal Baby kept in nursery. Fed bottle at night; feeds every 4 hours during day described by mothers. But some mothers went to nursery to give babies extra feed. Relaxed atmosphere; sisters 'kind' and whole emphasis on mother's rest. 'It is like a big, happy family.' Food 'good'. Visiting 11 a.m. to noon husbands only, 3–4 p.m., 7–8 p.m. If all is well 48-hour discharge can be arranged.

Southern General, Govan Road, Glasgow   MO

Spacious, airy, 'lovely' hospital.

Antenatal Doctors and midwives 'always busy but willing to answer questions'. But you do have to ask, or you may simply be told that everything is all right.

Labour Partner can stay, 'is made welcome by all', and provided with coffee. Woman has her own room for labour and delivery: 'Midwife made me feel like an individual and gave wonderful support throughout labour.' This is high-tech hospital though and 'all possible aids' are employed. Continuous electronic monitoring may be used and epidurals given so that labour can be accelerated. Caesarean sections done under epidural. One woman who had epidural Caesarean says she was able to touch baby before cord cut or placenta removed. Her husband, however, was not able to be present.

Postnatal Short-staffed, but plenty of help with breast-feeding. Woman whose epidural was spinal by mistake said she had severe headaches after and nurses did all they could to support her psychologically, look after baby for her and help with breast-feeding. Writers would have liked to have been better informed about babies' health. One woman, whose baby was in nursery, said, 'You have to assume no news is good news.' Smoking and non-smoking sitting-rooms. Food 'absolutely dreadful'; 'good food badly prepared and unattractively presented'; 'in no way entices woman with poor appetite to eat', and writers say it is cold after long journey from central kitchen. Plenty of baths/bidets. Waiting-room for visitors; only two allowed at each bed. This is not strictly adhered to, unless in woman's interest.

Suggestions Paediatric examination should always be done in mother's presence. Improve food and serve hot.

Stobhill General, Glasgow   MO

Big, up-to-date teaching hospital with 'heavy turnover of staff' and 'charming SNO'.

Antenatal Consultants 'interested', 'willing to answer questions' and some writers liked them very much. Care with GP possible; booking visit only at hospital, described as 'tedious'. Mothercraft classes run by 'efficient' sister, with 'good breathing exercises, but no liaison with labour ward staff'. Antenatal ward 'boring' but 'restful'; 'day is long'. 'Very good, pleasant nurses.' Sonicaid available and mother can hear her baby's heart. Visiting every afternoon and evening and own children welcome.

Labour Several writers thought that labour ward staff tended to wait for signs of distress as indications of progress and did not always know how advanced in labour a woman was. Electronic fetal monitoring used: 'It was faulty and not registering contractions . . . they believed the machine,' wrote a woman who was in strong labour and almost fully dilated. 'As I puffed and panted, midwife and auxiliary were discussing the latter's husband's pending redundancy.' The writer found this disturbing. Woman has to be wheeled to different room for delivery. Midwives described as authoritarian in second stage: 'Now you are going to behave yourself and do what I tell you and I won't have to cut you.' You can ask to see your baby's head as it is born and midwife lifts you up. Baby wrapped in towel and placed on mother's abdomen immediately.

Postnatal All babies go to nursery first 2–3 nights, but you can ask to be woken to feed. Excellent help with breast-feeding. Enormous varieties of nationalities amongst nursing staff apparently and some women cannot understand their accents. 'Extremely noisy' at nights on open-plan ward for spontaneous vaginal deliveries. Women woken at 5.30 a.m.: 'by the time I got back home I was exhausted'. One woman who found it difficult to sleep said, 'Some of night staff do not bother to lower their voices' and that mothers' rest hour in afternoon is 'a mockery'. Rule that 6 a.m. feed must be given by mother sitting *beside* bed and 10 a.m. feed *in* bed according to writers (1980). Breast-feeding mothers can have milk at any time. They say lavatories are not always clean, have no locks so doors do not close. 'You must throw your dressing-gown over door to let others know it is occupied.' 'Sleeping pills handed out like

Smarties', but breast-feeding mothers may refuse them. Food 'OK', 'not brilliant', 'surprisingly good considering numbers they cater for'.

Suggestions More liaison between sister teaching antenatal classes and labour ward staff. Reduce noise on postnatal ward. Improve lavatory, bath and shower facilities.

Ian Charles, Grantown-on-Spey, Moray HO

GP unit. Specialist unit 36 miles away. Nursing officer writes, 'Our unit is very well equipped, airy, light and peaceful, and the mothers who come to it find it quite a haven.'

Antenatal Relaxation and parentcraft classes available.

Labour Partner can be present. Occasional episiotomy and low-cavity forceps. But mostly normal deliveries.

Postnatal Nursing officer writes, 'Babies are with mothers all of the time, but not during the night unless the mother wishes to have the baby beside her.' She says 'It is easier for women to master the art of breast-feeding . . . as they can have almost individual nursing attention.' Women are transferred here from consultant unit for postnatal care and 'the mums are always glad of the peace and quiet of our maternity unit'. 'Husbands are encouraged to bring the other children, if any, to see mother and baby and maintain the family unit.'

Forth Park, Bennochy Road, Kirkcaldy, Fife MO

Bright, modern, busy teaching hospital, 'cheerful atmosphere', 'efficient staff' and 'high standards of care', in very pleasant surroundings.

Antenatal Long waits in clinics and some doctors 'very rushed'. Consultants described as 'patient', 'generous with time'. Everyone 'very helpful' and 'ready to work *with* me'. Antenatal care can be shared with GP. 'Good' relaxation classes and parentcraft talk on breast-feeding. Antenatal ward, in oldest part of hospital, is 'depressing', 'no windows and grey walls'. Writers felt lack of contact with outside world, lack of information contributing to anxiety. One woman compared it to police interrogation build-up. Said questions 'tend to be phrased rhetorically rather than inquiringly: 'A friendly stranger pops her head round a door saying, "No problems?" or "Slept well, did you?"' '

Labour She believes that such an environment institutionalizes women and prepares them for hospital takeover in labour: 'I let routine overwhelm me, the surroundings sapped me of my own emotional energy.' Writers felt that birth was something done *to* them rather than something they did for themselves and wished they could have been more involved. Women report seeing many different members of staff during labour. Drip to accelerate seems to be used frequently and may be set up without explanation: 'Doctors talked to one another, not me.' Ask if you want information and, if necessary, demand it, writers advise. Writers said they were alone much of labour: 'The bed was narrow and uncomfortable and I felt pinned down by the drip'; 'I felt I should almost apologize for being there.' They felt there was lack of personal contact between staff and women. Woman may be given pethidine without being told what it is or does, since it is put in drip. Mother is helped to sit up to see head at delivery.

Postnatal Breast-feeding has become much more flexible and there is postnatal support for breast-feeding mothers (1980). Writers felt they had too little information about their baby's health and say there was 'inadequate communication'. Mothers of jaundiced babies have been 'climbing the walls'. One is very much aware of being part of a system: 'Sometimes it is difficult to communicate emotional needs, even to sympathetic but busy staff'; 'Doctor whizzed round without actually talking to patients.' Writers stress it is very important to ask questions and say what you want. Nurses 'pleasant'.

SCBU One writer said she was not allowed to see her baby except at feeding times for first few days.

Postnatal check-up A woman who was depressed felt she could not say how awful she felt when faced by doctor, nurse and students, altogether six people, saying, 'No problems, are there?'

Suggestions Women should be able to feel they are more in control of their own labours. Postnatal check-up should not be 'public'.

Oban Hospital, Oban, Argyll   MO

Small, 'friendly' cottage hospital. Woman in labour may be with mothers who have had their babies.

Antenatal Classes 'not much help'.

Labour Midwives 'kind' but 'something of the atmosphere of boarding school'. Pethidine offered. It seems that large doses may be given; one woman says her mind was 'a complete blank' after. One woman in labour with three other newly delivered women longed for privacy, tried not to toss and turn or find more comfortable position, or even breathe in an audible way, because she was afraid of keeping other people awake.

Postnatal Lovely views. One bed in each ward in an enormous bay window overlooking Oban bay and westward to Isle of Mull. Baby can be with mother most of time. Conflicting advice given about breast-feeding. One said midwife advised her to avoid fruit and juices and another said it did not matter what she ate. Fathers, according to writers, only allowed to peer at babies through glass (1979). (Apparently there was a problem with a drunken father, so all fathers are treated as alcoholics.)

Paisley

Paisley Hospital, Corsebar Road, Paisley, Renfrew

Bright, modern in very attractive surroundings.

Antenatal Midwives 'friendly', 'helpful'; doctors welcome questions and are 'willing to discuss things'. 'One is always told why something is being done.' Ultrasound scan. Induction rate is still 30%; one woman described going 4 weeks past her original date and 2 weeks past revised date (after ultrasound). She says she asked not to be induced 'and the consultant was most understanding and sympathetic'. Daily oestriol tests done. Women who have been induced say they have not felt pressured. Antenatal classes 'helpful' and 'practical', but not much encouragement for breast-feeding and 'relaxation could have been much better taught'. Antenatal ward is 'pleasant'.

Labour Partner present throughout and made to feel welcome. One writer who was induced said she had ARM and asked to wait for a few hours to see if labour started without oxytocin drip, and this was agreed. One woman writes, 'every request for an epidural is considered and granted depending on the limitations of the anaesthetic service'. Doctors who come in are occasionally 'off-hand', 'tend to talk about you as if you weren't there'. Episiotomies not done routinely. Women said their babies were taken away for several hours after delivery.

Postnatal Mother can have baby with her by bedside all time except first night: 'But I didn't sleep anyway and ended up by going to the nursery to see how she was.' If baby does not settle can be taken to nursery if mother asks. Can breast-feed at night and if baby is in nursery someone will wake her when baby cries. Can feed whenever and wherever she wants to. DNO says that 43% of mothers leave hospital breast-feeding fully. Advise taking complete charge of own baby and going ahead with breast-feeding without consulting staff. 'Marked distinction between antenatal and postnatal wards . . . antenatal wards are much more relaxed. On postnatal ward staff are very concerned with routines.' Writers advise mothers not to be intimidated and suggest ignoring rules. If you do need help mothercraft sisters are 'marvellous' in helping with breast-feeding. 'One thing that upset me a lot was that I was sleeping in bed right next to the nursery and could hear the babies crying all night . . . the nurses ignored the babies completely. I could hear their comments, "You be quiet, it's not time for you to be fed yet"; "There's nothing wrong with him."' Bidets 'super'. DNO writes that 'in response from requests from patients, their children are now allowed to visit at all visiting times and by special arrangement at other times to meet individual circumstances'. Forty-eight-hour stay can be arranged.

Suggestions More relaxed atmosphere on postnatal wards, with less emphasis on routines.

Perth Royal Infirmary, Western Avenue, Perth

Cheerful, modern, very clean and SNO writes, 'We go out of our way to meet any special requests by patients.'

Antenatal SNO writes that 'all patients have full ultrasound screening'. One writer says that clinic is 'appalling in its distaste for toddlers . . . no suitable toys or books . . . one is segregated from the main waiting area'. SNO says that 'induction of labour rate is very low', but does not say what it is. Some women say that induction was done for no obvious reason on day baby was 'due'. Prostin used to ripen cervix: 'I was put under considerable pressure and didn't dare refuse.' Relaxation and parentcraft teaching programme and classes well attended. Visit to labour ward incorporated. Partners encouraged to attend.

Antenatal ward: staff 'pleasant', 'friendly', but some women said it was extremely difficult to get enough information and 'felt there was something drastically wrong about which I was not being told'. Some writers comment that some women got very depressed on antenatal ward.

Labour Writers describe full shave but at least one mother 'pleaded' for partial one. Writers say that when community midwives deliver their wishes are usually respected and mother can choose whether or not she has pain-relieving drugs. SNO says that monitoring equipment is very modern and is used 'when necessary'. Several writers describe being put on drip 'to get things going' once labour had started, without reasons for this being clearly given. Writers said they had 'strong encouragement' to have epidural; when one woman said 'No thank you,' and that she didn't want pethidine either unless felt necessary, she said doctors on round laughed at her. One writer who said she did not need any drugs 'at that time' said she felt her confidence threatened when midwife exclaimed: 'Oh, you want to conduct your own labour, do you?' Some writers had pethidine at end of first stage. Overall impression is that staff do not seem to have developed skill, for the most part, to help women trust their own bodies. Some women who are far from their own homes and have no companion especially need encouragement.

Second stage: hard, quick, repeated pushing may be advocated. SNO says that episiotomies are performed when necessary, others suggest they are done frequently. Leboyer-style delivery can be arranged and baby given to mother to hold immediately, according to writers. SNO writes, 'Bonding is encouraged from birth although it is now thought that, with the use of ultrasound a bond is established as soon as pregnancy is confirmed on scan.'

Postnatal Writers agree that there is lots of help with breast-feeding and that no complementary feeds are given. Women in amenity beds can feed on demand. One writer said that the babies were wheeled out if they cried during visiting times: 'I nearly went distracted hearing my baby cry.' Criticizing what she called 'antediluvian' attitudes, one woman said senior member of staff 'saw my light on at 4 a.m. and barged in to find me and the baby in bed together. (She had been feeding and fell asleep with me holding her.) ''What do you think *you're* doing?"' Women say they are told they should be resting if they are feeding or cuddling baby at night: 'They couldn't appreciate that I needed intimate contact with baby.' 'All wards, like clinic, grossly overheated.' Women say windows do not provide enough ventilation. 'No smoking' notices are not enforced and women say they were 'surrounded by fug'. There also seems to be a general feeling that there is not enough time for resting. Everyone agrees that 'all staff are very fond of babies'. Food is 'excellent'. One woman suggests that visiting hours are badly timed.

Suggestions Less reliance on technology and more help for giving birth naturally. Turn heat down a few degrees.

★ Daliburgh, South Uist, Western Isles   MO

'Ideal place to have a baby or go for a holiday.' Lovely views.

Atenatal If mother lives far from hospital she waits in it from time when baby due till actual birth.

Labour Induction may be offered, but if she says she is not keen, 'staff enthusiastically support her decision and it is not mentioned again'. 'Doctor reassured me that he had never seen a truly postmature baby.' 'Staff believe in no interference of any kind unless absolutely necessary.' Women can labour without drugs for pain relief if they wish, and can be up and about till they feel they prefer to be in bed: 'I really felt that the midwife was sharing in the experience with me.' Writers describe sitting up for delivery, midwives skilled at avoiding episiotomies and stitches. Mother given baby to hold and feed if she wishes. Father can hold baby too and can go to watch baby being bathed. (Why can't baby be bathed beside mother?)

Postnatal Each mother can decide what she wants to do with her baby. Encouraged to leave baby in nursery at night, welcome to feed if she wants to. Staff may suggest not feeding baby first 2 nights and giving artificial milk instead. One writer says this is a bad idea as it does not give enough stimulation to milk production. However, 'nobody forces anything on you'. Can pick up and cuddle baby and husbands are often given meals if they arrive at meal times. Fathers can help with looking after babies. Woman is not woken till 8 a.m. unless baby is crying and there is plenty of time to rest. Flexible visiting hours, visitors are welcomed and given cup of tea.

Stirling Royal Infirmary, Stirling   MO

'Efficient', 'well-organized' and staff 'very friendly'.

Antenatal Women say they often have to wait for up to 2 hours to be examined and doctors turn up late. Staff 'pleasant'. Parentcraft classes 'helpful', and include breathing.

Labour Most staff 'marvellous', but some 'authoritarian younger midwives'. Writers say there are too many examinations, often during contractions. Partner welcome and can be present throughout; 'is made to feel useful'. Women describe human monitoring in straightforward labours, rather than electronic monitoring. One writer said that young, inexperienced nurse told her to breathe deeply so as not to push (which would, in fact, stimulate pushing urge) while she was trying to pant: 'I did not feel happy left alone with her and demanded she get someone else.'

Postnatal Baby at mother's bedside 24 hours in 'very pleasant' wards. There is every encouragement to breast-feed, though writers say there are conflicting opinions. 'I was pleased to get home to listen to only one baby crying, do my own thing and not be upset by nurses telling me baby could not be fed for 2 hours at a stretch.' Women say there are far too many interruptions in early morning: 'noisy cleaners and nurses'; 'some auxiliaries seem to make as much noise as possible at 5 a.m. emptying bins'. Bidets appreciated. Food 'very good'. Hospital stay of 10 days considered too long.

Suggestions More consideration from some staff with understanding of distress caused by constant noise. Look again at early morning routines and the effect they can have on a mother who has been up all night with baby or awake listening to three others.

Eire

Erinville, Cork

Antenatal breast-feeding class and tour of labour ward.

Labour Women describe labouring without an enema or shave. The mother can have drugs for pain relief or not, as she wishes. Some writers would have preferred not to have had to lie down: 'I was asked to lie down on the delivery bed. The next contraction hit me like a vice grip as it was the first one I had had lying down.' Some writers objected strongly to being surrounded by a chorus of cheer-leaders: 'Nurses started piling in until there were about a half dozen standing around me . . . every time I started pushing all the nurses shouted "Push" in a chorus and in between shouting at me the rest of them were gossiping among themselves. I was lying on my back which caused me a lot of pain.' Several writers described intravenous oxytocin drip. Partner can be present all the time. Baby can be delivered straight on to mother's abdomen and cord not clamped or cut till it has stopped pulsating. One writer said her husband cut the cord. Some writers said they were not encouraged to breast-feed on delivery table and hospital gown made this difficult. Baby goes to ward with mother on trolley.

Postnatal Policy of rooming-in during day. At night babies are in nursery across hall from wards: 'The babies were screaming. Their distress was terrible and I could still hear their crying in my mind when I went home.' Writers say feeding is on 4-hourly schedule. 'I asked that my baby be brought to me at night. He was brought once the first night but not at all the second. I was unable to sleep worrying about him.' Several writers said they did not get much help with breast-feeding. One was told to let her baby cry if she thought he had had enough. Beds are 'high and narrow' and armchairs beside them 'hard and uncomfortable'. This makes it difficult to cuddle babies. Very 'utilitarian' interior decoration and furniture. 'The worst aspect was the noise. Every sound was magnified by the shiny surfaces. I couldn't sleep for the noise . . . By the time I got home I was shattered by the lack of sleep.' Visiting: 2 hours in afternoon and evening. Children not allowed, even in hall downstairs, apparently. Food 'not too good' for public patients, but 'very good, appetizing and nutritious' for private patients. Forty-eight-hour discharge can be arranged. One writer said she wrote to matron a few months after birth suggesting improvements but did not receive any reply.

Our Lady of Lourdes Hospital, Drogheda, County Louth

Voluntary hospital run by nuns, Medical Missionaries of Mary.

Antenatal Questions all answered and mothers say they do not feel rushed. Helpful antenatal classes, but held in afternoons so husbands cannot go. Tour of delivery suite, SCBU, newborn nursery, admission room and procedures explained.

Labour During admission procedures husband must stay in waiting room. Only one consultant allows fathers at delivery. Full shave. Soapy water enema routinely given, but some women choose to have suppositories instead. Membranes not routinely ruptured. Midwives 'cheerful' and each woman is assigned her personal midwife. 'The nurse sat on one side and V. was on the other and we chatted in between.' Mothers encouraged to walk around in first stage. Epidurals not available. If you want more pillows in delivery, ask for them. Mothers can deliver sitting up, legs flopped apart. Episiotomies not routinely done. Mother may not be allowed to hold her baby immediately after delivery. May only be handed baby already 'bundled up', after stitching completed. Partner asked to leave until after stitching. Baby to newborn nursery after parents have some time together.

Postnatal Baby stays beside mother all day, except for visiting hour of 4–5 p.m.; 7–9 p.m. for fathers only: 'I really enjoyed this time together. He got to know the baby before we got home.' At night baby is taken to nursery after last feed. Is brought to mother during night if breast-fed. Breast-feeding on demand: 'I never felt under any pressure to feed my baby at a certain time, or time how long.' But bottle of glucose appears at each feeding time. Mother need not give it. Babies are test-weighed 24 hours before mother goes home. 'This can cause great anxiety which can affect milk supply.'

Food lacking in roughage, though salads available. Writers advise getting fruit brought in. Last paediatric examination takes place in mother's presence, when she can ask questions. Children not allowed to visit, though they can be taken to waiting-room and mother can go down to them there. Forty-eight-hour discharge is 'just not on'.

Suggestion Stop doing full pubic shave. Fathers should be welcome not only during labour but also at delivery and at forceps delivery. More and better bathrooms needed. Include more fibre in diet. Visitors should never be allowed to smoke in postnatal ward. Children should be able to see and cuddle their new brother/sister every day.

The Coombe Lying-in, Cork Street, Dolphin's Barn, Dublin 8

Just off South Circular, modern buildings. Same doctor seen in antenatal clinic, but only after 32 weeks.

Labour Partners welcome. Women say they were put to bed on admission in a cubicle divided by curtains from others. Soap and water enema was given, it appears routinely, and perineal shave. Some were told that it was policy to rupture membranes on admission. They were offered standard dose of Pethilorphan, 150 mg, but mother may decline this. The master, in letter to an expectant mother, writes that: 'About 95% of couples are together, though the father may not be present if a problem arises' and 'occasionally if the labour ward gets very overcrowded'. 5% of women have epidurals; 17% electronic fetal monitoring. Woman is moved from labour to delivery room at second stage. Semi-reclining position for delivery with pillows. The master says 'We do not use the Leboyer method but . . . we do believe in gentle birth . . . the baby is usually given to the mother as soon as she delivers . . . The cord is clamped and cut immediately after delivery. Mothers who wish to suckle the baby immediately after birth may do so.' Fathers present if they wish and can be present for simple forceps delivery. Episiotomies not performed routinely. Mother and baby have time together in post-labour room, but then routinely separated for several hours. Babies under 5½ lb go to special care unit.

Postnatal 33% of mothers breast-feed. Two nurses work with breast-feeding mothers. Breast-feeding on demand allowed but not encouraged. Baby has to go to nursery at night unless mother is in single room, but she can ask to be woken to breast-feed if she wishes. Non-smoking wards were introduced a few years ago but some visitors and mothers ignore signs. Cigarettes no longer sold in hospital shops. Visiting: 1 hour in afternoon and 1 hour in evening, but flexible. Sibling visiting has been introduced on Sunday afternoons, though this is flexible for those travelling from the country. First-time mothers kept in for 6 days, others for 5 days, though when there is overcrowding this may be shortened. Food plentiful, but little roughage.

SCBU Babies can be visited at any time by parents, who are encouraged to do as much as possible for baby.

Material for this entry was partly contributed by Association for Improvements in Maternity Services, Dublin.

National Maternity Hospital, Holles Street, Dublin 2   M O

Antenatal Women see same doctor every time. No creche. Refreshments available. Antenatal classes for first-time mothers. Refresher for those who have already had babies.

Labour No shaving. No enema except on request. Partners welcome, but not for forceps delivery. One particular nurse assigned to each woman in labour. Women can walk around and/or choose position in bed. Can eat and drink in early labour. Epidurals not available on request. No choice of position in second stage. 80% episiotomy rate in first-time mothers, 10% in those having subsequent babies. Baby is delivered on to mother's abdomen and can be put to breast immediately. Cord cut when it has stopped pulsating. Goes back to ward with mother.

Postnatal Demand feeding if mother wishes. Glucose not given to breast-fed babies. No special help available for breast-feeding mothers. Special 'smoking' wards; otherwise smoking not allowed. Daily afternoon and evening visiting, husbands at any time by arrangement, children on Wednesday and Saturday afternoons.

The Rotunda, Parnell Square, Dublin 1

Very old building, parts dating from eighteenth century. Ground floor 'gloomy and depressing', especially entrance and corridors.

Antenatal Public clinic has benches and rows of chairs and women are weighed in front of others. Cubicles for examination separated by curtains. Writers say they see different doctors at each visit who 'volunteer no information as to progress, just the usual grunts'; 'When I did ask questions I got the distinct impression that I was considered out of order.'

Labour Partners often made welcome, including for forceps delivery, but master, in letter to woman inquiring writes, 'When our labour ward is very overcrowded we have to ask fathers to leave and wait outside.' Single mothers in a stable relationship can have partner present. No shave, no enema now. 'Lovely hot bath.' Can eat and drink in early labour. Women describe walking up and down corridor in first stage. 30% of first-time mothers have labour augmented with oxytocin drip, the induction rate is very low. There are very few epidurals, but available on request. Few forceps deliveries and low Caesarean section rate. No chatting or questioning during contractions; 'plenty of "You are doing really well" in the intervals'. Gas and oxygen offered, natural birth encouraged. Choice of epidural or general anaesthetic for Caesarean section. Delivery room 'bare' and 'open'. Delivery in left lateral or dorsal position. Master says, 'We do not encourage mothers to squat.' He writes that 'The baby is given to the mother immediately and the cord is not severed until it has stopped pulsating.' Writers, however, did not always hold their babies immediately: 'The cord was cut immediately and I stroked her. They then took her off to be weighed and towelled off and then brought her back to me to be suckled.' The baby may be taken away while the mother is stitched and washed. Episiotomy not routinely done: 80% first-time mothers have them and 30% others. Baby goes with mother to ward, may be put in bed beside her for a while, then in cot by bed.

Postnatal Breast-feeding on demand only if mother firm. She can be woken in night to feed if she asks. Glucose not given to breast-fed babies. Wards 'pleasant and airy', but mothers smoke. Food 'greasy'; not enough fruit or wholemeal bread. One woman said her 3-year-old came in every day encouraged by the staff. But sibling visiting is allowed only at discretion of ward sister. Staff 'friendly' but high annual turnover of junior staff because Rotunda is a teaching hospital. Postnatal wards modernized, 'bright' and 'cheerful'.

SCBU Mother is free to visit as often as she likes. No milk bank, but mothers can express their own milk. Sister in charge gives great support to mothers.

Suggestions Some mothers would like to have Leboyer approach to childbirth. (The master writes: 'We do not use the Leboyer method'.) At present only public patients can attend classes held jointly by physiotherapists and midwives, but other women hear these are good and would like to be able to attend them too.

St Columalle's, Lough Linstown, County Dublin   MO

No facilities to cope with complications. High-risk women go to National Maternity Hospital, Holles Street.

Antenatal Small clinic. Large 'No smoking' notice, but 'midwife told women they could smoke'.

Labour Geared to natural methods. Encourage father participation. Reluctant to do episiotomies.

Postnatal Baby is left with mother except at night and during visiting. Baby is given water. Smoking forbidden except in TV rooms.

Regional Hospital, Galway   MO

Antenatal Pleasant waiting-room, but sometimes overcrowded. No facilities for children. 'Seldom volunteer information.' Classes, but not for fathers. Tour of labour ward and delivery room.

Labour Part shave/no enema. Partner can stay throughout normal labour. Several writers described having intravenous oxytocin to stimulate labour a few hours after they had started. 'I was constantly reminded of my progress.' Midwives not familiar with relaxation techniques, according to writers. Midwife will wait for cord to stop pulsating before clamping and cutting it. Mother handed baby to hold. Writers do not seem to have breast-fed after delivery as a rule. Couple have extended time together with their baby; then baby to nursery.

Postnatal Breast-feeding on demand and help available. Mother is called during night. Some first-time mothers said they could have done with more help. Food 'adequate'. Visiting 2 hours in afternoon and 2 hours in evening; children 'always welcome'. Visitors tend to smoke, even though there are 'No smoking' signs.

Channel Islands

Princess Elizabeth, Guernsey

All women in Guernsey have their babies here, and apparently there is no choice of home birth. Clean, comfortable hospital with personal touch, 'friendly family atmosphere'. A policy of 'natural midwifery' and 'pleasant spirit of camaraderie'.

Antenatal 'A good meeting place.' Ultrasound. Facilities for amniocentesis.

Labour Women describe enema. Rooms are 'bright', 'sunny'. If woman says beforehand to doctor that she wants natural birth midwives may not offer drugs. Other writers have felt under pressure to have pethidine. One midwife assigned to each patient. Woman may sit on chair until she is ready to go to bed. Midwives are 'not authoritarian', 'calm', 'highly efficient', 'sympathetic', 'willing to cooperate with most things women may want to do'. Use first name and try to make woman comfortable with back-rubbing, etc. Partner may be 'hustled out' each time midwife examines. Electronic monitoring not used routinely. Woman who goes in in early labour at night may be given sleeping pills and pain-killers and partner sent away. Low rate of medical intervention generally. At second stage, back-support is offered but, according to some writers, not enough. Delivery bed is hard and brilliant strip lights are disturbing. Some women asked to sit up for delivery but say they were not allowed to. Ask midwife if you want to be told when the crown of baby's head appears. Episiotomies not routine. Mother given baby before cord cut. Couple have about an hour alone with their baby after delivery and mother can suckle baby. A patient was taken to ward 'starving hungry' but was only able to have toast as it was between meals, then a frugal tea because too late to order choice of food.

Postnatal Baby beside mother's bed during day except for afternoon visiting. Has her own feeding chart. Otherwise is left to do much as she wishes. First-time mothers may need more help than they sometimes get. Women say they are helped to feel 'special'. Baby in nursery at night. Mother encouraged to have 2 nights uninterrupted sleep and then women to feed in nursery, but you can choose to be woken from the beginning. Atmosphere 'friendly', 'relaxed'. Nurses 'patient', 'friendly', 'caring' and all willing to help with feeding problems *when asked*, but some have 'theoretical approach' to breast-feeding and some writers wish breast-feeding mothers had been available to help them. They said they felt nurses were not 'well-informed'. Heavy emphasis on breast-feeding mothers drinking lots of milk, mainly in form of milk-shakes. Some nurses not entirely happy with demand-feeding. Baby stays with mother when father visits in evening and he is encouraged to hold baby. Brothers and sisters allowed in nursery to see new baby. Leaflet states:

'Mum's other children taken to nursery by midwife to see and handle their new brother or sister.' Food 'delicious'. Writers say they enjoyed their stay, which was 'restful' and 'happy'.

Notes

I: The Medical Way of Birth

1. Pregnancy as a Disease State

1. Isobel Waterhouse, 'Dial-a-midwife', *Midwives Chronicle*, July 1977.
2. N. E. Page, 'Community experience in an integrated area', *Midwives Chronicle*, April 1978.
3. *Report of the Working Party on Antenatal Care*, London, National Childbirth Trust, 1980.
4. P. B. Terry, R. G. Condie, R. S. Settatree, 'Analysis of ethnic differences in perinatal statistics', *British Medical Journal*, 281 (1980), 1307–8.
5. Caroline Flint, 'A continuing labour of love', *Nursing Mirror*, 149 (1979), 16–18.
6. N. Fresco and D. Sylvestre, 'Psychological aspects of prenatal diagnosis' (Paper presented at 5th International Congress of Psychosomatic Medicine in Obstetrics and Gynaecology, Rome, 1977).
7. David Cox and Anthony Reading, 'Ultrasound scans hearten expectant mothers', *New Scientist*, 89 (1981), 143.
8. G. Chamberlain, *Lecture Notes on Obstetrics*, 4th ed., Oxford, Blackwell Scientific Publications, 1980.
9. *Annual Report 1980*, National Perinatal Epidemiology Unit, Oxford.

2. Childbirth as Clinical Crisis

1. 'William Goodell on the means employed at the Preston Retreat for the prevention and treatment of puerperal diseases', Philadelphia, 1874. Quoted in Richard W. Wertz and Dorothy C. Wertz, *Lying-In: A History of Childbirth in America*, New York, Free Press, 1977.
2. Harold Speert, *The Sloane Hospital Chronicle*, Philadelphia, F. A. Davis, 1963. Quoted in Wertz, op. cit.
3. Mona L. Romney and H. Gordon, 'Is your enema really necessary?' *British Medical Journal*, 282 (1981), 1269–71.
4. Mona L. Romney, 'Predelivery shaving: an unjustified assault?, *Journal of Obstetrics and Gynaecology*, 1 (1981), 43–5.
5. D. R. Ostergard, 'The physiology and clinical importance of amniotic fluid: a review', *Obstetric and Gynecological Survey*, 25 (1970), 297.
6. R. L. Schwarcz and others, 'Influence of amniotomy and maternal position on labour', *Proceedings of the VIII World Congress of Gynecology and Obstetrics*, Mexico, 1976.
7. E. A. Friedman, *Labor, Clinical Evaluation and Management*, New York, Appleton-Century Crofts, 1967.
8. R. L. Schwarcz and others, 'Fetal and maternal monitoring in spontaneous and inelective inductions', *American Journal of Obstetrics and Gynecology*, 120 (1974), 356–62.
9. S. G. Gabbe and others, 'Umbilical cord compression associated with amniotomy', *American Journal of Obstetrics and Gynecology*, 126 (1976), 353–5.
10. M. Martell and others, 'Blood acid-base balance at birth in neonates from labors with early and late rupture of membranes', *Journal of Paediatrics*, 89 (1976), 963–7.
11. The fetal heart records in this section are taken from Geoffrey Chamberlain, *Lecture Notes on Obstetrics*, 4th ed., Oxford, Blackwell Scientific Publications, 1980.
12. J. M. Beazley, 'The active management of labor', *American Journal of Obstetrics and Gynecology*, 122 (1975), 161–8.
13. P. J. Steer, *British Journal of Hospital Medicine*, 219 (1977), 17
14. I. Z. MacKenzie and Mostyn P. Embrey, *British Medical Journal*, 283 (1981), 142.
15. J. M. Beazley, 'The active management of labor, op. cit.
16. ibid.
17. I. Chalmers and others, 'Evaluation of different approaches to obstetric care', *British Journal of Obstetrics and Gynaecology*, 83 (1976), 921–33.
18. Introduction to Tim Chard and Martin Richards, eds, *Benefits and Hazards of the New Obstetrics*, London, Heinemann, 1977.
19. Kieran O'Driscoll and Declan Meagher, 'Active management of labour',

433

in *Clinics in Obstetrics and Gynaecology*, W. B. Saunders, 1980.

20. Roberto Caldeyro-Barcia, 'Some consequences of obstetrical interference', *Birth and the Family Journal*, 2 (1975), 2.

21. *The Dignity of Labour*, London, Tavistock Publications, 1979.

22. Editorial, *Lancet*, 2 (1977), 467–9.

23. R. A. Cole, P. W. Haowe, M. C. MacNaughton, 'Elective induction of labour', *Lancet*, 1 (1975), 767–70.

24. 2nd ed, National Childbirth Trust, 1978.

25. D. Richter and others, 'The advantage of elective labour by a psychosomatic approach' (Paper given at 5th International Congress of Psychosomatic Obstetrics and Gynaecology, Rome, 1977).

26. W. C. Chew and others, 'Influence of simultaneous low amniotomy and oxytocin infusion and other maternal factors on neonatal jaundice', *British Medical Journal*, 1 (1977), 72–3.

27. B. Yudkin and others, *British Journal of Obstetrics and Gynaecology*, 86 (1979), 257–65.

28. Quoted by Gary Stimeling, 'Will common delivery techniques ever become malpractice?', *Journal of Legal Medicine*, New York, May 1975.

29. R. J. Flaksman and others, *American Journal of Obstetrics and Gynecology*, 132 (1978), 885–8.

30. I. Chalmers, 'Obstetric practice and outcome of pregnancy in Cardiff residents 1965–73', *British Medical Journal*, 1 (1976), 733–8.

31. R. L. Goldenburg and others, 'Iatrogenic respiratory distress syndrome', *American Journal of Obstetrics and Gynecology*, 6 (1975), 617–20.

32. *The Dignity of Labour*, op. cit.

33. *Some Mothers' Experiences of Induced Labour*, 2nd ed., London, National Childbirth Trust, 1978.

34. In a lecture to the International Childbirth Education Association, Eastern-Southern Conference, June 1977.

35. Sir John Dewhurst, in address to conference on 'Pregnancy in the Eighties', Royal Society of Medicine, London, 1981.

36. Kieran O'Driscoll, 'An obstetrician's view of pain', *British Journal of Anaesthetics*, 47 (1975), 1053–8.

37. I. J. Hoult, A. H. MacLennan and L. E. S. Carrier, 'Lumbar epidural analgesia in labour: relation to fetal malposition and instrumental delivery', *British Medical Journal*, 1 (1977), 14–16.

38. *British Journal of Obstetrics and Gynaecology*, 88 (1981), 407–31.

39. Berry Brazelton, evidence to sub-committee on investigation and oversight of the house committee on science and technology, Washington, DC, 10.7.8.

40. Peter V. Scott and others, 'Intrathecal morphine as sole analgesic during labour', *British Medical Journal*, 281 (2 August 1980).

41. Sheila Kitzinger, *Some Mothers' Experiences of Induced Labour*, op. cit.

42. Charles D. Kimball, Commentary in *I.C.E.A. Review*, Vol. 4, No. 3, Dec. 1980.

43. R. Cogan, 'Endorphins and analgesia', *I.C.E.A. Review*, Vol. 4, No. 3, Dec. 1980.

44. M. Hughey and others, *Obstetrics and Gynecology*, 51 (1978), 634–7.

45. Joseph B. DeLee, 'The prophylactic forceps operation', *American Journal of Obstetrics and Gynecology*, 1 (1920), 34–44.

46. ibid.

47. ibid.

48. *British Births, 1970* (Survey under the joint auspices of the National Birthday Trust Fund and the Royal College of Obstetricians and Gynaecologists), London, Heinemann, 1975.

49. R. Caldeyro-Barcia and others, 'The bearing-down efforts and their effects on fetal heart rate, oxygenation and acid base balance', *Proceedings of 1st International Meeting of Perinatal Medicine*, Berlin, 1979.

50. *British Births, 1970*, op. cit.

51. Ann Oakley, *Women Confined*, Oxford, Martin Robertson, 1980.

52. Graham H. Barker, 'The unkindest cut of all', *World Medicine*, 8 August 1981.

53. *Some Women's Experiences of Episiotomy*, London, National Childbirth Trust, 1981.

54. 4th ed, Penguin Books, 1978.

55. A. E. Reading and others, 'How women view postepisiotomy pain', *British Medical Journal*, 284 (1982), 243–5.

56. *British Medical Journal*, 284 (1982), 220.

57. Ian Chalmers and Martin Richards, in T. Chard and M. P. M. Richards, eds., *Benefits and Hazards of the New Obstetrics*, London, Heinemann, 1977.

58. Rosenblatt, D., and others, *The In-*

fluence of Maternal Analgesia on Neonatal Behaviour: 11, Epidural Bupiracaine, Office of Research Reporting, Bethseda, Maryland, 1980.

59. *The Dignity of Labour*, op. cit.

60. *Nursing Mirror*, 147, 17 (1978), 18–22.

61. V. Smallpiece and P. A. Davies, *Lancet*, 2 (1964), 1349–52.

62. John C. Sinclair, 'Newborn thermal stress', *Perinatal Care* 2, 4 (1978), 30–40.

63. Ian Chalmers and others, 'The use of oxytocin and incidence of neonatal jaundice', *British Medical Journal* 2 (1975), 116–18.

64. Joel Richman and W. Goldthorp, in Sheila Kitzinger and John Davis, eds., *The Place of Birth*, London, OUP, 1978.

65. Julius A. Roth, 'Ritual and magic in the control of contagion', *American Sociological Review*, 22 (1957), 310–14.

II: New Ways of Birth

1. *The Century Illustrated Magazine*, February 1926; quoted in Richard W. Wertz and Dorothy C. Wertz, *Lying-in: A History of Childbirth in America*, New York, Free Press, 1977.

2. A. Measures, 'The nursing process', *Nursing Mirror*, 148, 24, 20 (1979); P. Ashworth, 'A way to better care', *Nursing Mirror*, 151, 9, 26 (1980); Rosemary Long, *Systematic Nursing Care*, London, Faber, 1981.

3. Margaret Adams and others, 'Trial run', *Nursing Mirror*, 7 October 1981.

4. R. J. Atwood, 'Parturitional posture and related birth behaviour', *ACTA Obstetrica et Ginecologica Scandinavica* (Sweden), 1976 (Supp. 57); R. W. Wertz and D. C. Wertz, *Lying In: A History of Childbirth in America*, New York, Free Press, 1977; Engelmann, *Labour Among Primitive People*, St Louis, 1882

5. P. Dunn, 'Obstetrics delivery today; for better or for worse?', *Lancet*, 1, 7963 (1976), 790–93; W. I. Hampton, 'Practical considerations for the routine application of left lateral Sims' position for vaginal delivery', *American Journal of Obstetrics and Gynecology*, 131 (1978), 129–33; M. A. Hugo, 'A look at maternal positions during labour', *Nurse-Midwifery*, XXII (1977), 26–7; Y. C. Lieu, Effects of an upright position during labor', *American Journal of Nursing*, 74 (1974) 2203–5; T. J. McManus and A. A. Calder, 'Upright posture and the efficiency of labor', *Lancet* 1, 8055 (1978), 72–4; C. Mendez-Bauer and others, 'Effects of standing position on spontaneous uterine contractility and other aspects of labor', *Journal of Perinatal Medicine*, 3 (1975), 89–100; I. N. Mitre, 'The influence of maternal position on duration of the active phase of labor', *International Journal of Gynaecology and Obstetrics*, 12 (1974), 181–3.

6. A. M. Flynn and J. Kelly, 'Continuous fetal monitoring in the ambulant patient in labour', *British Medical Journal*, 2 (1976) 842–3.

7. R. Caldeyro-Barcia, 'Some consequences of obstetrician interference', *Birth and the Family Journal*, 2 (1975), 2, and 'The influence of maternal position on time of spontaneous rupture of the membranes, progress of labor, and fetal head compression', *Birth and the Family Journal*, 6 (1979), 7.

8. Janet and Arthur Belaskas, *New Life*, London, Sidgwick & Jackson, 1979.

9. R. Caldeyro-Barcia and others, 'The bearing-down efforts and their effects on fetal heart rate, oxygenation and acid base balance', in *Proceedings of 1st International Meeting of Perinatal Medicine*, Berlin, 1979; R. Caldeyro-Barcia, 'Physiological and psychological bases for the modern and humanized management of normal labour', in *Proceedings of 6th International Congress of Psychosomatic Medicine in Obstetrics and Gynaecology*, 1980.

10. J. D. Bonica, 'Maternal respiratory changes during pregnancy and parturition', *Clinical Anaesthesia*, 10 (2) (1973).

11. B. Picci, 'Cardiovascular dynamics', in *The Physiological Basis of Human Performances*, Philadelphia, Lea & Febiger, 1967; V. Derbes and A. Kerr, 'Physiological mechanisms', *Cough Syncope*, Springfield, Illinois, C. Thomas, 1955; D. J. Ewing and others, 'Interaction between cardiovascular responses to sustained handgrip in the Valsalva manoeuvre', *British Heart Journal*, 38 (5) (1976), 483–90; P. I. Korner and others, 'Reflex and mechanical circulatory effects of graded Valsalva manoeuvre in normal man', *Journal of Applied Physiology*, 40 (3) (1976).

12. D. B. Scott, 'Inferor vena cava occlusion', *Clinical Anaesthesia*, 10 (2) (1973).

13. L. Thompson, 'Hazards of immobilization and effects on cardiovascular function', *American Journal of Nursing*, 702 (1967); H. Karlsson and others, 'Time courses of pulmonary gas exchange and heart rate changes in supine exercise', *Acta Physiologica Scandinavica*, 95 (3) (1975), 329–40.

14. *In British Births 1970* only 3% of women were recorded as receiving no drugs for pain in labour.

15. E. Noble, 'Respiratory considerations for childbirth', in P. Simkin and C. Reinke, eds., *Kaleidoscope of childbearing*, Seattle, Pennypress, 1978.

16. F. Leboyer, *Birth without Violence*, London, Collins (Fontana), 1977.

17. ibid.

18. Personal communication.

19. David A. Kliot and others, 'Parent-newborn bonding resulting from modification of traditional birth techniques using the Leboyer approach' (Paper given at 5th International Congress of Psychosomatic Medicine in Obstetrics and Gynaecology, Rome, 1977).

20. Leboyer, *Birth without Violence*, op. cit.

21. Gordon Stirrat, *Obstetrics*, London, Grant McIntyre, 1981.

22. N. M. Nelson and others, 'A randomized clinical trial of a Leboyer approach to childbirth', *New England Journal of Medicine*, 302 (1980), 655–60.

23. Aidan Macfarlane, *The Psychology of Childbirth*, London, Collins (Fontana), 1977.

24. Personal communication.

25. Jane Gillett, 'Childbirth in Pithiviers, France', *Lancett* II, 894, 27 October 1979; Michel Odent, 'The Evolution of Obstetrics at Pithiviers', *Birth and the Family Journal*, 8, 1, Spring 1981.

III: The Days After Birth

1. *Present Day Practice in Infant Feeding*, revised edition, London, HMSO, 1980.

2. Paul Buisseret, 'Common manifestations of cows' milk allergy in children', *Lancet*, 8059 (1978), 304–5.

3. Jean Ball, 'Stress in the postnatal period' (Paper given at the International Congress of Midwives, Brighton, England, 1981).

4. Jo Garcia, *Community Health Council News*, 70 and 72 (1981).

5. Sylvia Slaven, David Harvey, letter in *Lancet*, 8216 (1981), 392–3.

6. Marshall Klaus and John Kennell, *Maternal – Infant Bonding*, Mosby, 1976.

7. P. Du Chateau, 'The influence of early contact on maternal and infant behaviour in primiparae', *Birth and the Family Journal*, 4 (1976), 149–55.

8. Marshall Klaus and John Kennell, op. cit.; S. O'Connor and others, *Birth and the Family Journal*, 5 (1978), 231–4.

9. J. Lumley, *Birth Rites, Birth Rights*, Melbourne, Sphere, 1980.

IV: Planning Ahead for Birth

1. Margaret F. Myles, *Textbook for Midwives – with Modern Concepts of Obstetric and Neonatal Care*, 9th ed., London, Churchill Livingstone, 1981.

2. Mary Chamberlain, *Old Wives' Tales*, London, Virago, 1981, p. 154.

3. John Hargreaves, 'A little bit of Bradley and a lot of yourself', *The Birth Centre London Newsletter*, 17, 'The Assertive Issue' (Autumn 1981).

4. Penny Simkin and Carla Reinke, *Planning your Baby's Birth*, Seattle, Pennypress, 1981.

Organizations Concerned with Maternity Care

Active Birth Movement
Janet Balaskas,
32 Cholmeley Crescent,
London N6 5JR (01-348 1284)

AIMS (Association for Improvements in the Maternity Services)
Elizabeth Cockerell,
21 Franklin Gardens,
Hitchin,
Herts SG4 0NE (0462 2179)

Association of Radical Midwives
Lakefield,
82 The Drive,
Wimbledon,
London SW18

There are birth centres in some cities.
The London Birth Centre's address is:
48 Wroughton Road,
London SW11 (01-223 7076)

Maternity Alliance
Helene Hayman,
12 Park Crescent,
London W1 (01-267 5807)

National Childbirth Trust
9 Queensborough Terrace,
Bayswater,
London W2 3TB (01-221 3833)

Society to Support Home Confinements
Margaret Whyte,
17 Laburnum Avenue,
Durham (Durham (0385) 61325)

Index

Index

Your own experiences

Much of the information in this book has come from people who have recently used the hospitals concerned. To keep the record up to date for future editions of *The New Good Birth Guide* this form has been included in the hope that readers will want to share their experiences for the benefit of other mothers-to-be.

Please send your completed form to:

Sheila Kitzinger,
Standlake Manor,
Near Witney,
Oxon.

All information will be treated in confidence.

Name of hospital...

....

Address of hospital...

....

Date of baby's birth...

General impression of hospital

Antenatal care

The labour

Postnatal care

Things that could be improved in this hospital, and how

The best thing about the hospital

Signed ....

Name ....

Address ....

....

....

FIND OUT MORE ABOUT
PENGUIN BOOKS

We publish the largest range of titles of any English language paperback publisher. As well as novels, crime and science fiction, humour, biography and large-format illustrated books, Penguin series include *Pelican Books* (on the arts, sciences and current affairs), *Penguin Reference Books, Penguin Classics, Penguin Modern Classics, Penguin English Library, Penguin Handbooks* (on subjects from cookery and gardening to sport) and *Puffin Books* for children. Other series cover a wide variety of interests from poetry to crosswords, and there are also several newly formed series – *King Penguin, Penguin American Library* and *Penguin Travel Library*.

We are an international publishing house, but for copyright reasons not every Penguin title is available in every country. To find out more about the Penguins available in your country please write to our U.K. office – Dept EP, Penguin Books Ltd, Harmondsworth, Middlesex UB7 0DA – unless you live in one of the following areas:

In the U.S.A.: Dept DG, Penguin Books, 299 Murray Hill Parkway, East Rutherford, New Jersey 07073.

In Canada: Penguin Books Canada Ltd, 2801 John Street, Markham, Ontario L3R 1B4.

In Australia: Marketing Department, Penguin Books Australia Ltd, P.O. Box 257, Ringwood, Victoria 3134.

In New Zealand: Marketing Department, Penguin Books (N.Z.) Ltd, P.O. Box 4019, Auckland 10.

In India: Penguin Overseas Ltd, 706 Eros Apartments, 56 Nehru Place, New Delhi 110019.

Also by Sheila Kitzinger

THE EXPERIENCE
OF CHILDBIRTH

'For far too many women pregnancy and birth is still something that happens to them rather than something they set out consciously and joyfully to do themselves.'

A complete manual of physical and emotional preparation for the expectant mother. The physiology of pregnancy, the development of the foetus, and the successive stages of labour are described in detail. Moving on from the pioneer work of Grantly Dick-Read and later psychoprophylactic techniques, Mrs Kitzinger's research and teaching focus particularly on the psychological aspects of child-bearing, on the preparation of both wife and husband not only for birth but for parenthood and marital adjustment, and on a girl's changing relationship with her own mother.

THE EXPERIENCE
OF BREASTFEEDING

Happy breastfeeding depends both on what is right for *you* as an individual and on the emotional support and attitude of your partner.

This is why Sheila Kitzinger, an authority on childbirth who has herself breastfed five children, has written this sensible, comprehensive, up-to-date and thoroughly practical book for both of you. It includes all the recent research on the newborn baby's abilities and on the vital parent-child relationship, and explores sympathetically the stresses involved for both parents. She looks too at the mass of new evidence on the advantages of breastfeeding, at the constituents of breast milk and the effects of drugs upon it, and discusses the dangers of artificial feeding in Third World countries.

At the same time, Sheila Kitzinger firmly believes that the choice must rest with you. Too many people have spent too long telling women what they should do to be 'Supermums': the time has come to say unequivocally *'Your breasts belong to you'*.

Penguin N28170 Proof 1 24.3.83 Opus Photo 13691 F53-T1